Medical Practice
in Modern
England

The Impact of Specialization and State Medicine

Medical Practice
in Modern
England

Rosemary Stevens

With a new introduction by the author

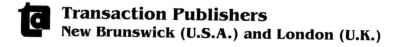

Transaction Publishers
New Brunswick (U.S.A.) and London (U.K.)

Library of Congress Catalog Number: 2002068483
ISBN: 0-7658-0956-7
Printed in the United States of America

Library of Congress Cataloging-in-Publication Data

Stevens, Rosemary.
    Medical practice in modern England : the impact of specialization and state medicine / Rosemary Stevens ; with a new introduction by the author.
        p. cm.
    Includes bibliographical references and index.
    ISBN 0-7658-0956-7 (paper : alk. paper)
        1. Medicine, State—Great Britain. 2. Social medicine—Great Britain.
    3. Medical policy—Great Britain. I. Title.

RA418.3.G7 S74 2003
362.1'0941—dc21   2002068483

Contents

List of Tables

List of Figures

Introduction to the Transaction Edition

Health and the State before the Mid-1970s: Structure, Power, and Rhetoric in England and the United States

In July 1946, the British government passed landmark legislation to create the National Health Service (NHS), which was implemented in 1948. In July 1965, almost twenty years later, President Lyndon Baines Johnson signed far-reaching legislation in the United States that is the basis for the present Medicare and Medicaid programs. Looking back from the early twenty-first century, both actions were successful in extending health services to previously underserved populations. Each country crafted legislation that drew on preexisting organizational patterns in medicine, on proposals for health reform formulated in earlier years, and on prevailing assumptions about the purposes and limits of government. In Great Britain, the NHS guaranteed health services that were largely free at the time of use, nationalized the hospitals, and built a top-down command and control health care system. In the United States, Medicare provided government-sponsored health insurance limited to the older generations (sixty-five-plus years of age) irrespective of income—individuals whom the private insurance sector demonstrably could not serve. Medicaid provided subsidy to the states to provide additional health benefits to elderly residents whose incomes fell below specified levels, as well as to disabled, blind, and deaf individuals, and to needy families with children.[1]

Nevertheless, in these, as in other countries, no one has been satisfied with the results. Massive organizational changes, problems, and expenses have accompanied the rise of each nation's version of the "health care state."[2] There is considerable unease on both sides of the Atlantic about how much medical care, and of what quality, should be accessible to all members of the population; which services should be subsidized by government; how best to stimulate private initiative and meet consumer preferences; whether co-payments and means testing are prudent or unfair social mechanisms; and how much tax money should be allocated to health care in light of competing social goods, such as national defense, public education, and controlling the overall rate of taxation. The recent history of the NHS has been aptly described as one of "continuous revolution,"[3] or, more gently perhaps, of "perpetual evolution."[4] The same can be said of health care in the United States, where "creative chaos"[5] is the kindest comment on the turmoil of the present. This is a good time to reconsider the historical baggage carried into each national health care system, and to take a new look at these huge national experiments in comparative perspective. It is in this spirit that *Medical Practice in Modern England* and *Welfare Medicine in America* are here offered to a new generation of readers and critics.

It is an honor and a privilege to see books one has written and that were published many years ago reissued. As an illustration of the time that has gone by since, my talented research assistant for *Medical Practice* is now the Rt. Hon. Michael Meacher, M.P., Minister for the Environment in the U.K. government. Why should anyone read these books today? Taken together, the two books describe English and American health care, their similarities and differences in providing health care to their respective populations, in an important period for health policy in both countries, between World War II and the early 1970s. Combined, they serve to emphasize how social legislation reflects past cultural practices rather than future expectations. In Rudolf Klein's apt phrase, this is the "politics of the second best."[6] The books show the impact of legislative action on powerful and potential players in health care organization and financing (often with unexpected consequences); illustrate the inertia and resilience of the social organizations involved in change; and emphasize the importance of implementation as a policymaking vehicle. All are useful messages for the present. "In any democratic system," writes Mark Peterson," a policy decision is always a beginning rather than an end."[7]

These books may also carry different meanings to today's readers than to their counterparts of, respectively, 1966 and 1974. They will, first, I hope, help to emphasize the importance of social/organizational history as a central explanatory technique for policy studies. The books were written at a time when historical studies with a wide sweep of subject matter and complex themes were thought unfashionable within the mainstream of the social sciences. Now, thankfully, the pendulum has swung. A new audience of social scientists in historical sociology and other fields may find these studies enlightening and helpful.

With the passage of time, these books have also become historical artifacts in their own right, contemporary documents of a rich, earlier period. It is a truism worth repeating that history reflects the ideas of the time in which it was written. Each of these books offers a unique view of the political, social, economic, organizational, and ideological issues influencing medical practice and health services as one informed observer (myself for the first book) and two (Robert Stevens and myself for the second) then saw them. Though they were not initially planned for this purpose, *Medical Practice in Modern England* and *Welfare Medicine in America* present today's readers with comparative historical case studies of the role of government in the two countries, the relationship between public and private sectors, and the relative choices made in bringing health services to the population. Old questions can be asked anew; specifically, how was the welfare state in medicine negotiated for health care in England, and with what results for the providers of care?; and, how did the implementation and reception of Medicaid shape America's version of a welfare state, and again, with what effects on the organization of care?

Medicaid provides an important window on health policy in the United States for at least two reasons. It demonstrates America's commitment to serve those in need, despite deep divisions about how best to serve the population as a whole; and it serves as a backstop and support of the private sector (insurance companies, for-profit and not-for-profit hospitals, medical practice corporations, etc.), through which it channels funds. As we showed in *Welfare Medicine in America*, Medicaid has also served, politically, to preempt broader proposals for national health insurance. Medicaid (like Medicare) poured money into privately run hospitals, making the old public hospitals seem marginal or irrelevant, though some great public hospitals survive to this day.[8] In contrast, both private and public hospitals were nationalized in Great Britain. Understanding the arguments, problems, and successes of those times does much to explain where the two systems find themselves today.

I look forward to bringing *Medical Practice* and *Welfare Medicine* to the attention of readers like my students, who were not born when these books were written but who live with the consequences of the policies and politics they describe. There is a new audience of historians and social scientists who are interested in the 1960s and 1970s, and indeed of the twentieth century as a whole. Younger readers also have a vested interest in the future of health policy. Current students in England who reach my present age will experience a very different NHS than the one originally designed, perhaps even different from what it is at present. American students will be Medicare and perhaps Medicaid recipients in the 2060s, one hundred years after the Medicare and Medicaid legislation—assuming those programs survive until then.

Author and Authors

Before considering the two books, comparatively and as scholarly studies, warts and all, some autobiographical comments may be helpful to set the stage. Like others who remember the 1960s, we are not the same persons, with the same thoughts, environment, or experiences, as we were then— young scholars probing the messiness, antecedents, and immediacy of what was then the present.

Medical Practice in Modern England was my first book, published when I was thirty-one years of age, and I have a special affection for and pride in it. Several of the British reviewers assumed I was American, though fortunately not holding this against me in their reviews of the book. I am a native Briton who became a U.S. citizen in 1968. Between

1957 and 1961 I was a graduate student in applied social science at the University of Manchester, trained for health care management in Sheffield and London, and worked in the NHS as a trainee and administrator. In 1961-62, while planning for the research that would lead to *Medical Practice*, I was a full-time public health student at Yale. All of my work, now as then, reflects the comparative perspectives that come from the shock of discovery. Through my English eyes, the American health system of the 1960s seemed illogical, contested, and impenetrable. Yet I was learning about the American system and its history with a cohort of American graduate students who seemed remarkably unfazed by its peculiarities, as indeed was I, at the time, about the NHS. Two pertinent understandings were thus made clear early on, equally relevant today: First, it is easy to accept familiar social structures without adequately questioning their rationale or roots; hence the importance of comparative perspectives. Second, the way in which any health system is organized and paid for can best (perhaps only) be understood through studying its own idiosyncratic history. In returning to England in the shadow of the Medicare debates of the early 1960s, I saw more clearly than before the anomalies, inconsistencies, and conflicts embedded in the NHS. Similarly, I turned to the research for *Welfare Medicine in America* in the early 1970s with the ability to dwell intellectually in both cultural systems.

I was then married to Robert B. Stevens, a distinguished historian/ lawyer at the Yale Law School, who was also a critical and valued mentor for the English book. Robert Stevens has focused most of his scholarly attention on the history of legal institutions. However, in 1970 he published an edited volume on the statutory history of social legislation in the United States.[9] We decided to join forces to work on Medicaid, aided by work done by graduate students in courses we were both teaching. I was then on the faculty of the Yale Medical School. *Welfare Medicine in America*, authored jointly and seamlessly, benefited from the mix of social science, public health, and legal perspectives that we brought to the project. The legal perspective was particularly important in the absence of strong national policy direction because, as is evident in the book, policymaking for Medicaid has been enmeshed in legal decisions, clarifications, wrangling, and rulings.

The Books in Comparative Perspective

I will present my own reactions to rereading these books in 2002 after a brief description and comparison, so as to place them in the environment in which they were written. *Medical Practice in Modern England: The Impact of Specialization and State Medicine*, first published in 1966, describes the invention and implementation of the National Health Service in England with special focus on the role of the national organizations of medicine and the implications of the NHS for the medical profession. My goal was to trace the history of specialization in medicine as a major trend after World War II, which affected, in turn, medical practice, the availability of health care, and the organization and costs of health services. Inevitably this meant analyzing the NHS as well as the formal organization and behavior of the medical profession. This book thus attempts to do two things: to provide a balanced historical analysis of the NHS as a central element in Britain's welfare state (as seen from the early 1960s), and to explore the role of medical organizations in shaping it and being shaped by it. I tried to avoid the divisive political rhetoric over "socialized medicine" that then distinguished health care debates on both sides of the Atlantic, in order to describe the practical realities that lay beneath; that is, the shaping of the health care system and power relations in it. As the book shows, the organization of the NHS solidified preexisting professional divisions in British medicine, between specialists and primary care doctors, and between primary care and hospitals.

In the United States, during the same period, the rapid specialization of medicine after World War II led to all-out competition among specialists for patients who could pay for their services in a largely private market. Private health insurance for the working population fueled increased demand for hospital and medical services. The quiet, American version of government aid for population coverage was tax relief, to encourage employers to organize and subsidize health insurance for employees. Federal funds were also made directly available in the 1940s and 1950s to help build a hospital and specialist infrastructure, through grants to states for building hospitals and the rapid expansion of biomedical research in increasingly specialized medical schools.[10]

While the NHS recognized general practitioners as having an essential structural role in England, with formalized relationships to both specialists and patients, there were no such protections for family doctors in the United States, where primary doctors and specialists competed for patients. At the very time the NHS was controlling the supply of medical specialists through salaried service and limited positions, the American system encouraged doctors to specialize. Indeed the proliferation of specialists, specialties, and subspecialties engendered professional and political concern about the decline of primary care, particularly evident in the 1960s.

In theory, Medicare and Medicaid could have required patients to have a primary care doctor with a gatekeeper role in the United States. By that time, though, the private market system was entrenched as a model of non-intervention by government agents. Thus Medicaid, as we showed in *Welfare Medicine*, introduced a huge system of government subsidy of services for the poor in the private sector in the late 1960s. The combined result of Medicare and Medicaid, implemented at the same time and along similar lines, was to pour additional money into the preexisting medical system, flaws and all. In stimulating demand for services (and paying for them), the two programs also encouraged additional private investment, notably in the nursing home industry.

Medical Practice in Modern England was published the same year Medicare and Medicaid were implemented. Both books have a strong comparative perspective. *Medical Practice* drew on my awareness of contemporary concerns about health and medicine in the United States and reflected my desire to bring the English experience to American readers, as well as to those in Britain and elsewhere. This strategy worked. *Medical Practice* was well reviewed in Britain, Canada, and the United States. Americans of the time tended to ignore or dismiss the NHS as an irrelevant, unacceptable aspect of a "socialized" state, or as the progeny of a poor, backward relative. "American physicians have been at once frightened of and fascinated by the British national health scheme," erroneously assuming that British traditions were similar to those in the United States, wrote a leading American commentator on the book.[11] Britons were equally toplofty about American health policy. It was easy to take the moral high ground, dismissing the American system for its lack of universal health coverage and its reliance on the crassness of the private market.

Yet even in the 1960s the two systems had much in common. For example, both countries had problems accommodating to the growing importance of hospitals as centers of medical treatment after World War II. In both there was concern about how to link an array of medical and community services to best serve those with chronic conditions. In both countries the future of primary care was on the national agenda. In both, too, there was surprisingly little information about the way medicine was actually practiced, and little was known about the quality of care. Consumers were not much in evidence as any form of driving force for change—as marked by their notable absence in each of these books. In both countries the high prestige of the medical profession was assumed to mirror uniformly high standards of clinical practice and behavior, without scrutiny from the public or the health care system.

At root these were organizational and managerial problems rather than strictly political issues, as later developments in both countries made clear. However, this sense of the commonality of organization and management across nations took a long time to become central to health care debates among academics and policymakers. The commonalities were obscured in politically-couched debates for and against state socialism, while comparative models tended to explain a nation's health services according to its place on a public-private continuum, with Britain and the Soviet Union at one end of the spectrum (the most socialist) and the United States at the other (the most market-oriented). I recall a talk I gave to an international audience of social scientists in Berlin in the early 1980s on comparative management of health care systems, without making reference to Marxism or any other ism, and this was received as a novel approach, even then. *Medical Practice* takes a pragmatic rather than an ideological position about the implementation of the NHS; even more so perhaps than does *Welfare Medicine*. Perhaps there were (and still are) things each country could learn from the other. The NHS of the 1960s might even be a possible harbinger of things to come in the United States, however horrifying or welcome that might be. Today many Europeans feel a rather similar fascination in contemplating health care in the United States as a model of privatization, managed and non-managed competition, and tolerance (however reluctantly) of 41 million uninsured residents.

Medical Practice in Modern England examines the antecedents and passage of the NHS Act in 1946, emphasizing concurrent developments in medical practice and the political roles of the profession; the emerging problems affecting administrative and medical hierarchies, ranging from determining medical incomes to planning for the future of family practice; and the interactions between the medical profession and the NHS in the early 1960s. The book shows how preexisting patterns of medical practice, already outmoded in the 1930s, were grafted into the NHS as a political compromise to ensure its passage and gain support from the medical profession in the 1940s, and beyond. Medical organizations were influential in shaping the service, particularly the institutional representatives of powerful specialties.

Not only was the division in British medicine between general practitioners and consultants (specialists) strengthened, with implications up to the present, professional leadership was also divided into two sets of institutions with separate goals. The British Medical Association largely represented general practitioners, who sought practice autonomy and private status in the new service. The Royal Colleges represented the consultants, who had no problem with salaried employment in the NHS hospital service, coupled as it was with their control of specified hospital beds and little or no regulation over their activities. In this critical implementation period, the specialists monopolized the hospitals, while general practitioners monopolized patients through controlling primary care. The NHS reinforced primary care as specialization was threatening it, and curbed the more general move toward specialism, as was happening in the United States in the 1950s and 1960s. Since there was no similarly (bi-modal) divided profession in the United States, the representative structures for medicine were different. In the 1960s, the American Medical Association represented the American medical profession writ large. However, a myriad of specialty associations were already rising to power. In the 1970s, as we note in *Welfare Medicine*, the AMA was losing members, again with ramifications to the present.

By the mid-1960s, the NHS had achieved its goal of providing a comprehensive, universal health service to the population, within overall budgetary constraints. The service was given virtually free at the time of delivery, was government-operated, and largely supported by general taxation. The administrative structures, though, were creaking. However good state medicine might be, the NHS was a vast bureaucratic system based on traditional institutions, whose virtue (at least then) was organizational stability rather than nimbleness in the face of change. Yet both the epidemiology of disease and the scientific and technological potential of medicine were changing fast on both sides of the Atlantic. General, specialist, and hospital practice were transformed after World War II with the advent of antibiotics and other powerful pharmaceuticals, together with new diagnostic and therapeutic techniques.[12] The population was aging, and the focus of health was shifting from acute to chronic conditions. Lasting themes were evident: how best to organize primary care; how to coordinate different aspects of health services; how to balance generalist and specialist care; and how to encourage teamwork, evaluation, up-to-date professional education, and medical efficiency. The medical profession had considerable authority within the service, but also had to negotiate with the NHS (and exerted pressure on government) in order to further the income of its own separate sectors. The book raises significant questions about power and authority in medical care, demonstrates that professional leadership may be *enhanced* rather than reduced under government programs (a still novel view in the United States), and stands as an early case study for asking a central question about the NHS: how (if at all) can any state (or perhaps any huge private corporation) own, operate, fund, and manage a health service, negotiate the power structures and economic tradeoffs inherent in each of these functions, and satisfy taxpayers, patients, physicians, and other health care stakeholders?

Welfare Medicine in America: A Case Study of Medicaid remains the only scholarly study to date of the implementation of the Medicaid program, from the enabling legislation in 1965 through self-evident problems by the early 1970s. The contested quest for national health insurance runs as a continuing background theme for the rapidly moving changes in Medicaid's program and direction, as does Medicaid's signal role in the late 1960s and early 1970s as an expression of the American welfare state. We were fortunate that this book, too, was welcomed at the time by reviewers in terms of its apparent objectivity, synthesis of social, economic, and organizational approaches, its ability to raise fundamental questions about the state and health care provision, and not least, its wealth of detail.

Welfare Medicine focuses more strongly on philosophical questions about the state's role in guaranteeing medical care than does *Medical Practice*, reflecting the fact that I regarded the NHS, not unreasonably, as a done deal philosophically in the 1960s. Its policy of universal, comprehensive services was established and, to American eyes, remarkably non-controversial. In contrast, American health care lurched along, sustained by the rhetoric of government-supported private enterprise but without clear policy definition. A central theme of *Welfare Medicine* is that Medicaid had no clear goals; hence the ease with which, on the one hand, it was heralded as the "sleeper" in the Medicare/Medicaid legislation, which might turn into socialized medicine for all in the United States, while on the other hand it was rapidly cut back to a traditional welfare program as costs rose. "What is the human good which medicine serves?" asked one reviewer, provoked to such questions by the book; "In what sense do the needs of some constitute rights which impose duties on others?" We describe "a social policy unable to settle on a distinct concept of welfare or of rights, wavering between a Rawlsian advantaging of the most disadvantaged and the reluctance of Nozick's minimal state to interfere with the liberty of individuals."[13]

Medicaid was (and is) a national program of federal grants to states to pay for medical services to needy families with children and to individuals who are elderly, blind, or disabled. Introduced into a culture of health care provision that assumed a central role for private enterprise in health insurance but recognized that government should support that market and act responsibly when the market fails, Medicaid stemmed from a long history of welfare policies and politics in the United States. The book begins with a brief history of the alternative and competing (if simplistic) philosophies for justifying the provision of health care to those who demonstrably need it—and who can be identified as "needy" through bureaucratic rules. These basic views were represented in the politics of "social insurance" versus "public assistance" approaches to social legislation in the 1960s. The former characterizes Medicare, which provides national health insurance with limited benefits to those sixty-five years of age and over, to disabled individuals, and to those who would otherwise die from kidney failure. Medicaid was built on American public assistance principles, and thus includes a means test as condition for entry, state rather than federal administration, and an eligibility structure that followed preexisting welfare provisions. Initially, as we show, it was not clear whether Medicaid was a "right" for potentially qualified beneficiaries or merely a state-dominated, churlish privilege. Medical benefits for those within the program could (and can) be quite generous, more so than for Medicare.

It was evident in the early 1970s that more needed to be known about the actual workings of the Medicaid program as implemented in the states. How, otherwise, was anyone to interpret the sometimes heady, sometimes alarmed expectations of Medicaid critics who saw the program as the "thin end of the wedge of socialized medicine?" Sociologist Michael M. Davis's much earlier comment on the importance of applied social research in health care in the United States bears repeating to this day, as a continuing refrain: "[W]here many people take sides and where more than two sides exist analysis is needed more than pronouncement."[14] We show, through state case studies, that implementation in the states demonstrated distinctive initial preferences, based on prior state experiences. Notably, California expressed a strong service commitment for those covered but put strict limits on Medicaid eligibility, while New York announced generous eligibility standards in a less organized service system. However, disillusion soon set in across the board as it became evident that costs were escalating far beyond expectation. The book traces the "euphoric demise" of Medicaid by early 1968, with the beginning of a period of political storm in Washington and the states, including finger-pointing, retrenchments, Congressional reappraisals, and new (though largely unimplemented) proposals from the Nixon administration.

The last five chapters cover the period July 1970-June 1973; that is, contemporary to the writing of the book. Federal administration was strengthened, but Medicaid costs continued to climb rapidly in the states. While the English system was reorganized in 1974 (largely unsuccessfully) around consensus management at the community level, Medicaid providers were being charged with fraud. From the 1970s to the present there has been continuing tension about Medicaid's role as a national program rather than as a diverse collection of State programs operating under federal rules; and there has been further tension as to whether, in any event, those rules should be tight or loose. Federalism remains a question central to American policymaking. At the same time, the hidden nature of the American welfare state, marked by opposition to a strong central governmental role for health care, threw many decisions to the courts. In retrospect, both lawyers and the legal system are remarkably absent as players in the NHS, as *Medical Practice in Modern England* demonstrates (though during the past ten years the courts have been more willing to intervene in the U.K.). Legal issues were sufficiently important in Medicaid implementation that we devoted a chapter of *Welfare Medicine* to the important role of the legal system (the courts) in crafting Medicaid as American social policy, in efforts to clarify its goals, eligibility, and basic rules.

Whether Medicaid was a "health" or a "welfare" program was an important issue in 1973. Today Medicaid is characterized as a right for state-specified health services for those individuals who are admitted to the program.[15] In the early 1970s, the question was open as to whether Medicaid was a stopgap alternative to universal national health insurance or a necessary piece of welfare reform. Today, after the failure of the ambitious Clinton Administration health reform proposals of 1993-94, and with the job-oriented, welfare reform movement trimming the welfare rolls since 1996, that question is no longer relevant. Medicaid, supplemented by a new federal-state program for extending health services to children, has its own established niche. It is a huge program of government purchase of health services for large segments of the population, paying the costs for a third of all births, a fourth of all health care for children under the age of five, and half of all nursing home care in the United States.[16]

Managing a system of public purchase of care in the private sector, problematic throughout the early years of Medicaid, remains a central challenge—not just for Medicaid, but for Medicare as well, and indeed for any proposals for extending the public role in health care in the United

States. At a core level *Welfare Medicine* raises fundamental questions as to what a much-sought single-payer insurance system might entail and what it might look like in the United States, at least as applying to those most in need of care. Today's practice is moving toward enrolling Medicaid beneficiaries in managed care, through contracts for specified services between the states and private insurers, which then contract with competing health care providers. The early days of Medicaid implementation, designed to bring the poor into the "mainstream" of middle-class medicine through paying middle-class fees, now seem naively optimistic—and have long since passed away. As the power of setting fees for privately insured patients moved from health care providers to the insurance purchasers in the 1990s, power relationships changed in American medicine. Today Medicaid managed care contracts often bring fiscal hardship to the private providers. Indeed, payment levels are so low for some hospital outpatient services that they are reportedly not worth collecting, taking into account the cost of billing for such services and the ever-present threat of a fine-tooth comb audit.

Both books vividly demonstrate the difficulty of implementing a single-payer system, even under the best of circumstances. Medicaid, like the NHS, exaggerated the weaknesses of the health care system, contributed to increased costs, and imposed new constraints on hospitals and physicians. Both books highlight the unintended consequences of legislative and regulatory action, and show how far health care policy has been made, and by extension continues to be made, through actions taken to correct problems generated at a previous stage of implementation. Hence the continuing reforms, slogans for mobilizing change, and new approaches that have marked health service provision in both countries to the present.

The basic attributes of each health service were in place at the time each book was written: England with its commitment to the whole population and seemingly intractable problems of organizing services; the United States committed to private health insurance for as many people as possible, based on the workplace, with some major gaps in coverage filled by government, and with the organization of services largely left to the private sector. In theory, either was a workable system. Why neither worked as well as expected is explored in these books, filtered through the times in which each book was written.

Reappraisals in 2002

If filtered through our own times, how might these books be written today? As dwellers in the present, we are irretrievably affected by the experiences of health care, more general aspects of the social, political, and economic environment, and the ever-changing language of debate since the 1970s. It would be impossible to write about the NHS up to 1966 or

Medicaid up to 1974 without taking the wisdom of hindsight into account; or perhaps, more accurately, a rather different set of cultural (temporal) biases. This more recent past includes debates about the failure of government action in health care in both countries in the 1970s, followed by reactive shifts toward private market solutions, including the virtues of competition and belief in better management in the 1980s; and then reaction in turn against such shifts in the 1990s and beyond—leading in England to the present upheavals of the NHS around consumerism, building primary care groups, and bringing private investment and management into the NHS; and in the United States to critiques and regulation of managed care corporations, and efforts to mobilize action around the quality of care. Doctors are dissatisfied in both countries, threatened by a perceived loss of clinical autonomy and increased surveillance of professional work through the move toward clinical governance in England and through practice guidelines and medical audits in the United States.

Today's language of debate is more attuned to business terms than to those of social service. Even though both books focus on structures, institutions, and management of health care, they assume that health services are different from other major economic enterprises; indeed, that as social services they are more akin to education than to (say) the banking industry. This was indeed a general view in the 1960s and early 1970s. Administrators were not educated for "management" in business schools, but for "administration" in schools of public health, public welfare, or (in England) social administration. Today in the United States, there is an army of health analysts in academia, banking, accounting, stock market analysis, business consulting, law, lobbying, think tanks, and elsewhere, drawn from many disciplines, each with vested interests in the system. Such roles existed thirty or forty years ago (we can see them in *Welfare Medicine*), but in nothing like today's profusion. The language of business has become ingrained as a vehicle for thinking about health care, infusing health policy in both countries—from the idea of internal markets in England to managed care in the United States. By the late 1980s it was natural for me, writing about the history of American hospitals, to frame my study in terms of their long, interweaving roles as charities and businesses.[17] Today I might say of the two books: In England, the good feelings engendered by the politics of egalitarianism overrode considerations of efficiency; while in the United States, belief in the efficacy of the market produced enormous social inefficiencies.

Today's policy questions focus more overtly than before on the role of government in the economy and in public budgets (of which health care is now a significant part), and as a manager of individual and social risk; on the future of professions as social institutions; on the impact of health systems on patients (and vice versa), and on consumerism more generally; on the moral value of a one-class system of health care (more like the NHS) versus a more stratified set of choices dependent on income and individual choice (more like the United States); on federalism and the relative authority of (and division of taxes between) the nation and states in domestic policy in the United States, a major theme for the future of Medicaid; on devolution and decentralization of authority for health care in Great Britain; and on the relationships between markets, professions, and states. While we touch on many of these questions in the books, there is now a large scholarly literature that would have to be taken into account in any new appraisal. On the other hand, because there was relatively little relevant secondary analysis (the work of other scholars) to draw on while we were doing the research for the books, we had the advantage of working in, and thinking across, relatively clear fields. We also had the privilege of doing contemporary fieldwork and conducting interviews with leading participants.

When the books were written, the literature of feminism was still quite young. It is disconcerting to read the then-common stylistic use of "he" to stand for an undifferentiated individual, including a doctor or a patient. Writing about these topics now, I would include a discussion of the role of health services for women and the role of women workers as a matter of course. Medicaid, for example, has a disproportionate effect on women, because of its primary role in serving mothers with young children at one end of the life course, and the elderly (predominantly female) at the other. On both sides of the Atlantic, too, increased cultural diversity has raised new themes. None of these comments changes the intrinsic value of the books as creatures of their time. But it is instructive, looking back, to see the embedded values they present.

For example, both books are remarkably, even quaintly, optimistic about the potential role of government to create better health care systems—too optimistic in the light of subsequent events. At the very least, I would now be much more critical of the NHS and the problems of a government service in England, and much less sanguine about the potential of the federal government to effect social change in the United States. I think I would also be more charitable toward those attempting to implement Medicaid in its early years, recognizing more clearly with the advantage of distance the complexities and uncertainties of those years. Moreover, national health insurance was demonstrably *not* just around the corner, as we sometimes seem to suggest.

My younger self accepted the nationalization of hospitals and the centralization of services in the NHS far more readily than I would now. Partly that was because it was a fait accompli, and seemed a natural parallel to other forms of nationalization after World War II, including that of energy corporations and the railways. Nevertheless, I could have been more critical. Most interesting, I think, from today's perspective is that the NHS centralized in one organization the means of production of health services (hospitals, specialists, family practitioners, and so on) *and* the means of paying for them. While the NHS could be seen as an incremental extension of the older national health insurance scheme, the combination of the functions of provider and guarantor of services (what we would now think of as seller and buyer) was actually quite radical. In theory, the NHS could have become a contractual service, with government buying services in the private sector, not unlike the health insurance systems of countries like Germany or France, or for the more limited sectors of the population covered by Medicare and Medicaid in the United States. Efforts by the Conservative government to create "internal markets" failed as one redesign of the NHS. In any event, the British government has been bedeviled by having to act as proprietor of a vast array of services and as employer of often obstreperous, disaffected groups, while also representing patients and fighting for budgets in Parliament. The sheer magnitude of the administrative tasks deserves scrutiny as a business proposition. Going the rounds in England in 2001 was the jest that the British NHS, with about one million employees, is the largest (public) organization in the world, with the exception of the Chinese army.[18]

The recent history of the NHS has been a saga of how to reorganize and reintegrate the organizations that were taken over on the "appointed day" for implementation of the NHS in 1948 into a more effective delivery system at the local level—and how far to go in separating the roles of buyer and seller. In recent years the pendulum has swung toward consumer satisfaction (a theme that was remarkably absent in the more paternalistic health service of 1966). Would this focus have come earlier if the health system had not been nationalized in the first place? Would the old public (local government) hospitals, taken into the NHS, have been abandoned in a more private system, like some formerly distinguished American public hospitals, or privatized like the California hospitals after Medicaid? Would previously charitable (voluntary) hospitals now behave more overtly as businesses, as in the United States? The answer to all of these questions is, perhaps. My purpose in raising such questions is merely to observe that these are the kinds of questions that would now infuse reexamination of the materials of *Medical Practice.*

Similarly, in *Welfare Medicine*, we would now, I think, give more emphasis to the management theme underlying the Medicaid program; that is, the problems inherent in any system of public purchase of health care from independent providers or through private insurers. These themes are now critical and current. We might also give less emphasis to the "philosophical"—actually, the rhetorical—bases for distinguishing public assistance and social insurance. Medicaid has taken on a new currency in the last five or six years, as efforts have been made simultaneously to get individuals of working age off welfare, but also to include health coverage to additional children (and sometimes immediate family members) through extended federal-state programs known as child health insurance programs, or CHIP.[19] Significantly, given the history of the negative rhetoric of "assistance," both Medicaid and the new programs are now called "insurance." Meanwhile, Medicare, like Social Security income payments, has been tarred with the new negative rhetoric of "entitlements." The basic dichotomy of insurance versus assistance is not a currently fashionable organizing theme, though it may reappear, of course, in the future.

It may still be possible to depict the history of American social policy for health services as one of intermittent efforts to extend medical technology to the masses. How to insure low-income workers who, through no fault of their own, are without health insurance is currently a vexing political question. So is extending out-of-hospital pharmaceutical benefits as an additional benefit for Medicare beneficiaries. Perhaps the United States will eventually attain universal health insurance coverage in some way or another, and for some or other level of service. However, it is not currently realistic to see Medicaid or Medicare as a step toward a universal national health insurance program, to be built in either of their images. We are older and possibly wiser through experience than when *Welfare Medicine* was written.

Future generations will bring their own, probably very different, perspectives to the history presented in *Medical Practice* and *Welfare Medicine*. The language of debate may well change again, and the research questions will reflect the predilections and experiences of that present. I hope these two books will be read with interest into the future, both for their materials and themes, and as a window into their times; and that they will provoke thought and stimulate original research by others.

The broad questions with which we began remain for exploration by younger scholars. Why do we have the patterns of organization, the health benefits, and the problems that we do? Why have we not been able or willing to design financing and organizational systems to bring the uncontroversial benefits of medicine efficiently to all members of the population, whether through government, the private sector, or a public-private mix? Why is there unease on both sides of the Atlantic about how much medical care, and of what quality, should be accessible to all members of the population? Given the very different cultural histories of each health system—a clear message of these books—how far are the systems actually converging? Which services are best subsidized by government, and why? What are the best ways to stimulate private sector initiative and meet consumer preferences? How much tax money should be allocated to health care in light of competing social goods, such as national defense, public education, or controlling the overall rate of taxation? And on what grounds do we judge any national system a success or a failure?

Rosemary A. Stevens
Philadelphia, 2002

NOTES

1. A primary characteristic of the U.S. health care system, then as now, is the multiplicity of ways in which the federal government funds and otherwise affects health services. One ramification of this has been to avoid strong central control; another has been to disguise the extent of government involvement. The latest figures show 10 percent of the U.S. population covered by Medicaid in 1999, 11 percent by Medicare, 64 percent by private health insurance (typically via place of employment), and 16 percent uninsured. Medicaid, with its 40 million enrollees, is now a larger program in terms of costs than Medicare. Medicaid is also the single largest source of federal funds flowing to the states. For state data see Kaiser Family Foundation, State Health Facts Online. www.statehealthfacts.kff.org. For general information on Medicaid see Kaiser Commission on Medicaid and the Uninsured, www.kff.org, as well as ongoing work by the Urban Institute, www.urban.org and the Commonwealth Fund, www.cmwf.org.

Official statistics generally credit government expenses as representing 45 percent of all health expenditures in the United States. However, these figures include government employees, whose health insurance is purchased in the private sector, under the heading of private rather than public expenditures. If included as public expenses instead, actual government expenditures rise to about 60 percent in the United States (Daniel M. Fox, Milbank Memorial Fund, personal communication). Better comparative statistics, based on common definitions, are needed for more precise cross-national analysis of the relative weight of government spending across different nations.

2. The useful term "health care state" has come into currency as a term to describe the contributions and the effects of public mechanisms to subsidize, provide, and regulate health services—in part as a successor term for the outdated term "welfare state" as applied to health care. See Michael Moran, *Governing the Health Care State: A Comparative Study of the United Kingdom, the United States and Germany* (Manchester and New York: Manchester University Press, 1999); Richard Freeman, *The Politics of Health in Europe* (Manchester and New York: Manchester University Press, 2000); European University Institute, European Forum, Centre for Advanced Studies, Conference, Opening Statement by the organizers, Maurizio Ferrera, Anna Guillen, and August Osterle, *Beyond the Health Care State: Institutional Innovations and New Priorities in Access, Coverage and Provision of Health Services,* Florence, Italy, February 20-27, 1999, www.iue.it, accessed March 9, 2002.

3. Charles Webster, *The National Health Service: A Political History* (Oxford and New York: Oxford University Press, 1998), 140.

4. Stephen Gillam, "Perpetual Evolution: A Stocktake," in *What Has New Labour Done for Primary Care? A Balance Sheet,* ed. Stephen Gillam (London: King's Fund, 2001), 1-29.

5. James C. Robinson, *The Corporate Practice of Medicine: Competition and Innovation in Health Care* (Berkeley: University of California Press, 1999), xii. A widely used term reflecting the often-perceived turbulence of health care as a negative movement is "destabilization." See Eli Ginzberg, "The Destabilization of Health Care," *New England Journal of Medicine* 315 (1986):757-61.

6. *Only Dissect: Rudolf Klein on Politics and Society,* ed. Patricia Day (Cambridge: Blackwell, 1996):319.

7. Mark A. Peterson, "Editor's Note," *Health Politics and Policy in a Federal System,* special edition of *Journal of Health Politics, Policy and Law* 26 (2001):1221.

8. See Harry F. Dowling, *City Hospitals: The Undercare of the Underprivileged* (Cambridge: Harvard University Press, 1982); Charles Brecher and Sheila Spiezo, *Privatization and Public Hospitals* (New York: Twentieth Century Fund, 1995); and Sandra Opdycke, *No One Was Turned Away: The Role of Public Hospitals in New York City Since 1900* (New York: Oxford University Press, 2000).

9. *Statutory History of the United States: Income Security,* ed. Robert B. Stevens (New York: Chelsea House Publishers in association with McGraw Hill, 1970).

10. I deal with these themes in *American Medicine and the Public Interest* (New Haven: Yale University Press, 1971; reissued with a new introduction, Berkeley: University of California Press, 1998).

11. Richard Magraw, book review, *Annals of Internal Medicine* 66 (1967):451.

12. I pay too little attention to these changes in the book, perhaps being too close to them at the time. For a more integrated (science/practice/organization) approach, see Irvine Loudon, John Horder, and Charles Webster, *General Practice Under the National Health Service, 1948-1997* (Oxford: Oxford University Press, 1998). On the relationship between health policy and the shift to chronic conditions in the United States, see Daniel M. Fox, *Power and Illness: The Failure and Future of American Health Policy* (Berkeley: University of California Press, 1993).

13. Albert R. Jonsen, book review, *Journal of Medicine and Philosophy* 1 (1976):283. The references are to John Rawls, *A Theory of Justice* (Cambridge: Belknap Press of Harvard University Press, 1971) and Robert Nozick, *Anarchy, State and Utopia* (New York: Basic Books, 1974).

14. Quoted by George Rosen, "Michael M. Davis (November 19, 1879-August 19, 1971): Pioneer in Medical Care," editorial, *American Journal of Public Health* 62 (1972):322.

15. Sara Rosenbaum, "Medicaid," *New England Journal of Medicine* 346 (February 21, 2002), 635-640.

16. ibid., 635.

17. Rosemary Stevens, *In Sickness and in Wealth: American Hospitals in the Twentieth Century* (New York: Basic Books, 1989; reissued with a new introduction, Baltimore: Johns Hopkins University Press, 1999).

18. This includes a notable exchange between Philip Hammond, M.P. and Alan Milburn, the Secretary of State for Health, during debate on the Health and Social Care Bill in the House of Commons. Hammond criticized the "hands-on control" and "micromanagement" of the NHS and asked if the Secretary of State "can point to a single successful productive enterprise on this scale...organized on a centralized basis..." Milburn replies, "The Chinese army." Hammond was not impressed. House of Commons Hansard Debates for 10 Jan 2001 (pts 29-30). www.parliament.the-stationery-office.co.uk/pa/cm200001/cmhansard/, accessed March 11, 2002.

19. Over time, Medicaid has diverged from its ties to cash assistance, allowing more individuals to be included for health benefits alone. In 1996 Medicaid was formally "delinked" from cash assistance. The descriptive rhetoric also changed. The federal-state programs formally known as Aid to Families with Dependent Children (AFDC) were renamed Temporary Aid for Needy Families (TANF). In 1998, of the almost 21 million children enrolled in Medicaid, about 8 million were "welfare related" and 13 million "poverty related" or "other." Congress enacted the State Children's Health Insurance Program (CHIP) under the Balanced Budget Act of 1997. The new program was designed to pay the costs of care for children under nineteen years of age who are not eligible for Medicaid and whose family incomes fall below 200 percent of the poverty line. Kaiser Commission on Medicaid and the Uninsured, "Health Coverage for Low Income Children," March 2001. www.kff.org, accessed December 20, 2001.

Preface

A considerable number of persons made this book possible by suggesting lines of research, offering encouragement, facilities, and information, criticizing the manuscript, and correcting errors of fact or interpretation. A study of this breadth is particularly dependent on goodwill and advice, and I cannot hope to do justice to all who willingly gave assistance. In singling out a relatively few to thank, I hope the others will in no way think I am not grateful for their contributions.

The original idea for the study came from discussions with I. S. Falk, Professor of Public Health (Medical Care) at Yale, to whom I owe an immense debt of gratitude. It was he who arranged the financing of the project, and it was he who has steered me away from many possible disasters. He has been ready with encouragement and advice throughout the whole life of this study, and he has managed to read most of the many drafts of this book.

For the research on this book I spent two academic years in England. Richard Titmuss, Professor of Social Administration in the University of London, generously gave his time to discuss innumerable aspects of medical care. He also made it possible for me to have the stimulating experience of a visiting appointment in the Department of Social Administration at the London School of Economics. Various other persons also made a major contribution by their reading and criticism of the manuscript. Professor Brian Abel-Smith (University of London), in the course of frequent discussions, prompted new lines of investigation and made particularly helpful suggestions on the organization of the book. He also read and commented on the whole of the manuscript at an early stage. Various parts of the same draft were also read by Roy M. Acheson, Professor of Epidemiology and Medicine at Yale. His comments were as informative as they were invaluable, and the chapters on the development of the specialties owe much to his help. For the historical background I owe a further debt to Edwin Clarke, formerly of Yale and now of the Wellcome Museum in London, and to Professor Charles Newman, whose book on medical education in the nineteenth century was an essential source of reference, and who gave me encouragement and assistance in the early stages of the project. I must also thank three practitioners—Drs. John Fry, R. C. Mac Keith, and D. M. Kellock—and two other academics— Dr. E. R. Weinerman, Professor of Medicine and Public Health at Yale, and Mrs. Margot Jefferys of Bedford College, London—for their painstaking review and thoughtful comments on parts of the manuscript at different stages.

Thanks to the generosity of the London School of Economics, I was fortunate in having Michael Meacher, now on the staff of the University of Essex, as my research assistant for three months. His diligence and enthusiasm made a considerable contribution on various aspects of the medical specialties, and he was a valuable critic of the whole of the study. Mrs. Naomi Burns and Mrs. Sheila Wellington ruthlessly pinpointed deficiencies in presentation: and two other friends, Drs. Joseph Sluglett and Robin Ilbert, read the entire manuscript from the view of the practitioner, and thereafter kept me in touch with GP attitudes. To all four I am most grateful.

The material was collected in England from three major sources: published materials, unpublished materials supplied by institutions and individual persons, and a wide spectrum of interviews with members of professional and administrative bodies. The cooperation of professional associations was crucial, and I was fortunate in their unfailing interest, courtesy, advice, and assistance. Drs. J. C. Cameron, S. J. Hadfield and Peter Wilson kindly answered questions on behalf of the British Medical Association, and Mr. T. Little allowed me access to the Association's statistical material. Miss I. Cook and Dr. Kenneth Robson generously gave their time to discuss the history and role of the Royal College of Physicians of London. Mr. John Lambert and other staff of the Royal College of Surgeons of England not only dealt patiently with my many requests, but also read and made invaluable comments on a large part of the manuscript; while Mr. Harold Edwards found time from his surgical and teaching duties to describe and evaluate the College's postgraduate training scheme. Mr. H. G. E. Arthure, Sir Arthur Bell, and Miss Ada Holloway were equally generous of their time in discussing the Royal College of Obstetricians and Gynaecologists. Mr. F. M. Stent, Secretary to the Examining Board in England, allowed me access to his records and facilities in which to study them.

Past and recent developments in the College of General Practitioners were described by Drs. R. M. S. McConaghey and John and Valerie Graves. Doctors E. M. Darmady, J. W. Howie, W. H. McMenemey and A. G. Signy spoke of the functions of the College of Pathologists; and the problems of the Royal Medico-Psychological Association, also in the process of becoming a College, were discussed by Dr. Brian Ackner,

Professor Desmond Curran, and Dr. A. Walk. Sir Terence Cawthorne and Mr. R. T. Hewitt explained the operation of the Royal Society of Medicine; if its role in the development of the specialties is not adequately emphasized in this book, this is my omission rather than theirs. I must also thank Mr. H. J. P. Arnold of the General Practitioners' Association, Doctors P. M. Elliott and P.S. Greaves of the Medical Practitioners' Union, and Dr. David Kerr of the Socialist Medical Association for analyzing the work of their organizations.

In the field of medical education I am particularly indebted to Dr. John Ellis and to Dr. A. A. G. Lewis, both of whom discoursed at length on several occasions on developments in the undergraduate and postgraduate fields. Sir James Paterson Ross, Professor G. A. Smart, Dr. A. W. Williams and Dr. A. G. W. Whitfield, all key figures in postgraduate medical training organized through university medical departments, were also very helpful on the nature and future of the programs in their respective hospital regions.

Numerous doctors and administrators gave their time to discuss committees of which they were chairman or secretary, or to expound on different aspects of medical planning and organization. I am especially grateful to Lord Brain (chairman of the Advisory Committee on Distinction Awards), Sir Robert Platt (chairman of the Platt committee on hospital medical staffing), and Sir Theodore Fox (then editor of the *Lancet*); to Mr. Robert Armstrong (secretary to the Standing Review Body on Doctors' and Dentists' Remuneration); and to Dr. Albertine Winner (deputy chief medical officer) and Dr. Frank Riley (senior medical officer) of the Ministry of Health.

For a large amount of official data I am indebted to the statistical division and other departments of the Ministry of Health. Information on the regional hospital services was made available at the Sheffield Regional Hospital Board by the Secretary, W. M. Naylor, and the assistant secretary, E. M. Sharman; and by Messrs. E. G. Braithwaite and A. J. Goldingay of the South West Metropolitan Regional Hospital Board. Two secretaries of hospital management committees, S. Hodkinson of Wolverhampton and John Williams of Ipswich, provided historical material on the development of the hospitals in their groups. Bryan McSwiney, administrator of St. Thomas' Hospital, London, allowed me regular access to that institution. Two senior administrative medical officers of regional hospital boards, John Revans of Wessex and R. H. M. Stewart of Newcastle, made special arrangements for me to visit hospitals and talk with staff in their areas so that my impressions would strike a balance between London and the provinces.

I am grateful to many other medical consultants, general practitioners, and administrators in London and in the provinces, who, by giving their time, their views, and often their hospitality, illuminated the statistics and the trends in terms of day-to-day hospital work and professional behavior. The staff of the hospital groups in which I stayed for several days wish to remain anonymous; as promised, I have done my best to make any of their quoted comments untraceable to source. All these persons helped to make the research, undertaken primarily in 1963 and 1964, an enjoyable as well as an instructive experience.

Mrs. Jean Sheppard, Mrs. Barbara Williams, Mrs. Grace L'Manian and Miss Kathryn Pettit typed, with considerable fortitude, successive illegible drafts of the manuscript. In its final stages the manuscript benefited from the tactful comments of Miss Jane Olson and Mrs. Anne Wilde of the Yale University Press, and from detailed suggestions by the press's reader. All this advice and help are gratefully acknowledged. The errors that remain are of course my own.

Finally, I should like to thank the United States Public Health Service for the generous grant which made this study possible.

R. S.

Yale University School of Medicine
New Haven, Connecticut
November 1965

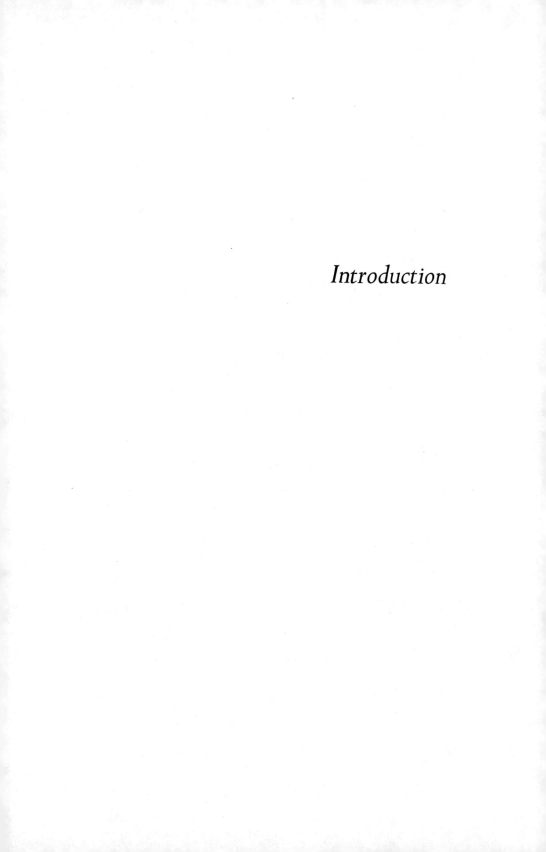

Introduction

Introduction

Before World War II, the great majority of practicing doctors in England and Wales were general practitioners. They had their own surgeries or offices, often in the front room of their own homes, and they were accustomed to dealing with a wide variety of ailments. Some GPs subsequently became specialists, but the majority did not. Specialists were few in number, tended to practice in the large towns, and to be associated with the larger hospitals. In 1939 there was only one specialist to every six or seven GPs, and they were highly concentrated: more than one third of them were in London alone.

But medicine was already changing rapidly under the impact of greater subdivisions in areas as diverse as physics, biochemistry, pharmacology, and genetics, whose span no general practitioner could hope to encompass. The search for new knowledge, the pursuit of greater efficiency and excellence, and an increasing public faith in expertise in all walks of life encouraged doctors to develop exclusive interests and to set themselves up as specialists in their chosen field.

Medical specialization itself was no new thing. Physicians had for centuries been differentiated from surgeons. Other fields, that were not previously considered within the scope of the recognized physician or surgeon, were firmly established as specialties practiced by medical men by the mid-nineteenth century. But the great acceleration of specialization was a product of twentieth-century science and technology. The emphasis in medical care began to shift from the general physician with a special interest—as in pathology, neurology, or cardiology—or a general surgeon interested in urological or ophthalmic surgery, to the full-time specialist exclusively engaged in a well-defined discipline. Specialists became a group of experts with special skills, training, and equipment and with a growing sense of their own specialist identity. Beside them the general practitioner, equally seeking specialist status, uneasily surveyed his future role. Whereas the theme of medical history in the nineteenth century was the integration of diverse skills into one medical profession, the theme of twentieth-century medical practice is a fragmentation within the profession.

In terms of the overall effectiveness of care rendered to the patient—the sole justification for the practice of medicine—the development of medical specialties marked an immeasurable increase in knowledge and skill. Specialization was prompted by those who sought excellence in particular areas within expanding fields; it was an inevitable and desirable accompaniment of scientific advance. But at the same time, the rapidity of change posed acute organizational problems. One immediate problem was the balance between general and specialist practice. A second was the obvious need for rational application of specialist skills so that the patient would benefit from the very technical advances that diversification was designed to achieve. There were problems of communication among the professional branches, there was a growing need for teamwork, and there were increasing but unspecific demands from the public for a personal or family doctor.

New strains were imposed on the organization of medical services and on the institutions of the medical profession. The hospital of the 1930s, still primarily a center for nursing care, became the cradle of new techniques; it rapidly expanded in facilities, equipment and staff, and consequently in cost, to become a major technical unit providing many services that could not be given elsewhere. In turn, the changing role of the hospital and the absence of an effective substitute raised major economic and social problems: the distribution and availability of specialist services to the population, the quality of those services, the ability of the patients to pay the hospital's ever-rising costs, and the balance between hospital and community medical care. Finally, the professional medical organizations were being forced to change. Not only were these bodies fragmented by the desire of specialists for independent status and their own training programs; they were also compelled, by the need to appraise wider questions, to take a strong public stand on the future development of medical care.

While these developments were the unavoidable accompaniment of the scientific improvements in medicine, pre-existing patterns of social and medical organization influenced the particular ways in which specialization developed in different countries. The problems were similar but, with different environments, medical planners were searching for answers from different points of view. Since the organization of medical practice continues to shape the impact of medical specialization, it seemed both appropriate and important to undertake a study of the medical practitioner in relation to various aspects of his environment, past and present.

This examination of patterns of medical care in England and Wales is the first part of a study designed to compare and contrast the medical care problems in England and the United States. A companion volume will trace the development and impact of specialization in the United States. A later work will undertake a comparison of the two countries, in an attempt to formulate general conclusions on past trends and suggest some professional and policy alternatives for future developments in medical care in both countries. The countries were chosen not only for their similar socioeconomic conditions and their common heritage but also because of their very different medical systems. By relating the current medical situation in each country to the historical development of its medical institutions, it should be possible to distil common organizational trends and at the same time to contrast and appraise particular, and possibly temporary, manifestations of unique national situations.

I began the research for this book by concentrating primarily on the relationship between specialism and generalism, on the development of the professional bodies, and on the growing involvement of the clinician in matters of public policy. But it soon became clear that many of the pressures already imposed on medical practice by specialization had affected the development and particular structures of the British National Health Service. That Service, introduced in 1948, was grafted onto accepted professional patterns; indeed, as will be described, it formalized and exaggerated their effects. Some of these patterns antedate the impact of either scientific specialization or state medical services; their origins were social rather than scientific and were due to professional rather than governmental behavior. The division of the profession into general practitioners and consultants survived the Act of 1858, which united physicians, surgeons, and apothecaries into one medical profession. The referral system was developed in the late nineteenth century in order to eliminate competition for patients between general practitioners and consultants. Hospital staffing patterns were evolved within the voluntary teaching hospitals primarily in the eighteenth and nineteenth centuries. General practitioners were excluded from staffs of the major voluntary hospitals at the beginning of the twentieth century; and the continued insistence on a monopoly of hospital beds by consultants merely followed an established trend.

Underlying professional tensions were also transferred into the National Health Service. The question of the differential status of consultants and general practitioners has been a cause of concern to both branches since the sixteenth century when the Royal College of Physicians was given oversight of apothecaries; and general practitioners were rising in social status long before specialization emphasized their new central role. Something of this ancient tension reappeared in the differential pay disputes of the early 1960s. The old divergence of interest between London and the provinces became, as the provincial medical schools developed, a divergence between the teaching and nonteaching hospitals. The National Health Service Act, as the culmination of discussions on the future of medical services carried on between the two world wars, reflected the needs of the 1930s rather than those of the post-World War II period. It came at a time when the response of professional structures to the pressures of specialization was, if not embryonic, at least incomplete.

One outcome of the efficiency of specialist medicine has been its increased social desirability. The specialist holds a kind of monopoly; his skill in his chosen field should be greater than the same skill practiced by anyone else.

This has led not only to increasing public demand for specialist care—one factor in the rapidly increasing number of specialists in the past thirty years —but also to questions of the availability of such services and of their augmented quality and value. Deprivation of specialist services to those needing their attention, for reasons of cost or inaccessibility, became an important social issue.

At the same time social mores changed. Even at the beginning of this century a child might die of malnutrition without a public outcry, although the death was socially preventable. Now both the medical profession and the general public pay at least lip service to the concept that no child should die of, say, an operable congenital abnormality—even though the cost of rectifying the deformity may be many times greater than was the cost of feeding a child in 1900. The change is partly a symptom of increased general affluence, partly of a different perspective of society; it may also reflect pride in the precision and effectiveness of modern medicine. Whatever the reason, there has been a growing acceptance that access to medical services is one of the modern social rights.

The National Health Service was one expression of this trend. The state was not obliged to intervene; large-scale voluntary prepaid programs might have provided a similar service. But involvement by government or insurance appeared to be the only logical answer to the need to reconcile the advances in medicine with the demands of the public. The individual relationship between one doctor and one patient remains the core of the medical function—but only the core. The doctor is involved in a rapidly expanding medical spectrum. He is increasingly dependent upon the advice of his colleagues and upon the facilities of the hospital. Behind the patient are all the expectations and resources of society for good medical care at a reasonable cost with the implications of efficient hospitals, rational planning, and well-trained professional and technical staff.

The basic social implications of modern medicine have been achieved under the National Health Service—the entitlement of the whole population to community-supported medical services, the regional development of hospital and specialist facilities, and the concentration of continuous care on the general or family doctor. But the traditions of the medical profession and the structure of the National Health Service have not of themselves led to adequate solutions for the organizational problems of modern medical care: how to reconcile the need for continued technological (and specialist) advance in hospital-based medicine with the provision of a comprehensive and coordinated family and community health service of high quality and ready accessibility. More positive and comprehensive planning is necessary to face the organizational problems of the future. A new coordination is required between general and specialist practice, between teaching and non-teaching hospitals and, above all, in professional education and training programs. The National Health Service has passed one stage; it is now entering another.

The crucial organizational questions of specialized medicine are, first, the changing role of the general practitioner and, second, the interdependence of hospital and nonhospital medicine. The overriding requirement is that all the patient's medical needs be met—whatever they prove to be, and whatever special skills they may require. The individual patient may have both a heart problem and an intestinal ulcer. Who is to decide whether he should first see a heart specialist, a radiologist, an abdominal surgeon, a specialist in internal medicine, or a psychiatrist? Who should link the various skills involved at each stage of treatment, and who should explain the alternatives to the patient? In England the general practitioner provides the coordinating function. If the GP did not exist he would have to be invented, for his central position as personal medical adviser to the patient has become more important as the specialties have proliferated.

But at the same time, as the boundaries of medical knowledge have widened, the old type of "general" practitioner has been quietly passing away. It has become impossible for one person to master all of medicine. The English general practitioner is in transition to a new, but as yet unspecified, role as a personal doctor with well-defined skills. Through the referral system, he sees all patients at first instance; thus, although the scope of his activities excludes year by year a larger proportion of total medical knowledge, the GP retains his central position, in which he must generalize over the whole of medicine, and select the specialized services he thinks appropriate.

Recognition of the GP as a *generalizer* rather than a *generalist* implies a much greater degree of interdependence of general practitioners and specialists than has customarily existed between them. No longer is medicine a matter of a general practitioner on the one side and a few specialists on the other in some kind of loose or arms-length relation; it must become a multidisciplinary team—at least a coordinated team and, better still, an integrated team—in which the personal doctor has an important place. The National Health Service has emphasized the *separation* between general and specialist practice at the very time that *coordination* and *integration* are becoming the essence of good medicine.

As the role of the general practitioner changes, the interrelationships among hospitals, specialists, and generalists have also to be modified. The hospital is the nucleus both of specialist practice and of specialist training. The general practitioner is focused on the patient within society. The two foci are not incompatible, but they demand realignments in two major areas: the role of the hospital in the organizational structure of medical care, and the development of professional education and training. The question is whether the hospital is or should be the core of all personal medical services, or whether it can best serve its purpose by retaining its traditional place at the fringe of medical care. Reports in the interwar period, notably the Dawson report of 1920, had assumed a medical system based on the second alternative, through primary and secondary health centers; and this concept was built into the NHS Act. A large-scale development of health centers might have linked general practitioners and specialists into one group-practice team, and removed to the health center many of the functions which are now being undertaken by hospital diagnostic and outpatient departments. But this plan was not put into effect. Consultative services were largely provided by the hospital, but the hospital did not expand to include the general aspects of medical care. On the contrary, it moved in the opposite direction, and the separations were widened. There was thus something approaching a divorce between the personal general doctor and the specialist, precipitating a continued question of the hospital's proper function in the future.

Changes in medicine are also reflected in the changing focus of education and training. The old assumption was that general practice was the prelude to specialized training, and thus of lesser technical status. The undergraduate years of medicine are now accepted as an introductory foundation for all who would be doctors. The two stages of "education" and "training" have been differentiated. As a result, the major responsibility for technical training of a practicing doctor—specialist or generalist—has been deferred to the postgraduate period. This is not peculiar or specific to Great Britain; it is as clearly evident, increasingly, in the United States. Indeed, it has to become more or less universal, because the underlying science and technology of medicine are universal; and the need for specialization and specialized training is pervasive. Questions of content and competence at the postgraduate level are similar to those that occupied much attention concerning undergraduate education and training more than a century ago. Indeed, if all doctors are recognized as specialists, and this would seem a logical trend whether their specialty is surgery, family practice, or administrative medicine, the standard of specialist training *is* the basic standard of medical practice. A more stringent supervision of postgraduate training may be necessary, whether this be through informal measures taken by the professional bodies or through an official licensing agency.

The questions posed by specialization concern the need to modify the institutions of medicine—the structure of medical services and the organization and function of the professional bodies—to adjust to scientific expansion and technical change. Each raises issues of social and professional responsibility for developing health services of good quality. This book has been written in the hope that understanding the social origins of medical organization will prompt discussion on its present relevance and future development.

I

The Professional Background

I

Foundations of Modern Medical Practice 1700–1858

Most of the basic characteristics of British medical practice were apparent in embryonic form at the time of the Medical Act of 1858 and were clearly in existence by 1900. These patterns include the development of the present system of undergraduate education and registration and of postgraduate examinations; the relative functions of the professional bodies and the universities; the operation of the referral system between general practitioner and specialist; and the staffing structure of British hospitals. They thus antedate the major influence on modern medicine—the vast and sudden strides in medical research that compelled a rapid growth of specialization, and the emergence of the National Health Service—and a knowledge of their origins is necessary to understand the structure and operation of current medical practice.

The Medical Hierarchy and the Growth of Hospitals

Until the Medical Act of 1858 established a single medical register for all medical practitioners with recognized diplomas or degrees, there were, besides the so-called quacks whose fields ranged from lithotomy to patent remedies, three separate categories of doctor: the physician, the surgeon, and the apothecary. Each group had its own professional body; each of these bodies had its own national institution in England, Scotland, and Ireland; and each had a distinct professional history. This division was to have a lasting impact on the development of medical practice. Physicians and surgeons were ancestors of today's consultants and specialists; apothecaries were the forerunners of today's general practitioners.

The Royal College of Physicians of London was incorporated by Henry VIII in 1518 to oversee the practice of medicine within a seven-mile radius of the City of London. Its primary purpose was to license recognized physicians who would thereby be distinguished from those who were unqualified; and it immediately established a monopoly. The function of the College of Physicians was overtly to protect the public: "to curb the audacity of those wicked men who shall profess medicine more for the sake of their avarice than from the assurance of any good conscience, whereby very many inconveniences may ensue to the rude and credulous populace." [1] But few of the "credulous populace" of the time can have received the benefits of the learned physicians' care; these early doctors attended only the Royal Family, the aristocracy, and the wealthy, and they were themselves drawn from the upper strata of society. The College thus began as an exclusive domain of upper-class medical practitioners. It was a professional guild of the elect, a college in the sense of providing a learned atmosphere for persons with similar interests and a joint determination to enhance the standing of their profession.

The Royal College of Physicians of Edinburgh (founded in 1681) and the Royal College of Physicians of Ireland (which began in 1654 and received its Royal Charter in 1667) were closely associated from their early years with the universities. At the time of their founding, university medical schools already existed in Ireland and Scotland, the earliest academic study of medicine in Britain having been at the University of Aberdeen. The Edinburgh physicians had close ties with the University of Edinburgh. In its early years, the president of the Irish College of Physicians was appointed by the Board of Trinity College, the only constituent college of the University of Dublin.[2]

There was, however, no university in London. Thus, although the Royal College of Physicians of London was the domain of Oxford and Cambridge graduates, it did not have the same kind of university focus as its counterparts. While the basic functions of the three Colleges were similar, each having the power to license physicians and to oversee apothecaries, their development was conditioned by local responsibility—originally metropolitan but gradually widening to influence the whole of each country. Until 1858, licentiates of the English and Irish Colleges of Physicians might not practice in Scotland, and Irish and Scottish apothecaries might not practice in London; and there was no general regulation of the requirements specified for each license.[3]

Surgery was an old and well-established trade long before the Colleges of Physicians were established, but it achieved the respectability of a profession only when surgeons were organizationally separated from their fellow barbers in the eighteenth century. With the extension of surgery as an intellectual discipline, under the influence of John Hunter and others, and the gradual development of surgical techniques, the surgeon gained in status; by 1800 he was beginning to approach the social level of the physician.[4]

1. Royal College of Physicians of London, *The Charter and Bye-Laws* (London, 1959), p. ix.

2. See Royal College of Physicians of Edinburgh, *Historical Sketch and Laws* (Edinburgh, 1925); J. D. H. Widdess, *A History of the Royal College of Physicians of Ireland* (Edinburgh, 1963); D. Guthrie, in F. N. L. Poynter (ed.), *The Evolution of Medical Practice in Britain* (London, 1961), pp. 45–60.

3. W. M. Frazer, *A History of English Public Health* (London, 1950), p. 74.

4. In 1800 the surgeons, in at least the most prestigious voluntary hospitals, were drawn from the same social backgrounds as physicians; both were likely to be the sons of professional men. Professionally, however, there was still a gulf between the

This development was reflected in the professional organizations: the Royal College of Surgeons of Edinburgh was incorporated in 1778, the Royal College of Surgeons in Ireland in 1784, and the Royal College of Surgeons of London (later of England) in 1800. Again, each body developed independently of the others.

The third and lowliest category of doctor was the apothecary. Originally general shopkeepers, apothecaries assumed a separate identity when they broke away from the Mystery of Grocers in 1617. In England the apothecary established the right to treat the sick during the plague of 1665, when many physicians, along with their rich patients, moved out of town to seek the more salubrious air of the country.[5] The House of Lords, sitting in its judicial capacity, upheld that right in the early eighteenth century, in spite of the objections of the Royal College of Physicians of London, which, through its powers (including that of visiting apothecaries' shops to destroy defective drugs), had repeatedly endeavored to limit the apothecary's authority.[6] From this time apothecaries gradually extended their medical function from keeping chemists' shops to compounding over-the-counter prescriptions and to prescribing for and treating patients in the home. Finally, in 1858, apothecaries were listed with physicians and surgeons in one register of medical practitioners.

There were not always clear lines of demarcation between the work of each group of practitioners, and their functions inevitably overlapped. Physicians invariably had university degrees from a Scottish, Irish, English, or foreign university; ideally they had a broad cultural background. They were concentrated in the major towns and cities: outside these centers, and for the lower rungs of society, surgeons and apothecaries predominated, and those who were both surgeons and apothecaries acted as general practitioners—a term that was in established use some time before 1830.[7] Most eighteenth-century surgeons and apothecaries had no diploma or degree, although some surgeons studied in Edinburgh, Dublin, or London, or in medical schools on the Continent. With the exception of a few ancient charitable institutions that had survived the Reformation, the only hospital in most towns was the infirmary attached to the workhouse, which accommodated the able-bodied and the sick poor of the neighborhood; students were apprenticed to practitioners in the town or to the surgeon attached to the infirmary.

---

learned physician and the practical surgeon. See Charles Newman, *The Evolution of Medical Education in the Nineteenth Century* (London, 1957), p. 16.

5. E. M. Brockbank, *The Foundation of Provincial Medical Education in England* (Manchester, 1936), p. 7.

6. A certain William Rose was prosecuted by the RCP of London for illegal practice. He was convicted by the trial court, but the House of Lords reversed the decision in 1703, holding that an apothecary could practice medicine and prescribe for a patient without the advice of a physician. The apothecary was allowed to charge for drugs only, not for advice. R. M. S. McConaghey, in Poynter (ed.), pp. 134–35. See also Zachary Cope, *Brit. Med. J.* i (1956), 1–6.

7. A.M. Carr-Saunders, and P.A. Wilson, *The Professions* (Oxford, 1933), p. 80.

This was the structure of the profession at the beginning of the hospital movement, and it inevitably molded hospital development. The early existence of professional associations rather than universities as the arbiters of standards distinguished the vocational rather than the academic aspects of medical education. Training was to develop through an apprenticeship system, medical schools were founded by practicing doctors, and hospital staffing was influenced by the needs of practical bedside teaching.

Voluntary general hospitals, and with them the beginning of teaching programs, began to be established in all parts of the country during the eighteenth century.[8] Westminster (1719), Guy's (1725), and St. George's (1733) represented the new movement in London. The Royal Infirmary in Edinburgh (1736), Leeds Infirmary (1767), Birmingham General Hospital (1779), and the "General Hospital near Nottingham" (1781) represented the trend in Scotland and the provinces. Between 1700 and 1825, 154 new hospitals and dispensaries were established in Britain[9] as charitable institutions for the sick poor—not for the middle class. They had their parallel in the foundation of charity schools—the result of humanitarian rather than scientific ideals. The rich were still cared for at home by a private physician or by a combination of apothecary and physician, the first responsible for day-to-day treatment, the second calling less frequently and acting as a consultant.[10] Indeed, home care for the wealthy continued until the late nineteenth and early twentieth centuries, when the combat against infection, the employment of aseptic surgical techniques, and the revolution in nursing evoked by Florence Nightingale had begun to create the modern hygienic hospital.

The ancient charity hospitals, often with monastic foundations, had employed physicians and surgeons to look after their patients on a cash-or-kind basis. But the physicians and surgeons who attended the new voluntary hospitals were expected to give their services free, as did the founders and board members of the new institutions. Subsequently, the older hospitals

8. Birmingham, e.g., with 40,000 people, accommodated a Town Infirmary with 270 beds and over 750 outpatients in 1766. Medical students were apprenticed to practitioners in the town; but the infirmary surgeon, a Mr. John Tomlinson (only physicians had university degrees and were entitled to be called "Doctor"), gave a weekly course of lectures, the first record of systematic medical teaching in that city. The establishment of a voluntary general hospital was approved in 1765, and opened 14 years later. Physicians and surgeons to the new hospital were allowed to take 12 apprentices. Birmingham University, *The History of the Birmingham Medical School* (Birmingham, 1925), pp. 1–12.

9. G.M. Trevelyan, *English Social History* (3d ed. London, 1948), p. 345.

10. Samuel Richardson's Clarissa Harlowe (1748) had the attendance in London of an apothecary, and a physician acting as consultant. "Her apothecary came in. He advised her to the air, and blamed her for so great an application, as he was told she made, to her pen; and he gave it as the doctor's opinion, as well as his own, that she would recover, if she herself desired to recover, and would use the means." *Clarissa* (Random House ed., New York, 1950), p. 579.

conformed and ceased to pay their attending physicians and surgeons.[11] A pattern of attending "honoraries" was established, drawn from the same social class as the lay members of the voluntary boards. This system was continued in voluntary hospitals established in the nineteenth and early twentieth centuries. It placed the physician and the increasingly respectable surgeon in a superior, noncontractual relationship with the hospital—and it naturally excluded from its attending staff the lowly apothecary.

The widespread development of voluntary hospitals coincided with great changes in medicine. Medical science in England followed the precepts of Sydenham. It was based on the careful observation of patients' symptoms rather than on experiment: when all the signs were observed, they could be classified into a distinct disease entity. This nosological approach to medicine was to have an enduring impact on the development of medical practice. It necessarily concentrated on the disease instead of the patient, and it was around the disease pattern that the nineteenth- and twentieth-century specialties were to grow. The eighteenth-century physician, like Linnaeus with his plants and butterflies, was able to collect his symptoms and analyze them from the conveniently increasing number of indigent patients found in the hospital wards. Hospital beds thus rapidly became valuable vehicles for individual observation and for teaching apprentices, and access to beds by physicians and surgeons was at a premium. The social structure of the medical profession had already ensured a small elite of consultants attached to the voluntary hospitals. The new medicine gave this elite a technological reason for limiting their number; it was in the interest of each industrious physician to attain responsibility for as many hospital beds as was consistent with his research activities.

The typical eighteenth-century voluntary hospital had a resident apothecary who acted under the guidance of the honorary physicians and surgeons. He was responsible for the daily bleeding, scarifyings, cuppings, and blisterings; he cared for the surgical instruments and was in charge of the baths and, where there was one, of the newfangled electrical machine. He might also be the collector of fees from any patient who could afford to pay, and act as secretary, pharmacist, or dispenser. He lived and ate his meals in the hospital, and he was allowed to have an apprentice. Attending surgeons rated higher than apothecaries on the social scale, but the physicians, besides being the epitome of elegance, were the source of all major medical decisions. No surgeon, for instance, might administer internal medicine, and no amputation or other major operation was allowed without the physician's approval.[12] The medical staff was "closed," appointment being made by the governing board, and the number of "honoraries" was relatively small. Hospital appointment therefore gained an exclusive reputation. Moreover, ap-

11. Brian Abel-Smith, *The Hospitals 1800–1948* (London, 1964), p. 6. I am indebted to this source for much of the hospital background in this chapter.

12. See Frank H. Jacob, *A History of the General Hospital near Nottingham* (London, 1951), pp. 95–99.

pointments to hospitals were the best advertisement any physician might have for promoting his private practice, and there were direct financial rewards in the apprenticeship fees to be gained from bedside teaching.

The teaching of medical students at the bedside was a direct outcome of the need for clinical observation. It gave a further dimension to hospital staffing in that each honorary physician or surgeon had his own retinue or "firm," to whom he expounded on the patient's condition. In addition, the study of particular diseases made it convenient to place patients with similar conditions in one ward, under one physician or surgeon. Hospital beds were assigned to members of the attending staff, sometimes equally, sometimes according to seniority—the more senior, the more beds. Each physician or surgeon (subject to major surgical decisions) was solely responsible for the treatment of patients in his beds. The "honorary," his apprentices, and his assigned beds functioned as a semiautonomous unit within the hospital. The modern pattern of English hospital staffing was thus apparent if, as yet, in embryonic form: a prestigious minority of medical practitioners had control of both the beds and the teaching in the major hospitals.

Not surprisingly, medical schools in England developed, chiefly in the nineteenth century, around the hospitals rather than the universities—in marked contrast to the system in Germany and countries that followed the German pattern, where medical education was to stem from university science departments.[13] While individual physicians and surgeons took paying pupils as apprentices, the gaps in academic knowledge were filled by a number of private schools outside the hospitals, perhaps the most famous being the Great Windmill Street School in London, founded by William Hunter in 1768. But gradually this casual system of "walking the hospitals" was replaced by organized courses and later by medical schools run by the voluntary hospitals. The private schools gradually withered away. Each major hospital founded its own school, staffed by the hospital physicians and surgeons. Teaching was necessarily subservient to practice; and English medical teachers were those with high professional standing rather than those with academic or teaching inclinations.[14]

Medical Education in the Early Nineteenth Century

The hierarchy of physicians, surgeons, and apothecaries and its relationship with the voluntary hospitals, well established by 1800, was dictated not by the nature of medical techniques, which were rapidly changing, but by

13. The first complete school of medicine and surgery in London was established in the London Hospital in 1785 by the physicians and surgeons attached to the hospital. In the United States, John Morgan, following the Continental–Scottish pattern, had set up a university medical faculty in Philadelphia 20 years earlier (1765). Charles Newman, *Evolution of Medical Education*, p. 34; R. Shryock, *Medicine and Society in America 1660–1860* (Great Seal Books, Ithaca, 1962), pp. 24–25.

14. George Newman, *Some Notes on Medical Education in England*, Cd. 9124 (London, 1918), p. 25.

the more tenuous divisions of social class. One speaker, defending the physicians as a caste in 1847, acknowledged great advantages to society of "a certain class of the medical profession having been educated with the gentry of the country, and having thereby acquired a tone of feeling which is very beneficial to the profession as a whole." [15] A physician was expected to hold the license of the Royal College of Physicians of London (LRCP) if he practiced within seven miles of the city, or the extra-license if he practiced elsewhere in England; but in fact few physicians outside London held this diploma.

In London, the license was essential for a position as a physician on the staff of a hospital. Those with the London license had, apart from their hospital work, to practice as consultants; they had come to expect those apothecaries who were employed by the middle class to refer difficult cases to them for their private attention. The license examination, in deference to the educational caliber of the candidates, was conducted in Latin until 1830. Physicians felt themselves to be the cream of society and the cream of the profession. Surgeons did their best to emulate this attitude; giving their services free and surrounded by their pupils, they too "looked upon the hospitals as theirs, not the public's." [16]

Over the years, the scope of the London College of Physicians increased. Compilation of a pharmacopoeia occupied the College until the Act of 1858, when this function was taken over by the General Medical Council. In the eighteenth century, the College played a major role in public health through its efforts to bring under control the sale of gin, which led to the Gin Acts of 1736, 1751, and 1752. Later it played an important part in collecting evidence and making reports on vaccination; and at the turn of the nineteenth century it was responsible for supervising the care of the insane in the London area.[17]

In the nineteenth century, however, the College suffered a long decline. Apothecaries, relentlessly rising in status, were feeling the need for their own licensing examination and for raising their standards and status. Many apothecaries by this time were often also surgeons, and the Royal College of Surgeons was forced to improve its own training requirements through the apothecaries' activities. The rapid growth in educational programs in the first half of the nineteenth century concerned these two groups which were outside the sphere of the College of Physicians. The programs centered, first, on upgrading the apothecary and the surgeon–apothecary and, second, as a direct result of this, on the rapid development of teaching outside London.

Systematic training of apothecaries was achieved through the Apothecaries Act of 1815, the first medical landmark of the nineteenth century.

15. *Report of the Select Committee on Medical Registration* (London, 1847), quoted by Carr-Saunders and Wilson, *The Professions,* p. 75.

16. S. Sprigge, *The Life and Times of Thomas Wakley* (London, 1897), p. 110.

17. Charles Dodds and L. M. Payne, in Poynter (ed.), *Evolution of Medical Practice,* pp. 43–44.

This act gave power to the Society of Apothecaries for the first time to examine and license apothecaries throughout England and Wales. Candidates had to be competent in Latin; to produce certificates of attendance at lectures and of six months' attendance at a public hospital, infirmary, or dispensary; and to have completed a five-year apprenticeship. Apothecaries who practiced without a license could be, and were, prosecuted by the Society. Within a generation the Apothecaries Act created a body of relatively well-trained and informed medical practitioners who were, nevertheless, still educationally and socially inferior to the small elite of physicians.

The license of the Society of Apothecaries (LSA) rapidly became the most popular of the medical diplomas. Coupled with the basic membership examination of the Royal College of Surgeons (MRCS) it was the usual goal of medical students in the new hospital schools. By the 1840s, five out of every six students in the London hospitals were working for the LSA and the proportion was probably higher outside London. The Royal College of Physicians remained exclusive. Until 1858, its rules did not allow the simultaneous possession of its basic diploma (LRCP) and that of the Surgeons or Apothecaries. It was possible to practice medicine as well as surgery by holding the MRCS alone; one fifth of those with the MRCS in the 1850s are believed to have practiced as general practitioners with no diploma other than that.

But the great majority who had diplomas in the middle of the nineteenth century held both the LSA and the MRCS.[18] These were not only rank-and-file country doctors but men who were both eminent surgeons and teachers. A legal decision in 1829 enabled apothecaries to enhance their status still further. They were now allowed to claim payment for their medicine or for their skill and attention (but not for both), where previously they had been allowed to charge for medicine alone: apothecaries were competing successfully with physicians.

The traditional structure of the profession was clearly under enormous strain. The Royal College of Physicians was restricted in numbers because its members had to be M.D.s, whereas the Society of Apothecaries and the Royal College of Surgeons were not so limited. The Royal College of Surgeons had some 200 fellows and 8,000 members by the middle of the century; many of these were also apothecaries. The Royal College of Physicians was left behind. In 1834 it could boast only 274 licentiates and 113 fellows.[19] The two routes to medical practice now diverged widely, and the surgeons and apothecaries, with diplomas from their professional bodies, appeared about to swamp the relatively minute flow of physicians from the universities.

At the same time, teaching programs for the diplomas of the surgeons and apothecaries in the provinces began to counterbalance the power of the London Colleges. Typically, the provincial medical schools were estab-

18. Charles Newman, *Evolution of Medical Education,* pp. 78 and 230.
19. Abel-Smith, *The Hospitals,* p. 2; Carr-Saunders and Wilson, p. 72.

lished by surgeons who had been trained in London or abroad before returning to their native cities. The first school of anatomy *and medicine* outside London, Oxford, and Cambridge was the Mount Street School in Manchester (1814), although there was an earlier school of anatomy in Bristol (1807). Schools quickly followed at Liverpool, Leeds, and Birmingham; it was claimed that local training for the MRCS and LSA was necessary to save students from the "distractions and allurement" of London.[20] To be effective, each school had to be recognized as a teaching body by the Society of Apothecaries and the Royal College of Surgeons. The apothecaries readily approved the schools but did not hesitate to delay or withdraw recognition where the standards were considered insufficient; undoubtedly this had a major impact on the quality of the schools. The surgeons, because of their teaching regulations, were more reluctant to approve the provincial schools. Their material concern was bound up with the "firm" system of hospital teaching. Since each student paid substantial fees directly to his mentor, and since the Council, teachers, and examiners of the Royal College of Surgeons resided in London, there was every incentive for leading surgeons to insist on the continuance of a compulsory period of training in London for each provincial student.[21] The ensuing battle for recognition between the Royal College of Surgeons and the provincial schools led to a Select Committee on medical education in 1834, but not until 1839 did the College drop its London requirement. Provincially-based registrars for the LSA had been appointed several years before (1831). The new schools, although they still trained for London examinations, were becoming relatively unfettered.

As each provincial city continued to grow in size and prosperity—the prolonged result of the Industrial Revolution—it developed its own university of which the medical school became an early and integral part. Although not formally recognized until the late nineteenth or early twentieth century when the "redbrick" universities received their charters, the links between medical schools and general colleges in these cities had been effected much earlier. Manchester's medical school, for example, became the medical department of Owen's College in 1851. In this, the development of the provincial schools was clearly different from the London medical schools whose hospital affiliation, even up to the present, has in many ways remained more intimate than their relationship with the University.

University College, London, the nucleus of London University, was

20. *History of Birmingham Medical School,* p. 20.

21. "The hospital surgeons appointed the lecturers to the medical schools—that is, they appointed themselves, their relations, and the gentlemen who had paid them large fees to become their apprentices. The hospital surgeons were also the authorities at the College of Surgeons, that is, they were the men who decided that the lectures of certain gentlemen should be compulsory for all medical students in London. The compulsory lectures were delivered by themselves, their relatives, or their apprentices." Sprigge, p. 172.

opened in 1828 as a nonsectarian college for students who could not pass the religious tests imposed by Oxford and Cambridge. It had facilities for teaching candidates for the LSA and MRCS. The medical department of Kings College, London, was founded in 1831. In 1833 the Royal College of Surgeons unsuccessfully petitioned the Crown against allowing the proposed University of London, including University College and Kings College, to grant medical degrees. A second petition, also to no avail, was sent in 1834, and in 1836 the University of London was incorporated as an examining body for conferring degrees. The views of the Royal College of Surgeons however, prevailed. The degree in surgery, it was announced, would not carry with it the right to *practice* surgery. Although the University degree and the College diploma were made legally equivalent in 1858, the struggle between the Royal Colleges and the University continued for the next sixty years, until the attempts by the Colleges to institute a joint examination in medicine and surgery with the University of London, and even to found a rival university, were finally abandoned.[22]

For many years the establishment of London University did not affect the position of the medical schools attached to the London teaching hospitals. Students in these schools, as elsewhere, normally took the professional rather than the university examinations. This situation continued through the nineteenth and well into the twentieth century. The rulers of the Royal Colleges and the teachers of the schools were one and the same. The development of medical schools had therefore extended, rather than reduced, the influence of the professional bodies.[23] Even now, the basic medical examinations may be taken either at a university or through the Royal Colleges, which continue to have no university affiliation.

Hospital schools flourished in England because medical instruction in the universities was weak. Dr. John Haviland, appointed Regius Professor at Cambridge in 1817, had finally instituted medical lectures and an examination in that university. Reform at Oxford gained momentum only when Henry Acland became Regius Professor in the second half of the century. The foundation of the medical faculty at Durham in 1856 added a further source of university medical teaching, but these moves were too late to

22. The Royal Colleges wanted the degree of M.D. to be granted to those who became LRCP and MRCS, because the title "Doctor" was thought to be desirable. Discussions on the ways and means of attaining this end lasted from 1885 until 1908 and was raised again, abortively, in 1938. Instead, the Colleges moved farther from, instead of closer to, the university educational centers of medicine. Zachary Cope, *The History of the Royal College of Surgeons of England* (London, 1959), pp. 157–64.

23. A prominent London doctor and medical reformer said in 1857, "Few persons, unless they have lived in London, could form any idea of the power of the ruling body of these Colleges, not so much in their corporate capacity, as in that of individuals. They were the medical attendants of nearly every member of both Houses of Parliament, and they were frequently consulted by those members with regard to particular Bills which came before them." *Brit. Med. J. i* (1857), 673–74 (Dr. Lankester).

change the locus of English medical teaching. At the time of the Medical Act of 1858, all of the present twelve undergraduate medical schools of the London hospitals were in existence, and there were rapidly rising medical schools in nine provincial towns elsewhere in England; all of these originated outside universities from the interests of local hospital clinicians.[24]

At Oxford and Cambridge the basic Bachelor of Medicine degree followed an Arts degree. The medical degrees of London University, and later of the provincial universities, grew from hospital training programs. These had not been designed, as in the old universities, for philosophical inquiry and study of the classics but for practical apprenticeship and instruction. The new M.B. and B.S. (surgery) degrees that were developed at London University and the provincial universities naturally evolved as undergraduate programs, qualification for which, as for the LSA and MRCS examinations, was determined by educational background alone. The M.D. was a higher degree, somewhat on the level of a Ph.D. In England, unlike Germany and the United States, the M.D. did not develop as the cachet of all medical men, and today only a minute proportion of practitioners in England has a valid claim to the title of "doctor."

The Profession and the Act of 1858

The structure of the medical profession was linked with the organization of the professional bodies. The Royal College of Physicians was governed by its fellows (FRCP), chosen from those who were licentiates, and thus of higher professional standing. At the beginning of the nineteenth century the Royal College of Surgeons had only one grade of membership. But it too was forced to introduce a second tier of association when the MRCS had become so popular as to signify a certain surgical competence rather than a higher expertise, a diploma for general practitioners rather than for surgical consultants and teachers.

After its abortive battle with the provincial medical schools and its opposition to London University in the 1820s and 1830s, the Royal College of Surgeons turned to the more fruitful activity of providing a cadre of surgeons who would be of sufficient caliber to teach MRCS candidates in the burgeoning schools. It was decided to establish a special college examination under the Court of Examiners, which would confer the status of fellowship (FRCS) on successful candidates. The creation of fellows was permitted by the new Charter of 1843 and the first fellowship examination was held in 1844. The two-part examination—a primary test in the basic medical sciences and a final in surgery—was similar to the examination of

24. The provincial towns were Birmingham, Bristol, Hull, Leeds, Liverpool, Manchester, Newcastle, Sheffield, and York. Apart from Newcastle, where there were two schools, one teaching in connection with London University and one with Durham University, these schools did not give degrees. They still prepared for the College of Surgeons, the Society of Apothecaries, and also for the armed forces. Newman, *Evolution of Medical Education*, pp. 116–17.

today. Six years of professional study were required (or five years for those with an arts degree), and the candidate had to be at least 25 years old and of certified good character.[25] By this decision, later followed by the Royal College of Physicians, the structure of modern professional medical education was established: a basic and relatively common diploma followed by one with more prestige, both awarded by a professional College. The first was suitable for general practitioners; the second was desirable for the surgical consultant of repute with his own hospital beds and his own retinue of students. Appointments in voluntary hospitals were jealously guarded and eagerly sought. In London these appointments, together with the examining and teaching systems, remained largely under the influence of the doyens of the Royal Colleges.

Outside the London voluntary hospitals, and beyond the sphere of the Royal Colleges, general practitioners (usually with the LSA and MRCS diplomas) were rising in importance with the growing affluence of the industrial cities. By about 1860 the GP was firmly established as the doctor of the rising middle classes.[26] It was typical of the growing influence of the provincial centers at this time that the most powerful medical association in Britain originated outside London—at a meeting of fifty doctors in Worcester in 1832. The Provincial Medical and Surgical Association which resulted from this meeting was largely set up to counteract, in the provinces, the power of the Colleges. London members were not invited to join until 1853, and three years after that the society was renamed the British Medical Association. The Association prospered, despite the jibe of the rambunctious Thomas Wakley of the *Lancet* that its founder, Dr. Hastings, was being bribed with the prospect of a fellowship in the Royal College of Physicians to extinguish provincial reform.[27] By 1848, eight branches had been established in different areas of the British Isles; in 1852 there were fourteen; and by 1882 the present contours of the BMA were visible.

Because of the existence of the Royal Colleges and the Society of Apothecaries, the British Medical Association was to have less long-term influence over national medical education and standards than its counterpart, the American Medical Association (established 1847) in the United States. Moreover, the higher echelons of practice in Britain were represented in the colleges. The BMA thus quickly developed as the champion of the average, often underprivileged, practitioner, for whom it became the spokesman for higher recognition.

By the middle of the last century the medical profession was ripe for

25. See Cope, *History of the RCS*, pp. 57–69.

26. Of about 15,000 practitioners registered to practice in 1860, fewer than 1,200 were working in 117 of the larger voluntary hospitals. Of these, only 579 were described as "physicians and surgeons who have charge of inpatients." The remainder of the 1,200 were juniors and assistants. By far the majority of all registered doctors were general practitioners, working chiefly outside the large voluntary hospitals. Abel-Smith, pp. 19–20.

27. E. M. Little, *History of the British Medical Association* (London, 1932), p. 34.

reform. There was no reliable list of medical practitioners; there were still two without diplomas for each practitioner who had one,[28] and the diploma and degree situation was hopelessly confused. With the exception of physicians and leading surgeons, doctors were held in relatively low social repute. Reports of the committees on medical education of 1834 and 1847 had exposed gross deficiencies in medical training and made adverse comments on the efficiency of the Royal Colleges. Three kinds of doctors were still being produced by the three regulating bodies: the Physicians, the Surgeons, and the Apothecaries. Although various proposals had been made in the first half of the nineteenth century to organize joint (conjoint) examining schemes, these had repeatedly fallen through because of the sectional interests involved. The idea of a common medical registration was particularly repugnant to the numerically small but highly influential physicians; they feared that, while it might raise the prestige of the profession as a whole, it would reduce the physician's status to a common norm. Reform was of most immediate interest to the large and increasingly vocal body of general practitioners.

The debates on reform centered on two broad alternatives. Given the professional interest in creating one recognized and registered medical practitioner from the three kinds of doctor, either an official council could be set up over the existing examining bodies or there could be a "single portal of entry" to the profession. The first would imply the supervision of all examinations—the university M.B. and M.D., and the professional bodies' LRCP, MRCS, and LSA (together with their counterparts in Scotland and Ireland). The second would recognize one examination, and one only, as a licensing requirement; this could either be an examination for a designated university degree or a special examination under some kind of state board system. Fifteen consecutive bills were discussed and rejected by the Houses of Parliament. The sixteenth—a compromise version of the first alternative —was passed in 1858.[29]

The Medical Act of 1858 created an official council, now the General Medical Council, whose membership was appointed by the medical corporations, the universities, and the Crown to regulate the standards of existing examining bodies. The Council was deliberately made independent of the Colleges and the universities, although it was naturally manned by distinguished members of the profession. Its responsibility was (as it still is) to the Privy Council, and thus to the Crown. The Council was to supervise medical education, but not to examine, and to maintain a medical register and a pharmacopoeia.[30]

The Act of 1858 marked the beginning of the modern system of medical

28. Ibid., pp. 5–6.
29. For the politics of the various bills, see Charles Newman, pp. 134–93.
30. Those not familiar with the function of the General Medical Council and the British registration process may find it helpful to refer to the additional notes at the end of the book, pp. 369–70.

training. Under the General Medical Council the provincial medical schools were emancipated from the London examinations. The Act was to give great power to the universities; it provided recognition for the large body of practitioners outside the teaching hospitals; and it forced the Royal Colleges to modify their examining structure. In 1861 the Royal College of Physicians of London reorganized its license examination; it was no longer a monopoly examination for physicians but a primary examination, legally equivalent to the license of the Society of Apothecaries, which could be combined with membership in the Royal College of Surgeons as a fully registrable license to practice under the Medical Act; and similar moves were made by the Scottish and Irish Colleges. The Physicians also introduced a new grade of membership (MRCP) as a higher diploma, somewhat similar in status to the FRCS. Candidates for the London MRCP were to hold an arts degree or pass an examination in general education, to be over the age of 25, to have studied medicine for five years, and to produce a certificate of moral character. Candidates for the Edinburgh MRCP examination (instituted in 1881), unlike its London counterpart, were allowed to be examined in a special subject as well as in general medicine—a difference that remained until the London College altered its regulations in 1964.[31] Although the FRCS and MRCP examinations remained within the preserve of their repective Colleges, the two English Royal Colleges formed a conjoint board in 1884 to grant the MRCS and LRCP diplomas jointly. Similar arrangements were made between the professional examining bodies in Scotland (Scottish Triple Board, 1884) and Ireland (Irish Conjoint Board, 1886), also overseen by the General Medical Council. Under an Act of 1886, all students had to pass examinations in both medicine and surgery from either a university or a conjoint board to become eligible for the Medical Register. The Society of Apothecaries, excluded from the Conjoint Board, gradually declined. The LSA was transformed into a dual medical and surgical diploma, but it could not compete with the glamor of its rivals. After the passing of the 1858 Act, the final triumph of the surgeon–apothecary, the Society lost its leadership in the medical world.

Both the London Royal Colleges thus had two grades which were entered by examination and were more or less comparable in status. The MRCS

31. The MRCP regulations included a "grandfather" clause to enable physicians with the old and superior license to transfer to membership merely on payment of a registration fee. The new LRCP contained a similar clause. The London College extended for one year the privilege of becoming a LRCP without examination to all graduates or licentiates of universities in Great Britain. The Edinburgh College interpreted the LRCP more liberally as a general practitioner diploma and granted it within one year of grace to men of "mature age" who had begun as surgeons or apothecaries but had no degree. A large number of applicants—including GPs from England—flocked to Edinburgh, and on return erroneously entitled themselves "Doctor" (as was the custom of London licentiates who held university degrees). The Edinburgh College was accused of selling licenses. However, the new license examinations of both colleges, like the GP diplomas, did not require a university degree.

and LRCP were basic registrable diplomas in surgery and medicine, which qualified the holder for the Medical Register. Combined, they would be suitable for the general practitioner. The FRCS and MRCP required higher general education and greater experience and were additional examinations for prospective consultants. In addition, the Royal College of Physicians had a third category of fellows (FRCP), elected on the basis of esteem. All these grades exist today. The higher diplomas were linked with government of the Colleges. Only fellows might elect the governing body of the Royal College of Surgeons; and it was from the members (not the lowly licentiates) that the governing fellows of the College of Physicians were drawn. The concept of rank, of the lower and the higher category of doctor, was thus retained, but ironically it was now within the Royal Colleges.

Instead of simplifying the structure of the medical profession, the 1858 Act consolidated its complexities. There were marked variations in standards among the examining bodies. At the end of the nineteenth century, the great majority listed in the Medical Register in England were those with conjoint board diplomas; in Scotland, however, the university degree was the more general qualification. The individual took one examination, either at a university in the United Kingdom or in the examination hall of a conjoint board or Apothecaries' Society. A pass simultaneously permitted a candidate to use letters after his name—a university degree or Royal College affiliation—and legal entitlement to practice. The GP was content with this; but the aspiring consultant looked forward to higher things. In London the MRCP was a prerequisite for appointment as a physician to a voluntary hospital; outside London the university M.D. had more status. The aspiring consultant surgeon had to pass the fellowship examination of the Royal College of Surgeons.

The three streams of medical practice had been integrated, but the old divisions continued to exist at the postgraduate level and in medical practice. There were still three kinds of practitioner: the consultant physician and the consultant surgeon with access to beds in the major voluntary hospitals, and the general medical practitioner without such access and of inferior professional status. Specialization and state intervention in medical practice were to be built around these basic divisions.

2

Medical Practice 1858–1914

From Paris, the center of medical learning in the first half of the nineteenth century, the scientific study of disease entities was exported to all centers in the western world. This was a time of discovery, of pushing back the boundaries of medicine, of correlating the pathological findings of anatomists at dissection with those observed through symptomatology at the bedside.[1] There was a growing need for facilities in which appropriate studies could be made of particular organs, lesions, conditions, or diseases. From this compelling movement were to grow special hospitals—for the eye, the ear, the skin, for children, or for nervous diseases. Around these hospitals the education and the identification of the specialist developed, and, toward the end of the nineteenth century, specialized departments were established in the general hospitals. At the same time, the growth of cities and towns fostered the formation of specialist private practices, which could survive only in large populations.

Rise of the Specialties

The staffing system of the voluntary hospitals did not encourage innovation. Competition for admission to the honorary staff meant years of anxious waiting for the aspiring physician or surgeon while he performed junior work in the hospital and hoped to attract the favorable notice of his seniors. Vacancies arose only through the retirement or death of an incumbent. The aspirant could not afford to be an innovator; he was compelled to pay at least lip service to the practices and beliefs of his seniors. This meant adherence to the concepts of a wide generalist medical culture rather than to the new specialized scientific medicine which was emerging from the empirical research and diagnostic practice of the early and middle nineteenth century. The physicians who were fellows of the Royal College and ran the hospitals were general physicians; the most influential surgeons were the general surgeons. Throughout the nineteenth century and afterward the great proportion of beds in the large voluntary hospitals was, not unnaturally, allocated to general medicine and general surgery. Physicians and surgeons

1. For an analysis of factors that led to the development of specialization, see George Rosen, *The Specialization of Medicine with Particular Reference to Ophthalmology* (New York, 1944).

already on hospital staffs might develop special interests, but they were not appointed in their specialist capacity.

The younger generations, interested in particular aspects of medicine or in particular techniques, had no means of breaking into the charmed circle. In the first half of the nineteenth century the number of hospital beds in England and Wales had risen from about three thousand to nearly eight thousand. Despite this expansion, the demand for beds for teaching and research far outran the supply. The only alternative to the frustrated junior or the aspiring specialist was to found his own hospital.[2] The specialist hospital movement, which gained momentum during the century, developed concurrently all over the country. Despite the complaint of one critic that "Specialization has not become popular with the medical profession, it was sneered at by the medical corporations," by 1900 there were 128 special hospitals in England and Wales;[3] and these, especially in London, were the centers of specialist teaching and research.

Some of the reluctance of the older generation to recognize specialties was undoubtedly due to the association of these fields with quacks. This was particularly true of ophthalmology, ear, nose, and throat diseases, bone-setting, and urology. The foundation of the first new type of special hospital by J. C. Saunders—Moorfields Eye Hospital in London (1804)—was in more than one way the beginning of a new era of medicine. It was a sign, recognized by the new specialists, of the incorporation into the body of medicine of long-practiced nonmedical arts, and it provided a new focus for medical education. As Sir William Lawrence claimed of Moorfields in 1825, "you may see more of diseases of the eye in this institution in three months than in the largest hospital in fifty years."[4] Similarly, Joseph Toynbee (1815-66), the pioneer British otologist, vowed he would "rescue aural surgery from the hands of quacks";[5] and urology developed from the old practice of

2. Abel-Smith, *The Hospitals*, pp. 16, 21.
3. Richard Kershaw, *Special Hospitals* (London, 1909), pp. 28, 43.
4. Ibid., p. 28.
5. The first hospital devoted to the ear was the Royal Ear Hospital, London (1816), but it was founded by a man described as "profoundly ignorant of the anatomy of the ear," and it was only with Toynbee and pioneers of the same generation that aural surgery began to gain eminence. Both Saunders and Toynbee were respected anatomists and general surgeons and are exemplars of medical practice of the time. Saunders (1773–1810) was apprenticed to a surgeon in Barnstaple, dresser to the famous surgeon Astley Cooper, and demonstrator in anatomy at St. Thomas' Hospital, London. Toynbee at 17 was apprenticed in Soho, attended the Little Windmill Street School and St. George's and University College hospitals. He became a MRCS in 1838, and a fellow in 1843; he built up a large private practice in London and was on the staff of St. Mary's Hospital. Ophthalmology and otology antedated both general anesthesia and antisepsis. Morton's famous demonstration of ether anesthesia took place in Boston, Mass., in 1846; ether was used in England the same year. The first attempt at surgery with carbolic as an antiseptic was made by Lister in Glasgow in 1865. D. Guthrie, *Brit. Med. Bull.* 2 (1944), 372; *The Dictionary of National Biography;* Arturo Castiglione, *A History of Medicine* (New York, 1947), pp. 719, 723–26.

"cutting for the stone." Suspicion of these new fields only slowly evaporated. As late as 1860, a surgeon appointed to the staff of St. Mary's Hospital, London, was forced to resign for simultaneously accepting an appointment at St. Peter's Hospital for the Stone: "He knows," said the medical committee in condemning his action, "that special hospitals in general and special hospitals for stone in particular are not only useless but worse than useless." [6]

Nevertheless, as the nineteenth century progressed, an increasing number of hospital staff held dual appointments with a special hospital. Of 195 physicians and surgeons attached to the London general hospitals in 1889, only 31 did not also hold office in one of the special hospitals, and almost every special hospital had a fellow of the Royal College of Physicians or Surgeons attached to it.[7] The existence of specialization could no longer be denied. Modern instruments such as the ophthalmoscope and laryngoscope were difficult to use and required special training. Ophthalmology and otolaryngology, which developed around these instruments, were therefore easily accepted; it is recorded that two of the original staff of St. Mary's Hospital confined their practice to these specialties in 1851. Dermatology had emerged as a specialty through the work of Willan and Bateman at the beginning of the nineteenth century. The first demonstrators in dermatology were Andrews and Southey, appointed to St. Bartholomew's Hospital in 1867.[8] But already dermatology, then a branch of surgery, was a flourishing field for private practice. Thomas Wakley is supposed to have advised the young Erasmus Wilson:

> Hang anatomy; stick to skins. Read about skin, write about skin, speak nothing but skin, and that as publicly and as often as you can. Get your name so closely associated with skin that directly the name of Erasmus Wilson is mentioned in any drawing room everybody present will begin to scratch.[9]

Wilson happily followed this advice and became a wealthy man. By 1869 he was able to found with his own money a Chair of Dermatology and, despite such costly endeavors as erecting Cleopatra's Needle on the Thames Embankment, *Sir* Erasmus left on his death in 1884 the large sum of £200,000 to the Royal College of Surgeons, of which he had been made president in 1881. By this time, belated respectability for these specialties and others was being achieved by the foundation of specialist departments and outpatient clinics in the voluntary general hospitals, chiefly in the 1870s

6. Zachary Cope, *The History of St. Mary's Hospital Medical School* (London, 1954), pp. 35–36.

7. *Brit. Med. J. ii* (1889), 620.

8. G. E. Gask, *Brit. Med. J. ii* (1935), 816.

9. Kershaw, p. 30. Biographical details from Kershaw and *Dictionary of National Biography.*

and 1880s. St. Thomas' Hospital set up outpatient departments for ophthalmology in 1871, for otolaryngology in 1882, and dermatology in 1884,[10] and other leading hospitals were developing simultaneously along similar lines.

Not all specialties, however, advanced as rapidly as these; nor were there many such colorful figures as Erasmus Wilson to defend them. Professions tend to be conservative in relation to new methods and fields developed by amateurs. For a long time the specialties were regarded by regular doctors as doubtful additions to knowledge, much as hypnotism is regarded today; they were also potential competition. Medical obstetrics, advanced by the pioneer work of Smellie and William Hunter in the eighteenth century, was excluded from general hospitals because of the dual dangers of puerpural sepsis and the effect of such an immodest subject on the tender souls of medical students. St. Thomas' Hospital, for fear it might encourage immorality, did not establish a department of gynecology until 1888. Efforts made by obstetricians from the early nineteenth century to set up an examination in their field within the curricula of the Royal College of Surgeons were successfully resisted by the College until the new Committee of Management of the Conjoint Board (1884) set up an examination in midwifery as part of the basic examination.[11] Attendance at a dozen confinements was not enforced by the physicians and surgeons on the General Medical Council as a condition of registration until 1888. But there was still reluctance to recognize obstetrics as a medical subject, and nonmedical midwifery continued to thrive. It was (and still is) only in Ireland that proficiency in obstetrics and gynecology was shown in a university degree by including a Bachelorship of the Art of Obstetrics.

Dentistry was another potential medical specialty that was not fully incorporated into medicine. Tooth-drawing, like eye diseases and obstetrics, had for long been a flourishing nonmedical field. It gained respectability in the eighteenth century, and by the nineteenth was practiced by a small group of medical men as well as by a large group of untrained practitioners. Unlike other medical specialties, however, dentistry achieved respectability outside medicine. The Royal College of Surgeons granted a license in dental surgery (LDS) in 1859, perhaps indicating that dentistry was part of surgery. But the Dentists Act, 1878, set up a separate register for dentists (although under the General Medical Council), admitting to the register all those then engaged in dental practice. General dental practitioners were thus distinguished from general medical practitioners. They had a different training program, a different profession, and a different organization—the British Dental Association—founded in 1880.[12] Although a number of surgeons

10. E. M. McInnes, *St. Thomas' Hospital* (London, 1963), pp. 147–48.
11. Cope, *History of the Royal College of Surgeons*, pp. 146–55.
12. A College of Dentists was formed in 1857 but was merged with the Odontological Society in 1863, after arrangements had been made for a dental department within the Royal College of Surgeons. The Dentists Act of 1878 set up a register

continued to be interested in dental problems, consultant hospital dentistry was not established until World War II.

It is tempting to speculate what would have happened if psychiatrists had also set up as a separate profession; for psychiatrists, practicing in geographically remote mental hospitals, were as divorced as dentists from the developments in the prestigious voluntary hospitals in London and other major cities. But psychiatrists, unlike the majority of dentists, were medical practitioners. They were thus committed to developing their field inside rather than outside medicine. Public mental hospitals, or county lunatic asylums as they were known, built under a permissive act of 1808, developed rapidly in the second half of the nineteenth century. The public hospitals employed medical practitioners as "asylum doctors," who as early as 1841 organized themselves into the society that became the Royal Medico-Psychological Association, the major spokesman for psychiatry. The association set up a certificate of its own in 1885, thus launching postgraduate education in psychiatry. But the certificate was unpopular. It had no administrative significance, it was vocational and narrow in scope, and it took no account of the basic sciences.[13] At the same time psychiatry was being half-heartedly introduced into certain voluntary hospitals. In 1865 London University recommended that medical schools hold a special course in psychological medicine; but the teaching hospitals, where they did eventually co-opt a psychiatrist, allowed him no beds or outpatient clinics.

Charing Cross Hospital appointed a psychiatrist in 1902. By this time it had departments for obstetrics, children, skin diseases, electricity, radiography, ear, nose, and throat, ophthalmology, anesthesiology, and orthopedics.[14] It was probably typical of the state of outpatient departments in the large voluntary general hospitals, both in London and in the main provincial centers. Despite the creation of these departments, specialization was still on the fringe of medical practice. Specialists in the general hospitals "were looked upon, more or less, with jealousy"; [15] and the officer in charge of the so-called special department was often a junior staff member, chiefly or entirely confined to outpatient work. Patients admitted as inpatients were handed over to the generalist, who "was not always as enthusiastic in the special branch as his colleague by whom the patient was referred." This

---

of dentists, also kept by the General Medical Council. This arrangement was modified by the Dentists Act of 1921, when the rules and benefits of registration were strengthened, and a separate Dental Board was set up under the General Medical Council. Under the Dentists Act, 1956, dentists were given an independent General Dental Council. A registered medical practitioner is, however, still fully entitled to practice dentistry, whether or not his name is also on the Dentists' Register.

13. Aubrey Lewis, in D. L. Davies and M. Shepherd (eds.) *Psychiatric Education* (Institute of Psychiatry, London, 1964), p. 10

14. H. C. Cameron, *Mr. Guy's Hospital 1726–1948* (London, 1954), p. 345; and W. Hunter, *Historical Account of Charing Cross Hospital and Medical School* (London, 1914), pp. 169–72.

15. Kershaw, p. 44, and passim.

state of affairs did not begin to change until the first decade of the twentieth century, when the general hospitals made a real effort to reorganize departments "in an active spirit" by appointing specialists who had been trained in a special hospital. The London special hospitals retained their position as postgraduate teaching centers, connected in no way with the undergraduate hospital schools. Although formal postgraduate education was barely developed, the twenty-two major special hospitals in London—out of which were to grow the present postgraduate institutes—were visited by well over 5,000 doctors and 500 students in 1907.[16] In the provincial cities the special hospitals tended to be integrated with the rising university medical departments.

Medical societies—the next stage in professional consolidation of specialist fields—developed in the last quarter of the nineteenth century around the special hospitals. The Ophthalmological Society of the United Kingdom, founded in 1881, evolved from informal discussions in the house surgeons' room at Moorfields.[17] Sir Morell MacKenzie, who founded the Hospital for Diseases of the Throat and Chest, in Golden Square, London (1863), was also responsible for founding the *Journal of Laryngology and Otology* (1887), and the British Laryngological and Rhinological Association (1888). By 1905, when suggestions were being made for an amalgamation of certain specialist societies, sixteen separate specialties in medicine and surgery could be distinguished; these became the first specialist sections of the new Royal Society of Medicine.[18]

The "Referral" System is Established

The growth of specialized hospitals provided the ammunition for a conflict of interest between the general practitioner (the old surgeon–apothecary) and the hospital physician and surgeon. Although these were now in the same Medical Register, the social and professional differences survived, and the last half of the nineteenth and the first part of the twentieth century were years of bitter rivalry between the two kinds of doctor.

Traditionally, the physician was practitioner to the upper classes and the hospitalized poor, while the GP cared for the remainder of society; their functions were distinguished by the social class of their patients. The increasing urbanization of society in the nineteenth century was accompanied by the rise of the suburban middle class and the development of new professions. This bolstered the position of the general practitioner at a time

16. Conference of Deans of the Metropolitan Schools of Medicine, *Medical Education in London* (1908), p. 165; and Kershaw, p. 48.

17. R. R. James, *Brit. Med. Bull. 1* (1943), 159.

18. The sections were: anesthesia, clinical practice, dermatology, diseases of children, epidemiology, otorhinolaryngology, internal medicine, psychiatry, neurology, obstetrics and gynecology, odontology, ophthalmology, pathology, state medicine, surgery, and therapeutics. Maurice Davidson, *The Royal Society of Medicine* (London, 1955), pp. 31–32.

when medicine was increasingly hospital-based. Both GPs and "consultants" (the physicians and surgeons) found themselves competing for the prosperous middle classes; and the special hospitals fanned the flame. "Many of the cases treated at these special hospitals are of the most ordinary nature, and not in the least requiring the skill of a specialist, but could be quite well treated by a general practitioner," wrote one critic in 1900. More materially, it was complained that special hospitals were being used by a class of the community "quite above the general run of those who go to general hospitals," and were undercutting the GP's practice.[19] Complaints of such "hospital abuse" sprinkled the pages of the *British Medical Journal*—which came out strongly for the GP—from the 1850s. They reached their climax with the increasing development in general hospitals of special outpatient clinics which, originally set up for the destitute sick, were being used increasingly by middle-class patients. The practitioner foresaw his practice jeopardized and his patients diminishing until the hospitals, so clearly associated with the Royal Colleges, would swallow up the bulk of his living.

The issue was central to the development of medical practice. If the general practitioner and the hospital "honorary" were to be fused into one kind of doctor—as the British Medical Association appeared to favor—then the outpatient department could either be limited to the care of the sick poor or could be used by all doctors alike for special purposes. Instead of having the physician and surgeon for the rich and the general practitioner for the middle classes, with a continuing scramble of borderline cases, all doctors would be available to see all kinds of patients. One corollary, as the BMA was not averse to pointing out, was open access by all practitioners to hospital beds. If this had gone through, the present system of medical practice in England might have been akin to that in the United States; and the arguments on the justification for, and functions of, the hospital outpatient department vis à vis the private consulting room might have been delayed by over half a century. There was, however, every advantage to the consultant to continue to exclude the general practitioner from the large voluntary hospitals; and the latter's attempt to intrude upon the preserves of the consultant inevitably failed.

Instead, the "referral" system was evolved. By the late nineteenth century, hospital staff who specialized were acting as consultants to other doctors on cases of particular interest. At the beginning of the twentieth century, almost a third of the outpatients and over half the inpatients seen in the Central London Throat and Ear Hospital—to take one example—were referred there by other doctors.[20] The picture was complicated by doctors who worked as part-time specialists and who thus competed with both branches for patients. Articles appeared on consultant etiquette in which it was suggested that GPs should send their patients for a second opinion only to full-

19. Horatio Nelson Hardy, *The State of the Medical Profession in Great Britain and Ireland in 1900* (Dublin, 1901), pp. 53–54.
20. Kershaw, unpaged appendix.

time consultants who were not also general practitioners. Consultants were to be called in for a second opinion by general practitioners, but the latter would retain a continuing relationship with the patient. This is what eventually happened—the result of informal professional agreement rather than anything inherent in the educational or organizational system. At the same time, hospital outpatient departments gradually became extensions of specialized inpatient units instead of general clinics. *The physician and surgeon retained the hospital, but the general practitioner retained the patient.*

Hospital Practice in the Early Twentieth Century

The referral system was established by the end of the nineteenth century. By this time two medical archetypes had been developed: the hospital consultant, a brilliant bluff empiricist, impressing his group of students at the bedside with a barbed, self-conscious wit; and the kindly omnicompetent general practitioner who knew and loved all his patients. These images were to linger long after what shreds of fact they represented had passed away, but they were perhaps true of many men who were in practice at the turn of this century. Diagnostic aids and advances in techniques have lessened the mystique surrounding the consultant; they have at the same time devalued the art of general clinical observation that was the hallmark of the nineteenth-century consultant.

Despite the impact of specialized hospitals and departments, the typical consultant was still a generalist. Following the bedside tradition of English medicine, with its emphasis on general clinical observation, he was only incidentally concerned with scientific material. Abraham Flexner, visiting from the United States, wrote in 1910:

> Once on the hospital staff, the typical English clinician gives up the laboratory and with it the laboratory state of mind. He contributes no longer to theoretical literature; his world changes. He fraternizes with another social set.[21]

The technological specialties were well behind the clinical fields. The study of anesthetics had not even a place in the medical curriculum in 1900. The pathologist, where he existed, was ill-paid and badly served with equipment. Radiology was in its infancy and could not be counted as a full specialty. At Nottingham General Hospital X-ray equipment was under the care of the honorary dentist; at St. Mary's Hospital, London, X-ray pictures of fractured limbs were taken by the theater beadle. Obstetrics was still an "out-patient affair."[22] General physicians and surgeons reigned supreme. In Germany, a concurrent leader in the development of medical science and clinical arts, the structure of medical practice was more conducive to medical specialization; efficiency was being increased by setting up specialist depart-

21. *Medical Education in Europe* (New York, 1912), p. 193.
22. Jacob, *History of Nottingham General Hospital*, p. 230; Cope, *History of St. Mary's Hospital Medical School*, p. 100; Flexner, pp. 204–05.

ments in the hospitals, each team headed by a professor. In England, characteristically, the bacteriological revolution appeared to have made little impression on the practice of medicine.

In 1900, as in 1800, appointment to the staff of a voluntary hospital represented "the prosperous culmination of a successful professional career." Physicians and surgeons served voluntarily on the staff of both general and special hospitals, "the *kudos* of being on the staff of the hospital being supposed to recompense them sufficiently." [23] Most consultants never strayed outside their teaching hospitals during their struggle up the ladder; and teaching hospital staffs were therefore inevitably inbred. Teaching was still undertaken by the hospital staff and not by university professors. There were no chiefs of medicine or surgery; each man's allocated beds (perhaps 30 or 40) were his own preserve. There was still a gulf between the GP and the consultant, and it was still more fashionable to be a generalist than a specialist, or a physician than a surgeon. The surgeon took himself to see his private patients by train, horse vehicle, bicycle, or on foot, but the physicians "stuck to their carriages." [24]

The categories of surgery and general practice, the usual combination of the mid-nineteenth century, were clearly differentiated in the 1880s and 1890s, following the great advances in anesthesia, asepsis, and operative techniques. Thomas Jones of Manchester, appointed as honorary surgeon in 1880, was one of the first surgeons in that city to set up purely for consulting and operating. At Nottingham, which was not a medical teaching center, although three of the four honorary surgeons to the General Hospital were also general practitioners in 1899, no GPs were appointed after that date.[25] In their turn, however, general practitioners increasingly had access to small voluntary hospitals outside the main centers. These "cottage" hospitals, first established in the 1850s, had become by the beginning of the twentieth century important adjuncts to the average general practitioner. But the three kinds of voluntary hospital—general, special, and cottage—were to cause planning headaches which have existed to the present.

Outside the charmed circle of the voluntary hospital, important changes had been effected in public medical services. The first Medical Officer of Health had been appointed in 1847. In 1848 the first Public Health Act had set up the General Board of Health, and an act in 1871 had created a combined poor law and sanitary authority in the local government board; the Public Health Act of 1872 made the appointment of medical officers of health compulsory in the reconstituted local sanitary authorities. The Public Health Act of 1875, codifying existing public health law and embodying new provisions, heralded the wide development of fever hospitals for infectious diseases and of sanatoria by local authorities. By the early 1900s there were

23. Hardy, p. 54.
24. G. Grey Turner, in British Medical Journal symposium, *Fifty Years of Medicine* (London, 1950), p. 280.
25. Jacob, pp. 233–34.

nearly a thousand isolation hospitals and other institutions under the public health service.

The poor-law medical service, despite its many defects, was also reaching large dimensions. In 1910, over 3,700 general practitioners were working for at least part of their time in the poor-law service—probably one sixth of all doctors practicing in England and Wales.[26] Most of them were also public vaccinators, and many of those in the rural areas were also part-time medical officers of health. These developments gave rise to demands for specific training in state or public medicine and, under the Local Government Act of 1888, a diploma in public health became mandatory for the large body of practitioners entering the public health field. Public health and its foreign equivalent of tropical medicine became the first special branches of medicine with recognized postgraduate diplomas from a university or the Royal Colleges' Conjoint Board.[27]

This was not the sum of the medical practitioner's public responsibilities. Legislation in the last quarter of the nineteenth and the early years of the twentieth century involved him in certification of births and deaths and in the notification of infectious diseases, as well as in a myriad of other duties under acts relating to factories, vaccination, children, public health, workmen's compensation, and housing. The doctor, and in this case particularly the general practitioner, had become increasingly involved in social organizations and in matters of social policy. He was an adviser on public committees dealing with nonmedical services. His organization, the BMA, had campaigned in the nineteenth century not only for the material needs of its members—such as upgrading the Poor Law Medical Officers and army doctors—but also for smoke abatement and, despite the limitations it would impose on its members, for the adoption of procedures for registering disease.

In the voluntary hospitals, expanding medical knowledge had effected great changes, but they had a recognized ancestry. For the GP there had been a revolution; he had become central to the administration of public health and sanitary services and was acknowledged as a responsible public servant.

26. Sidney and Beatrice Webb, *The State and The Doctor* (London, 1910) p. 11, and passim.

27. The first Diploma in State Medicine in the United Kingdom was instituted by Trinity College, Dublin, in 1870. In England, a Diploma in Public Health (DPH) was established by Cambridge University in 1875, which provided a prototype for other universities and licensing bodies, including the Conjoint Board of the Royal Colleges (1887). The diploma was recognized by the General Medical Council and in time was provided by almost all universities and licensing bodies in Great Britain and Ireland. Tropical medicine was based on the health needs of Englishmen stationed in India and other territories of the British Empire and in the armed forces. A chair of tropical medicine was set up in Liverpool, whose port was the gateway to the tropics, as early as 1902. Both Liverpool and Cambridge Universities established diplomas in tropical medicine at the beginning of the twentieth century, and the diploma of the English Conjoint Board followed in 1911.

National Health Insurance; The Act of 1911

Specialization and public medicine developed side by side with different foci and different reasons for their existence. The extension of public medicine was a social rather than a scientific phenomenon, stemming largely from public-health and welfare legislation of the late nineteenth and early twentieth centuries. Throughout Europe public health systems had been introduced and, following Bismarck's example in Germany in 1883, compulsory national health insurance was being enacted for all employed persons under a certain income limit. The English response to this movement was the Health Insurance Act, 1911, which provided for the insured free medical care by general practitioners, but not by hospitals or specialists.

The 1911 Act established the first clear example of state financing of medical services. At the same time, the health insurance system, by focusing solely on general practitioner services, emphasized still further the division between general practitioners and consultants. The Act was to consolidate and strengthen the position of the general practitioner. It gave the average doctor a much better income, it rapidly increased the number of general practitioners, and it brought the mass of wage earners into contact with doctors. It established throughout society the concept of the "family doctor," and it bolstered the referral system. In many ways, therefore, it was the ultimate climax of the cycle of general practice initiated by the 1815 Apothecaries' Act.

Doctors entered service under the scheme largely on their own terms. Through insistence on its "Six Cardinal Points," the BMA had a profound influence on the health insurance system and ultimately, as a result, on the structure of the National Health Service which superseded it thirty-seven years later. The six points were insistence on an upper income limit (£2 per week) for those entitled to medical benefit; free choice of doctor by the patient, subject to the doctor's acceptance; benefits to be administered by local health committees and not by the friendly societies; choice of their method of remuneration by doctors in each district; medical remuneration to be what the profession considered adequate for the work performed; and adequate medical representation among the insurance commissioners (who administered the scheme and were replaced by the Ministry of Health in 1919), in the Central Advisory Committee, and in the local health (later called insurance) committees, with statutory recognition of a local medical committee representing the profession in the district of each health committee.[28] In its original form the Bill had placed the control of medical benefit in the hands of friendly societies, did not allow for choice of doctor, and did not give the profession representation on administrative committees. All

28. See R. M. Titmuss in Morris Ginsberg (ed.) *Law and Opinion in England in the Twentieth Century* (London, 1959), pp. 299–319; G. F. McCleary, *National Health Insurance* (London, 1932), pp. 71–93.

36

these points were reversed after conferences between the BMA and the government.

The payment mechanism chosen by the profession from four alternatives, including salary, was that of capitation fee for each person in the GP's practice who was eligible for benefits. Only two areas, Manchester and Salford, chose a fee-for-service system, and these cities eventually changed to capitation. Thus, whereas other public medical practitioners—the poor-law doctor, the asylum doctor, the medical officer of health, and the doctor employed by the Colonial Service or the armed forces—were employed on a salary, the health insurance scheme instead introduced "panel" practice at the volition of the profession: payment according to the number of people on the doctor's list or panel. This decision was to have important consequences on the status of general practice, the full implications of which are being seen only today.

The BMA emerged from the negotiations on health insurance as a formidable power. It succeeded in strengthening the organization of GPs at district level, for the local medical committees (although not part of the BMA) were to be used as vital supplementary organizations. At national level the BMA set up its own Insurance Acts Committee, which was recognized by the government to represent the general body of doctors engaged in insurance practice. The GP, although not directly employed by the state, thus found himself a part of a large-scale organizational complex.

According to one view in 1905, the BMA was "very largely officered by the West End consultants in London, and the consultants in the big towns." [29] But most of its activities made little impression on consultant practice. Almost all the BMA's reform movements of the nineteenth and early twentieth centuries, including the fights against contract practice and quack remedies, had primarily affected the status of the general practitioner. The Health Insurance Act emphasized still further the role of the BMA as spokesman for general practice; yet despite its rising power in its dealings with the government, the Royal Colleges continued to be the arbiters of professional standards and the focus of consultant interests.

The 1858 Medical Act had created one profession, but the rise of special departments in hospitals forced a dichotomy of general and consultant practices, eventually resolved in a referral system. By the outbreak of World War I, GPs were organized within the National Health Insurance scheme. They were rapidly becoming family practitioners. The hospital staffing structure remained as before. Consultants attached only to voluntary hospitals, as honorary unpaid staff, were entirely dependent on their private fees; GPs increasingly had the secondary resource of capitation fees for their panel practice. The great acceleration of specialization was still to come, but all the basic patterns of modern medical practice were already well established.

29. Quoted by Brian Abel-Smith, *A History of the Nursing Profession* (London, 1960), p. 75.

3

Development of the Specialties
1914–1939

The First World War stimulated the development of special skills and special interests, particularly in psychiatry, orthopedics, and plastic and thoracic surgery. At the same time, advances applicable to medical practice were being made in nonclinical fields—biochemistry, bacteriology, and endocrinology—and in the social services. Radiotherapy was being adopted in a number of hospitals; diagnostic radiology was expanding. By the early 1920s medical specialization, although deplored by those who saw that medicine was irrevocably disunited,[1] was generally accepted as necessary and inevitable. Many specialties were gradually evolving from a peripheral interest in a particular sphere of general medicine or general surgery to bodies of knowledge in their own right. Medical practice between the two world wars reflected the struggle between the Royal Colleges which wanted to retain medicine as a unified whole, with the emerging groups which wanted to raise standards in their own special fields and to advance their own status. Not surprisingly, no clear pattern emerged from the struggle.

The historical division between practitioners of medicine and of surgery, although they had been united at the level of registration, survived at the postgraduate stage. Consultants—even though they were specialists—aligned themselves through their training and diplomas with one branch or the other. The aspiring consultant in any specialty was expected to have the MRCP or

1. "The specialists of the new generation," wrote one complainant in the mid-1920s, "are gradually including parts of the body other than those to which they were originally limited. A modern gynaecologist operates on everything connected with the female. I cannot see anything that is excluded by the modern orthopaedic surgeon; and the modern urologist appears to be gradually claiming all the surgical diseases that affect the male in the same way as a modern gynaecologist is claiming all the diseases that affect the female. Even the modern laryngologist is beginning to include within his ambit diseases that are extra-laryngeal—such as goitre, carcinoma of the tongue, and glands of the neck—and thus he appears to be encroaching on the realms of the modern gynaecologists and urologists. . . . Why break up surgery into specialties that are becoming only names, and which have no physiological, pathological or technical reasons for their existence?" G. L. Cheatle, *Brit. Med. J. ii* (1925), 959.

FRCS or the university M.D. or M.S. degree before he would be considered for an appointment to a major voluntary hospital. Some specialties had crossed the boundary lines between medicine and surgery. Dermatology had become a subspecialty of general medicine, laryngology and gynecology subspecialties of general surgery. Leading obstetricians and gynecologists of the late nineteenth century were Fellows of the Royal College of Physicians; at the turn of the century young London gynecologists became Fellows of the Royal College of Surgeons as well; but by the second decade of the century they took the FRCS alone.[2] Other specialties included narrow ranges in both fields. Ophthalmologists, otologists, laryngologists, neurologists, and urologists of World War I required specialized knowledge of both medicine and surgery in a functionally limited sphere. But the alliance with one branch (and thus with one College) largely remained.

A second major result of the power and prestige of the Colleges was the continued division of the medical profession into consultants and general practitioners. The referral system put the GP on one side of the fence and the consultant on the other. Although the impact of specialization was beginning to break down this barrier by the late 1930s—so that it was not always easy to distinguish the general practitioner, the specialist, and the consultant—the basic division inhibited the development of large specialty groups in which GPs and consultants were united by a common interest. The consultant pediatrician was professionally and emotionally closer to the consultant general physician than to the GP who also had a special interest in children. The consultant's primary allegiance was to his Royal College, not to his specialty. Because of the existence of the Colleges, the pattern of specialty organizations that grew up in England in the 1920s and 1930s was far different from that of the United States where in the same period independent boards to certify specialties were being established.

Without specialty boards the definition of a specialist remained ambiguous. In general, a specialty was born when practitioners interested in that field formed a specialist hospital or society, consolidated by the foundation of a specialist section of the Royal Society of Medicine and the BMA; and academic respectability was added when a university chair was named. Only two specialties (obstetrics–gynecology and radiology) formed organizations complementary to the two Royal Colleges: that is, with an exclusive membership attained through postgraduate examination. A number of specialties made no demand for their own diplomas or degrees. Yet others compromised by establishing postgraduate diplomas under universities or the Conjoint Board of the Royal Colleges, parallel to those already set up for those specializing in public health or tropical medicine. Such diplomas did not, however, have the cachet of the MRCP or FRCS, and were not considered of a comparable standard.

2. William Fletcher Shaw, *Twenty-five Years—The Story of the Royal College of Obstetricians and Gynaecologists 1929–1954* (London, 1954), p. 4.

The Postwar Period

Two specialties which early set up their own postgraduate diplomas were ophthalmology and otolaryngology (ear, nose, and throat). Both were firmly established as specialties in the nineteenth century, and both had hospitals devoted to their fields in almost every major city in the country. The chief concern between the two world wars was not the standard of practice in these hospitals—which was recognized as high—but in the quality of treatment of these diseases by general practitioners. The Diploma in Ophthalmology had been established by Oxford in 1907 after a comment by the General Medical Council on medical students' lack of knowledge in this field. The social aspects of eye diseases had been brought into prominence through the increasing, and increasingly efficient, social services of the early twentieth century. A steady advance was being made in the alleviation and prevention of blindness through the establishment of pensions for the blind and of special schools and hospitals; the school health service (established in 1907) enabled the early detection and isolation of conjunctivitis, and spectacles were provided for school children having errors of vision. Maternity and infant welfare service facilitated notification and treatment of ophthalmia of the newborn. The Council of British Ophthalmologists (founded in 1918) engaged in discussions over a wide range of problems, including the vision of drivers of heavy vehicles, the dangers of eyestrain in cinemas, and the urgent need for improved medical education in ophthalmology. Yet general practitioners with an interest in eye diseases were ill-prepared to treat them. Medical students were still not examined over the whole spectrum of ophthalmology when the Conjoint Board of the Royal Colleges introduced its postgraduate Diploma in Ophthalmic Medicine and Surgery (DOMS) in 1920.[3]

Similar problems were presented in ear, nose, and throat conditions. Before the war, otolaryngology was a branch of surgery, and its exponents competed with each other in inventing instruments and devising operations. Between the wars, attitudes were distinctly more conservative, partly (as with ophthalmology) because earlier and more careful treatment of acute infections had reduced the need for surgery, especially in children, and partly owing to the introduction of the sulfonamides. The specialty was therefore largely the concern of the general practitioner. A special diploma in otolaryngology had been proposed several times before one was set up by the Conjoint Board in 1920 (DLO). A precipitating factor at this time was apparently criticism by the American Medical Association and American specialty

3. *Brit. Med. J. i.* (1920), 647. The General Medical Council had agreed in 1910 that all students be examined in "some branch" of ophthalmology, but not until 1922—after expressed anxiety at the lack of compulsory ophthalmic training for future general practitioners by the BMA and the ophthalmic associations—did it recommend that each student be instructed in diseases of the eye, refraction, and the use of the ophthalmoscope. *Brit. Med. J. i* (1919), 416; *ii* (1923), 195.

societies on the standard of otolaryngology in that country, which led to the formation of a specialty board in the United States.[4]

But perhaps the single most important factor in this as in other specialties was the increasing number of GP specialists, particularly in the larger northern industrial towns and in the rural areas. They had access to cottage hospitals (many developed as war memorial units) or nursing homes, and they combined ordinary panel practice with special work such as tonsillectomies, anesthesiology, or pediatrics. The new diplomas, which required a modest training period (typically six months), were of particular use to this kind of specialist, who would not normally aspire to the FRCS. There were thus two kinds of specialists developing side by side around the general practitioners and general consultants.

The GP specialist was limited to specialties that could be undertaken in conjunction with his insurance practice and the hospital facilities that were available to him. It was comparatively easy to be a part-time anesthesiologist, because of the relative shortage of these specialists, or an obstetrician or pediatrician. It was less easy for a GP to undertake orthopedics, neurosurgery, or cardiology—fields that were developing within the major hospitals as sophisticated disciplines. Such specialties were the domain of the consultant on the hospital staff, who already held a higher diploma or degree and had no need of specialist diplomas to show his competence or advance his practice. In none of the new subspecialties of general medicine and general surgery developing in the teaching hospitals was there a call for a Conjoint Board diploma.

Orthopedics was transformed during World War I. Before the war it specialized in lateral curvature, flat feet and knock-knees, and a few congenital deformities; there was comparatively little operating. Orthopedics emerged from the war as a sophisticated branch of surgery. A degree in orthopedics, the M.Ch. Ortho., was established at Liverpool University in 1924, largely through the efforts of Sir Robert Jones, the leading orthopedist at this time. The requirements for this degree were far in advance of those for diploma courses in other specialties. By 1933, the year of Sir Robert's death, orthopedic hospitals were distributed throughout the country, and specialists in charge devoted all their time to orthopedic surgery. This development was complemented by the foundation of specialty societies. The British Orthopaedic Association (BOA) was founded in 1918 and the International Society of Orthopaedic Surgery in 1929. The Royal Society of Medicine established orthopedics as a subspecialty of surgery in 1913 and as a full section in 1922; the BMA formed an orthopedics section in 1935. Yet orthopedics remained a relatively small specialty in terms of size. In 1939 there were less than half as many orthopedic surgeons as otolaryngologists and less than a third the number of ophthalmologists.[5]

4. *Brit. Med. J. ii* (1920), 711.

5. In a study of specialists practicing in Britain in 1938–39, A. Bradford Hill recorded that 4.1% of full-time specialists were orthopedic surgeons. Otolaryngology

Thoracic surgery, plastic surgery, neurosurgery, and cardiology were also advanced by the war, but they remained small elite specialties within the major hospitals. No diploma or degree was called for; training was by practical experience following the FRCS. Both cardiology and neurology, which were medical subspecialties, were penalized by the sharp division of consultants into physicians or surgeons. The MRCP produced the chest and neurological physicians, the FRCS the chest and neurological surgeons— each with their own beds and clinics. By now (and in contrast to the nineteenth century) any conflict between the physician and surgeon over the superintendence of cases tended to resolve itself in favor of the surgeon: "He was no longer content to act the plumber for the physician." [6]

Neurology was further complicated by the need to redefine its boundaries. Applied anatomy and applied physiology, which had proved a fruitful field of research for many years, were becoming exhausted, and new regions into which neurology might expand were in danger of being claimed by other branches of medicine. Neurology was being encroached on by general medicine, biochemistry, and bacteriology, and the nervous system could no longer be treated in isolation from the remainder of the organism. Some held that all nervous and mental disorders were within the province of the neurologist. Others stressed that all psychiatric problems were outside the province of the neurologist and that his work should consist only of the study of conditions produced by organic lesions of the nervous system [7]—a view that was largely to prevail. Neurology had never limited itself to the study of purely organic disease, but the division was accentuated by the physical separation of psychiatric from other kinds of hospitals. British neurology was dominated by the London hospital devoted to it: the National Hospital for Nervous Diseases. Psychiatry had developed in the mental hospitals and was still regarded more as a public service than a respectable clinical subject. In 1938 there were only nine psychiatric beds in the London undergraduate teaching hospitals, of a total bed complement of 6,700. [8]

The Conjoint Board set up a Diploma in Psychological Medicine (DPM) in 1920. A major effort was made by the Medico-Psychological Association in 1923 to advance the teaching of psychiatry within the universities. In the same year the Maudsley Hospital, an independent school of London University, was opened as an institution designed to provide early psychiatric treatment and research and teaching in psychiatry. The move marked a decisive step toward full "consultant" status for psychiatrists, but there was still a

---

accounted for 9.6%, ophthalmology 15.1%. *Report of the Interdepartmental Committee on the Remuneration of Consultants and Specialists* (Cmd. 7420, 1948) (Spens Report on Consultants and Specialists), pp. 22–25. Figures for all specialties are given in Table 1, chap. 8.

6. Prof. George Gask, reported in *Brit. Med. J.* ii (1935), 816.

7. *Brit. Med. J.* ii (1934), 725; ii (1936), 395.

8. A. M. H. Gray and A. Topping, *The Hospital Services of London and the Surrounding Area*, Hospital Survey (HMSO, 1945), p. 82.

long way to go. Moreover, for psychiatry the question of its relevance to other branches of internal medicine was more evident than for the branches of medicine that had developed in the general and voluntary specialist hospitals. When the Mental Hospital Department of the London County Council decided in 1938 to make promotion dependent on obtaining the MRCP, objections were raised that if a higher academic degree were wanted at all, a specific psychiatric diploma such as the Diploma in Psychological Medicine should be instituted.[9] The question remained open. Most psychiatrists in the country continued to favor the DPM and did not attempt the MRCP. They thus continued outside the mainstream of general medicine, represented by the Royal College of Physicians, a factor of marked importance in the debates over a college for psychiatrists more than twenty years later.

Obstetrics and Gynecology: A New Professional College

Obstetrics proved a prime example of the difficulty in establishing effective relationships between hospital and community services where none had been before, and of the problems involved in having both consultants and general practitioners who considered themselves experts in the same field. The specialty was in some ways also still marked by the old disfavor for the "man-midwife" and the dictum of an earlier president of the Royal College of Physicians that "obstetrics is no calling for a gentleman." [10]

Meanwhile midwifery was developing as an independent discipline. The Central Midwives Board, set up by the Act of 1902, introduced a register for nonmedical midwives and produced regulations that were much more strictly drawn up than those of the medical qualifying bodies. Midwifery became a skilled and highly respected profession, with the midwife performing the actual deliveries for the general practitioner—not only of the poor but also, in the course of time, of the middle and upper classes of society. The midwife became the practical obstetrician, while medical obstetrics weltered in a climate of indecision, self-interest, and delay. In the 1890s, 70 per cent of confinements were thought to have been attended by doctors. By 1912, in contrast, 80 per cent of the confinements in many urban areas were attended by midwives; and even where doctors were present the medical fees were less than before.[11] As a result, even today in England a substantial propor-

9. The president of the Medico-Psychological Association had written to all medical examining bodies in 1910 urging establishment of a diploma in psychological medicine, and five universities had responded. Nevertheless, by the end of World War I fewer than 20 candidates had taken the diploma. Psychiatry was unpopular for both professional and social reasons. One social objection after World War I was that assistant medical officers in mental hospitals were doomed to celibacy, being "merely perpetual house-surgeons, living as bachelors in rooms." Teaching in the mental hospitals was almost nonexistent. Lewis, in *Psychiatric Education* (Davies and Shepherd, eds.), pp. 12–17; *Brit. Med. J. i* (1938), 1071 ("A.M.O."); *ii* (1919), 328.
    10. Shaw, p. 5, passim.
    11. Comyns Carr, Stuart Garnett, and J. H. Taylor, *National Insurance* (London, 1912, p. 53.

tion of obstetrics is undertaken in family homes rather than in hospitals, and in both places the deliveries are normally by a midwife rather than an obstetrician.

By 1920 the failure to raise the standard of medical teaching in obstetrics had become a scandal. By far the most serious effect was the maternal mortality rate. Deaths from childbearing in Great Britain and Ireland were almost stationary in the period 1891–1914; and despite frequent reiteration of the value of antenatal care, the great majority of pregnant women had none of any kind. Efforts to improve the maternity and child welfare services developed through social action rather than professional reform. Local authorities set up maternity clinics, and the Ministry of Health suggested the minimum length of training suitable for medical officers attached to maternity hospitals.[12] Less than one bed in twenty was allotted to lying-in cases in the principal London hospitals, a grim heritage of the maternal mortality of earlier times. Now the hospital was relatively aseptic, but the rigid system of bed allocation in the voluntary hospitals obstructed change. Physicians and surgeons would not give up the beds necessary for the proper teaching of obstetrics and gynecology until they were required to do so by the examining bodies—and neither these bodies nor the General Medical Council, dominated by consultants from the teaching hospitals, were willing to assert the necessary authority.[13]

Separate special hospitals for obstetrics and gynecology had been established throughout the country. Midwives and general practitioners dealt only with obstetrics, not gynecology. One problem therefore to be resolved was whether obstetrics and gynecology were one field or two. A second was whether or not midwifery ought to be considered, as had traditionally been done, a logical part of general practice or whether it should be limited to specialists. The second problem was easier to solve than the first, since general practitioners had a strong interest in maintaining obstetrics as part of their work. A report from the section of obstetrics and gynecology of the Royal Society of Medicine (1919) and the statement of the profession to the 1926 Royal Commission were agreed that a woman should normally be attached to her general practitioner in pregnancy. It followed that institutional provision should be reserved for cases requiring serious obstetrical surgery, for those with antenatal complications, and for those whose home conditions were dangerous or unsuitable or for whom isolation because of septic infection was indicated.[14] Consultant and GP obstetrics were to exist

12. *Brit. Med. J. i* (1920), 303; *Lancet i* (1926), 451.
13. *Lancet ii* (1920), 25–26.
14. See *Brit Med. J. ii* (1919), 276, 347. Perhaps the most telling factor however, was that general practitioners enjoyed maternity work. A suggestion by Prof. Munro Kerr of Glasgow University in 1926 for a specialized public maternity service was, for example, vehemently opposed by the *British Medical Journal* not only for a "too restricted specialism" but also for "compulsory interference with the patient's choice and liberty" and "bureaucratic regulation"—comments that more than once have indicated professional reluctance to embark upon a course of action. *Brit. Med. J. i* (1926), 1000.

side by side, with hospital confinements for many years continuing to be the exception rather than the rule.

The need to solve these problems, and the growing numbers and authority of the consultant group, led to demands from leading obstetricians and gynecologists to found their own separate college, since it was felt that the Royal College of Physicians and the Royal College of Surgeons had failed to initiate the necessary measures to upgrade education for and practice of these specialties. This movement was led by Blair Bell of Liverpool (who had founded the national Gynaecological Visiting Society in 1911) and Fletcher Shaw of Manchester. The Royal Colleges were faced with a dilemma. Up to this point, the specialties had been contained within their walls—either because specialization naturally followed from the MRCP or FRCS diploma, or through the new specialty diplomas arranged by the universities or through their own Conjoint Board. University diplomas did not present a problem of authority to the Colleges, but the creation of a new professional college challenged their traditional supremacy as the great leaders of medicine. Not surprisingly, the Royal Colleges objected to a new foundation. Fortunately for the obstetricians, maternal mortality was made a plank in the political platform of Baldwin's second administration (1924–29). The Minister of Health (Neville Chamberlain) personally intervened to arrange a meeting between Blair Bell and the presidents of the two Colleges. The Colleges insisted that any diploma given by the obstetricians should carry no legal qualification to practice, and then reluctantly agreed to the new foundation.[15]

The British College of Obstetricians was duly established in September 1929. The Royal Colleges had moved too late. Although they set up a rival obstetrics diploma in the same year—which, the president of the Royal College of Physicians loftily pronounced, was a "guarantee of a high standard of attainment" in the subject[16]—their diploma quickly failed. The College of Obstetricians established a diploma for GPs in 1931 (now the Dip. Obst. RCOG) and a membership examination (now the MRCOG) for consultants in 1936. Membership in the College became a sine qua non for consultant appointments in obstetrics and gynecology, as the MRCP and FRCS were for medicine and surgery. The practice of obstetrics and gynecology was combined. Hospitals improved their facilities to the standard thought necessary for adequate training, and the College at once became a center for consultation on midwifery matters. Last, but not least, the College brought an elevation of status to the specialty and its practitioners, symbolized most clearly in the granting of the title of *Royal* to the College in 1938, although the outbreak of war prevented the charter from being approved until 1946. The number of professional Colleges had increased from two to three, and the traditional supremacy of the older Colleges was at last being challenged.

15. Shaw, pp. 37–38.
16. "Annual Address Delivered to the Royal College of Physicians of London by the President" (Royal College of Physicians, 1930).

Specialty Developments in the 1930s

Radiologists also considered founding an independent college. Like obstetrics, radiology was not clearly medicine or surgery; neither the MRCP nor the FRCS was directly relevant to it, and it was closely linked with advances in the physical sciences. But it was a specialty that was developing rapidly. X rays were used in World War I to detect foreign bodies, compound fractures, and gas gangrene. In the 1920s explorations were made in a number of radiological fields, and as a result X-ray departments expanded rapidly. The radiologist was usually also the physiotherapist and was in charge of all electrical equipment in a combined department. Radiotherapy, which began with attempts to treat lupus, rodent ulcers, and the removal of superfluous hair, was also developing; and in 1920 electrotherapeutics and the remedial use of X rays were generally recognized. Radiology was rising in status, full hospital rank being increasingly given to radiologists in hospitals.

The professional aspects of the specialty advanced in concert. The British Association for the Advancement of Radiology and Physiotherapy (BARP) had been set up in 1917 to sponsor the teaching for a new Diploma in Medical Radiology and Electrology (DMRE) to be set up by the University of Cambridge; the first examination for the DMRE was held in 1920. In the same year the Society of Radiographers was founded (with the assistance of the Institute of Electrical Engineers and the BARP) to give professional status to certified nonmedical assistants in X-ray and electrotherapeutic departments. The amalgamation of the BARP with the Roentgen Society in 1927 aided the interests of radiologists through the formation of representative special committees to express authoritative opinions on behalf of the specialty. The central question—which was to be raised again in specialties such as anesthesiology, pathology, and physical medicine—was whether the radiologist was to be regarded as a full medical consultant or as a mere technician. A closely associated problem was whether radiographers might make diagnostic reports directly to the clinical staff or whether they must always work through a medical radiologist. Some consultants held that "it is the pictures which are paid for, not the opinion." [17] In 1929, no hospital, cottage or otherwise, considered itself properly equipped without an X-ray department, but many did not have a trained radiologist in charge of the department. The place of the radiologist in the hospital was thus of immediate importance.

In 1930, London University established a chair in radiology. Three universities now offered diplomas—Cambridge, Edinburgh, and Liverpool—and radiology could be taken as a special subject for the Edinburgh MRCP. These were augmented by the Conjoint Board's Diploma in Radiology (1932); and an Academic Diploma in Medical Radiology was instituted by London University in 1933. The British Association of Radiologists was

17. *Brit. Med. J. i* (1929), 778.

founded in 1934, and the Society of Radiotherapists in 1935, both bodies including only full-fledged practitioners among their membership. Despite this progress there was still pressure for a college to afford the ultimate level of prestige on a par with the physicians, surgeons, and now obstetricians and gynecologists. The title "College of Radiologists" was opposed by the older Colleges, and finally the new organization, by amalgamation of the Association of Radiologists with the Society of Radiotherapists, was called "the Faculty of Radiologists" (1939), with two sections, to accommodate the two branches of the subject.[18] The faculty, although independent of the Colleges, did not try to compete with the existing radiology diploma from the Conjoint Board. Instead, it created its own fellowship (FFR) above the standards of the existing diplomas; this became a more advanced examination in its specialty than the FRCS, MRCP, or MRCOG.

Meanwhile, physical medicine was developing as an independent specialty, although it was more a collection of individual methods of treatment than a unified discipline; it included balneology (the therapeutic use of baths), actinotherapy (the use of rays), electrology, massage, and exercise. Nonmedical physiotherapists, who had already had a society for over twenty years, received their Royal Charter in 1920. Medical physiotherapists had no specialty examination. The demand for physical treatment in the 1920s and 1930s came forcibly from the lay public; and gradually departments of physical medicine were established in hospitals and equipped with modern installations. But to the orthodox physician, there were obvious dangers in physical medicine: "With the public's childlike love for machinery, the temptation so to apply it was very great." [19] There was a danger that the physiotherapist would not keep closely in touch with the physicist on the one hand and the clinician on the other; or, even worse, he might wander away from the bedrock of pathology and lose himself in a sea of speculation. Last, there was the very real danger of commercial exploitation of patients by untrained men.[20] For all these reasons the status of physical medicine as a medical specialty was hotly debated in the midwar years. The physical medicine group at the BMA, concerned about their status in 1938, did not find their request for a diploma supported by the other members of the BMA. Altogether there was an atmosphere of discontent, and, not surprisingly, the specialty remained relatively small.

While these developments were affecting practice in the larger hospitals in the late 1920s and early 1930s, GP specialism was increasing. In 1935 two more diplomas were added by the Conjoint Board for the use primarily

18. Cope, *History of the Royal College of Surgeons,* p. 195.
19. Lord Horder, reported in *Brit. Med. J. i* (1936), 808.
20. " A type of pseudo-scientist was accustomed to go around an apparently well-equipped room and turn on one switch after another in the hope that at last the patient would say he felt better." *Brit. Med. J. i* (1937), 884. Others felt that physical medicine was no more than a "rather despised adjunct to the department of surgical orthopaedics." *Brit. Med. J. i* (1938), 46.

of GPs. These were the Diploma in Child Health (DCH) and the Diploma in Anaesthetics (DA).[21]

Pediatrics did not really develop in England before the interwar period. This was partly because, through the operation of the "referral system," the common diseases of children were seen by general practitioners; partly because it was hard for a beginner to establish himself when pediatric specialists were expected to be unpaid consultants to the voluntary hospitals; and partly because it had been unusual for a physician to a large general hospital, who had a special interest in children, to resign all his other work and to concentrate on pediatrics alone.[22] Although a large number of general physicians treated children in their adult wards, there were few consultant pediatricians, the focus of pediatrics as a specialty being the Great Ormond Street Hospital for Sick Children, in London. Pediatrics inevitably was thus largely a GP specialty. The British Paediatric Association (founded in 1928) was the driving force behind the establishment of the child health diploma, stimulated by an increased social interest in the health and welfare of children and possibly by the impetus given to study of the newborn by the activities of the College of Obstetricians. The content of the diploma was widely based. "It is no secret," said the *Lancet,* "that the establishment of the new diploma was prompted by a feeling on the part of pædiatricians that medical officers of child welfare centres had often received no special training in the recognition and treatment of diseases in infancy and childhood." [23] Hospital pediatricians however continued to rely mainly on the MRCP. They allied themselves with other medical consultants rather than with the general practitioners of their subject—a clear example of the old division between GPs and consultants inhibiting the development of separate specialty groups.

The Diploma in Anaesthetics was set up to provide a gauge of competence in GP anesthesiology; for even in the large towns anesthetics was widely practiced as a sideline by local practitioners.[24] Partly because of this, partly because of its brief existence as a separate specialty (at the beginning of the century it was largely an adjunct of surgery), and partly because of the distrust by general clinicians of the technician, anesthetics had a low status. In fact, however, it was developing advanced technical skills. New

21. Since its foundation in 1884 to provide the joint diploma of LRCP and MRCS, the Conjoint Board had developed eight postgraduate specialty diplomas: public health, 1887; tropical medicine, 1911; ophthalmology, psychological medicine, laryngology and otology, 1920; medical radiology, 1932; anesthesiology, child health, 1935. Others followed: medical radiodiagnosis, medical radiotherapy, physical medicine, 1944; industrial medicine, 1946; pathology, 1950. In most of these subjects diplomas were also offered by universities. Cope, *History of the RCS,* p. 155.

22. Pediatrics, it was remarked in 1931, "supplies rather a restricted field for the interests of a first-class intelligence." *Brit. Med. J.* ii (1931), 997. The development of pediatrics is described in H. C. Cameron, *The British Paediatric Association, 1928–52* (London, 1955), from which this section is largely drawn.

23. *Lancet ii* (1935), 773.

24. The diploma was reportedly to protect the public from incompetent practice and the individual doctor from "unfair competition." *Lancet i* (1935), 1451.

techniques in anesthesia were introduced in the 1920s, and it was only their adoption, together with the discovery of sulfa drugs, penicillin, and other antibiotics as powerful defenses against infection, that was later to enable the exploration of the heart, lungs, and other comparatively inaccessible organs. But the effect of these techniques on the status of the practitioner was to be delayed until after World War II. A speaker in 1938 acidly reminded the profession that there had been a change in anesthetic practice in recent years and it was no longer a matter of "a bottle and a rag." [25] The Association of Anaesthetists remained dissatisfied with their status and their emoluments. Anesthesiologists still felt they were looked upon as little better than assistants at operations. Anesthetics did not develop as a nursing specialty, as in the United States; there was thus no problem of nonmedical assistants reporting directly to surgeons. Nevertheless, the same questions applied as to radiology. Was the anesthetist primarily a technician, who need not be of consultant status or even medically trained, or was he a clinician?

This question was equally applicable to the third rapidly growing specialty. Pathology encompasses four disciplines: bacteriology (which, after the rapid scientific advances in that field from the 1880s onward, constituted the bulk of the work), hematology, biochemistry, and morbid anatomy. In the smaller nonteaching centers, the clinical pathologist practiced all four aspects of his specialty, as his clinical colleague still practiced as a general physician. In the larger hospitals, however, separate departments were devoted to the separate subjects. In both, pathologists suffered from the clinicians' concept of them as "purely hewers of wood and drawers of water for their particular benefit." [26] Courses leading to a postgraduate diploma in bacteriology were established at Manchester University by Professor Topley in 1923 and served as a pattern from which Topley developed courses for an academic Diploma in Bacteriology at London University. But there was no specific training for the general pathologist.

An important unifying influence between bacteriology and other aspects of pathology in England was the Pathological Society of Great Britain and Ireland, founded in 1906 to provide a valuable stimulus to experimental pathology and to keep morbid anatomists and bacteriologists together. The Association of Clinical Pathologists came into being in 1927, started by a group of men who were drawn largely from the nonteaching hospitals and the provinces, who felt the need of a society emphasizing the practical aspects of pathology as a bedside specialty. Recent scientific advances had stressed the clinical aspects of the subject. The discovery of insulin in 1922 brought the chemical pathologist to the patient; hematology had also changed from an interesting laboratory subject to a bedside procedure for the accurate diagnosis of pernicious anemia and for exercising exact scientific control upon the effects of treatment. But most pathological work con-

25. R. Scott Stevenson, *Brit. Med. J.* Suppl. *ii* (1938), 73.
26. *Brit. Med. J. ii* (1925), 554.

tinued to be routine drudgery, and much of it was undertaken by specialist technicians, the Institute of Medical Laboratory Technology having been incorporated in 1912. By the mid-1930s the pathologist was becoming the administrative head of a busy, relatively large, and increasingly better-equipped department. But like the radiologist, he was still of lesser status than the general physician and general surgeon. He was often employed on a salary; he had little or none of the trappings of private practice; and he lacked the ultimate status symbol: responsibility for a specified unit of hospital beds.

The Patterns of Specialism

These specialties were not the only ones to develop in the interwar period, but they aroused the greatest organizational activity. Dermatology, for example, continued to advance in parallel with the general advance in housing and cleanliness, the better education of the community, the improvement in medical inspection of school children, and the cooperation of workers in this branch with those in other branches of medicine; but it lacked energy and direction. Urology was somewhat similar, although three London hospitals as well as numerous special departments in large general hospitals were dedicated to this specialty. A specialist journal had been founded in 1929, but there were no demands for a special diploma. Dermatologists, like cardiologists and neurologists, were content with the MRCP. Urologists, like plastic surgeons and neurosurgeons, were happy with the FRCS. They were both part of a relatively small elite of consulting physicians and surgeons—and they were also both relatively small specialties.

Taking the specialties as a whole there was no clear pattern of development. Some saw the rapid growth of specialization in the 1920s and 1930s as a temporary phase, destined to advance research and technique in particular areas of medicine and then to retreat. "Young men were learning to use the cystoscope and other methods of diagnosis as they learned to drive a car. When they in turn became senior, they would not need a specialist for these purposes." [27] Others, more accurately, saw specialization as the inevitable accompaniment of a scientific advance that would continue to accelerate. Specialties were no longer merely indications of scientific interest, marked by attachment to a special hospital and attendance at after-dinner discussion clubs or the appropriate section of the Royal Society of Medicine. They had become professionalized groups, each conscious of its own particular needs: inclusion of their subject in the undergraduate curriculum, raised standards of training (and simultaneously the status of the specialty), and representation on appropriate administrative and professional bodies.

The specialties which were particularly concerned about their education and status were the rapidly increasing nonclinical and "service" specialties (anesthesiology, radiology, and pathology) together with those which were not associated with the eminent London special hospitals founded in the

27. Gask, *Brit. Med. J.* ii (1935), 816.

nineteenth century, or which were by the midwar period associated with public health needs or general practice. Both the Royal Society of Medicine and the British Medical Association had sections in which the scientific and organizational future of each specialty could be discussed and which provided platforms for reform. But they did not have exclusive rights over admittance to each specialty. Equally, the diplomas set up by the universities and the Conjoint Board were in most cases permissive, not prescriptive, to practice in the specialty. Medical officers of health were expected to hold the DPH, but otolaryngologists were not expected to hold the DLO. One difference was between public and private employment. Local health authorities could specify requirements for medical officers employed by them in the increasingly important municipal hospitals. Voluntary hospitals were not so organized, although they were unofficially committed to recognition of the MRCP and FRCS as the major postgraduate diplomas, which the Conjoint Board's new diplomas were not of a standard to rival. Thus, with few exceptions, the diplomas set up in the 1920s and 1930s bore no social status and gave no practicing privileges; they were evidence of a purely vocational attainment.

It could have been argued that the time had come for a state register of specialists, just as there was a state register for all practitioners with the basic diplomas or degrees. In this case, it would not matter where the actual specialist diploma was taken—at a university or through a college—provided both were registrable. The university, with its wide facilities, its acknowledged links with teaching hospitals, and its full-time staff, would have seemed the more logical alternative for the provision of specialist training, and, indeed, it had been at the universities that the first special diplomas were evolved. But the Colleges were the traditional arbiters of consultant status. The question of such certification, however, makes assumptions that were not valid at the time: first, that the profession as a whole was concerned at the fragmentary process of the specialties; second, given the division of English practice into consultants and GPs, that it was necessary or desirable to test the competence of specialists; and, third, that the government was interested in the problem. As the 1858 Act had shown, legislation followed, rather than forecast, professional intent. In the absence of a specialist register, there was only one viable alternative that would satisfy the increasing demands of groups for recognition. Only a college, or similar association, could assume representative or autocratic power over the individuals in the specialty and only where admittance was by examination could its authority be complete.

In England, the existence of a small consultant group and a large group of general practitioners inhibited the development of specialty groups; friction between the specialties might have undermined the distinction between the two branches of practice. Much of the impetus for special examinations was aimed at general practice. But, as the obstetricians and radiologists had shown, the urge to split off was apparent, even among consultant groups, when it was felt that the Royal Colleges were offering too little. Size of specialty was clearly one factor affecting the desire to separate. An estimated 8 per cent of specialists in 1939 were gynecologists, and over 7 per cent were radiologists.[28] Other relatively large specialties were otolaryngology, ophthalmology, and anesthesiology, and these were to be the next specialties to demand their independence, after World War II.

28. Spens Report on Consultants and Specialists, pp. 22–25.

4

Problems of Medical Practice
in the Late 1930s

The simultaneous success of the National Health Insurance scheme (1912–48) and the effect of increasing specialization in medicine focused public and professional interest on the organization of medical services. The advances in medicine in the interwar period raised questions on the role of the hospital, the status of general practice, and the future organization of general and specialized services.

By the end of the 1930s, after a long period of discussion, a number of ideas had crystallized on the need for reform and redefinition of medical services. First, it was evident that the insurance scheme, by now fully accepted, ought to be extended in both population coverage and scope of benefits. Second, a solution had to be found for the chaos in hospital development, and for the specialist services that were associated with them. Third, there was the question of the most efficient organization of general practitioners, who had already begun to move from the traditional one-man practice into small partnerships. Finally, there needed to be a precise definition of "general practitioner," "consultant," and "specialist."

The Impact of National Health Insurance

National Health Insurance had reinforced general practice at the very time that specialization was threatening it. In 1938, 40 per cent of the total population of England and Wales were covered by the scheme, and 90 per cent of all general practitioners were participating in it. Well over a third of the income of these "panel" doctors in the years 1936–38 was derived from insurance capitation payments and it was claimed that health insurance work took two thirds of the GP's time.[1] State-financed medicine had thus become an important facet of the GP's professional life.

General practitioners were on the whole favorable to the system. The twenty-first birthday party of National Health Insurance was celebrated in

1. The average size of the GP's "panel" was 1,072 per principal, and more than 7% of panel doctors had over 2,500 insurance patients on their lists. See Hermann Levy, *National Health Insurance* (Cambridge, 1944), p. 123; Austin Bradford Hill, *J. Roy. Statistical Soc. A cxiv* (1951), 23; Spens Report on General Practitioners, p. 11.

1933 by a luncheon organized by the BMA and other organizations concerned with the insurance administration: Lloyd George (the scheme's originator) was the guest of honor. The BMA had set its unequivocal seal of approval several years earlier in a memorandum of evidence to the Royal Commission on National Health Insurance, which reported in 1926; its memorandum left no doubt of the general benefits believed to have been conferred on the community.[2] The BMA also had cause to be proud of the rights built into the system as a result of its efforts. These included the right of all practitioners to enter or leave the scheme at will, the close approximation of insurance service to private practice, and the considerable share the profession had in the scheme's administration. As the *British Medical Journal* said, the attitude of the profession was one of "willing acceptance." It exhorted the American Medical Association to be encouraged by the fact that "the much greater experiences of the British Medical Association in collective negotiation and bargaining indicates that the power of the organized medical profession, reasonably exercised, is very effective." [3]

Indeed, both the BMA and other medical and lay organizations testifying to the Royal Commission recommended a broad extension of health insurance. Coverage had been increased since the 1911 Act came into effect, but wives and dependents of insured persons in Britain were still excluded, as were the self-employed and those above a certain income. Moreover, even for those who were covered by the scheme, the medical benefits were limited. They applied only to *general practitioner* care and associated drugs and appliances, a limitation that was increasingly noticed as specialist care became more frequent. There was a strong case for including complete consultant and specialist advice and treatment, laboratory service, hospital and institutional care, dental care, and full supporting services to insured persons and their family dependents. If it had been accepted, the basis of the present National Health Service might have been entirely different. But in this the BMA was more progressive than the Ministry of Health and the Commissioners who signed the Majority Report in 1926. They commented that if specialist services were to be provided for insured people at home and in hospitals, they would feel seriously concerned about the position of noninsured persons of moderate means. The only remedy would be to make a

2. "(a) Large numbers, indeed whole classes, of persons are now receiving a real medical attention which they formerly did not receive at all, (b) the number of practitioners in proportion to the population in densely populated areas has increased, (c) the amount and character of the medical attention given is immensely superior to that formerly given in the great majority of clubs, (d) illness is now coming under skilled observation and treatment at an earlier stage than was formerly the case, (e) the work of practitioners has been given a bias towards prevention that was formerly not so marked, (f) clinical records are being provided which may be made of great service in relation to public health and medical research, (g) cooperation among practitioners is being encouraged to an increasing degree, (h) there is now a more marked recognition than formerly of the collective responsibility of the profession to the community in respect of all health matters." H.B. Brackenbury, *New Engl. J. Med. 210* (1934), 851–54. The BMA memorandum is quoted in this source.

3. *Brit. Med. J. i* (1935), 365.

similar benefit available also to the middle classes. Although convinced that this problem "must ultimately be faced," the Commissioners did not feel equal to the task;[4] the decision to provide comprehensive medical services through the agency of government was to be delayed for twenty years.

Throughout the 1930s and in the early years of World War II, the BMA continued to be an advocate of an extended health service organized through the state;[5] but nothing was done. As a result, the voluntary hospitals did not receive the financial transfusion that compulsory hospital insurance might have provided. Consultant and specialist services remained outside health insurance until it was abandoned in 1948.

The division of GP work into panel and nonpanel practice affected the form in which specialist practice developed. There was no financial incentive for the panel doctor in a working-class area to specialize. His insurance capitation fees were for general medical care only. As a specialist he would have to develop his own private practice in a highly competitive and, in the early stages, a financially unrewarding market. The patient exercised free choice of doctor only at the general practitioner level; for choice of consultant or specialist, he was invariably guided by his panel doctor. Thus under the system of referral, specialization could not be used to attract new patients as self-diagnosed walk-ins from the street. On the other hand, the insurance system provided a useful financial foothold for the prospective full-time specialist on his way up the career ladder. A period in general practice as a young man was a not uncommon experience of those who were appointed as consultants in the 1940s and early 1950s. The panel system thus encouraged doctors to remain primarily generalists, although many developed some part-time specialist practice and later became full-time specialists.

There was also a development of partnerships among GPs to share expenses and organize off-duty rotas. One survey in 1938 indicated that 45 per cent of general practitioners were in some form of partnership.[6] In market towns such as Stratford-on-Avon, Banbury, and Winchester, there were embryonic specialist group practices, in which general practitioners built up their specialty interests and combined to offer a variety of services on the American pattern.[7] But this was comparatively rare. As a general trend, specialty group practice of this kind was barely observable. Professional ethics and the traditions of the referral system also prevented con-

4. *Report of the Royal Commission on National Health Insurance,* Cmd. 2596 (HMSO, 1928), pp. 30, 125–26.

5. The BMA's report on a general medical service, published in 1930 and revised and reissued in 1938, again recommended a modified health insurance scheme on the basis of which a comprehensive medical service would be established. Dependents of insured persons would be covered, together with all others of equivalent economic status, and it would include consultant and specialist services as well as full dental and ophthalmic benefits and full maternity services. BMA, *The British Medical Association's Proposals for a General Medical Service for the Nation* (London, 1930).

6. Spens Report on General Practitioners, p. 19.

7. See *Lancet ii* (1964), 360 (E. O. Evans).

sultants and GPs from practicing together in common partnerships. Fellows of the Royal College of Physicians for example, were (and still are) specifically debarred from practicing in any kind of partnership without special permission of the Censors' Board of the College; nor were they allowed, as was the custom among general practitioners, to buy or sell the goodwill of a practice.[8] In theory the referral system precluded the need for group specialist practice, since the general practitioner was the central coordinating figure who directed a patient to a specialist as he thought necessary. "Without the mediation of the doctor," Lord Horder inquired in 1938, "how were the common folk to link up with the health services?"[9] Specialism in medicine was thus admittedly the complement of the family doctor and not a substitute for him.

The insurance scheme had a profound impact on hospital practice. When the benefits were first made available in 1913, a number of hospitals had refused to accept insured persons unless referred by their panel doctor.[10] The voluntary hospitals gradually ceased to be open institutions for the poorer sections of society and the outpatient clinic became a center for specialist practice, to which patients came bearing their doctor's letters. At the same time, since there was no longer the fierce competition between general practitioners and outpatient departments (for the insurance system reinforced the concept of basic continuity of care by a general practitioner) and since the general practitioner received his capitation fee whether he referred the patient to the hospital or not, there was every incentive for him to send complex cases to the hospital. This was particularly true in the cities where large voluntary hospitals were easily available, and it became more so as both voluntary and municipal hospitals expanded and improved their facilities. There was the very real danger that the GP in the shadow of the great hospitals would become merely a signer of certificates and a signpost to the hospital.[11]

In being restricted to GPs, the health insurance system thus furthered the dichotomy of GPs and consultants. About one out of three senior practitioners had access to hospital beds in the late 1930s. Of these probably half were general practitioners, with or without a specialty interest, to whom beds in cottage hospitals or in small hospitals in the market towns were available; almost all of the remainder were exclusively engaged in consultant or specialist practice. Although no precise figures are available, it seems likely that there were about 2,800 full-time consultants and specialists in Britain in 1938–39, compared with some 18,000 general practitioners.[12]

8. Under Bye-Law 157 of the Royal College of Physicians of London.

9. *Brit. Med. J.* Suppl. *i* (1938), 37.

10. Abel-Smith, *The Hospitals,* pp. 244–46. The insurance scheme came into operation in July 1912, but benefits were not paid until January 1913.

11. See P. E. P. (Political and Economic Planning) *Report on the British Health Services* (London, 1937,), pp. 161–65.

12. The figures are tentative because no authoritative national records were kept, and definitions of practice categories varied. The BMA figures for Britain in 1937 showed

At the same time, as the GP's income was raised by his panel practice, consultants and general practitioners drew closer in social position.[13] Under National Health Insurance the GP became a well-established figure. While most general practitioners were not well-to-do, they were comfortably situated, with a net average income in 1936–38 of about £1000 a year.[14] "Medicine gives to those who follow it an honourable position," proclaimed the *British Medical Journal:* "The well-educated doctor stands high among his neighbours." According to the same source, National Health Insurance had induced a "better class of man" to enter general practice;[15] and indicatively, the *Journal* addressed its remarks exclusively to those prospective medical students attending the public (i.e. preparatory) schools.

The dean of at least one London medical school proudly emphasized personal selection of students, over proficiency in examinations, according to the three basic criteria of the public school man: "High intelligence, outstanding character, and considerable skill at games." Interhospital rugby football (sport of the public schools) reached its zenith in popularity. While it was undoubtedly true, as the *Journal* had claimed in the late 1920s, that "the culture which in past centuries belonged to the physician alone has spread to all ranks of the profession," this had been largely achieved by drawing medical students from a homogeneous social group. The group was staunchly middle-class. In 1938–39 almost 90 per cent of the students at one English medical school were entirely self-financed—a much higher proportion than students in other university faculties or medical students in Scotland where medicine was still a means of raising one's social status.[16] The great majority entered general practice, and accepted insurance patients.

There was no specific training for general practice. Probably half the students left hospitals immediately on graduation to set up their plates as independent GPs, to buy a vacant practice, or to be taken into an established partnership. The prospective consultant, if he did not have a period in general practice, struggled his way up the hospital ladder, from house officer (intern) to registrar (resident) until he was appointed to the hospital

---

2,797 "consultants and specialists," 285 consultant teachers, and 2,381 other hospital staff. Hill's figures would indicate about 2,860 full-time consultants plus about 570 doctors who were predominantly in consultant practice in 1938-39; he found a total of 6,868 names on the part-time visiting staffs of voluntary and municipal hospitals; Hill, *J. Roy. Statistical Soc.* (1951), pp. 25, 27, 30; BMA personal communication.

13. One example of the increased standard of living was the opposition by doctors to a proposed new tax on motor vehicles in 1920, because it would fall on them unfairly. In some parts of the country, it was claimed, doctors had to keep two cars, "as they could not afford to wait if their ordinary car broke down until it could be repaired." *Brit. Med. J. i.* (1920), 648, 660.

14. Hill, *J. Roy. Statistical Soc.* (1951), p. 26.

15. *Brit. Med. J. ii* (1937), 445.

16. Cope, *St. Mary's Hospital Medical School*, pp. 69, 71. *Brit. Med. J. ii* (1929), 386. Ministry of Health and Department of Health of Scotland *Report of the Interdepartmental Committee on Medical Schools* (Goodenough report) (London, 1944), p. 101.

staff. If he were lucky, consultant status could be attained by the age of 30; but he could be unsuccessful at any stage of the ladder since all posts—including consultant appointments—were limited in number. Consultant posts were only for those who were willing to chance the system. Moreover, successful private practice depended on hospital staff status since professional custom ensured that GPs refer patients only to those consultants who had achieved the respectability of a hospital appointment. It was thought that many potential specialists who did not have private incomes were diverted by marriage into the financial security of general practice.[17] There was thus neither a distinct social gulf nor necessarily a difference in ability between those choosing general practice and those who became consultants.

A consultant appointment, once reached, brought comparative affluence through its associated private practice. Even in the early years of his private practice (between the ages of 35 and 40), although the general practitioner already had a long start on the newfledged hospital doctor, the average consultant was thought to earn more in the late 1930s than the average general practitioner. By the time both were in the 55–64 age group, the consultant was earning almost twice as much as the GP. The most lucrative consultant fields were gynecology and general surgery. At the bottom were the least fashionable specialties—anesthesiology, pathology, and psychiatry. Medical remuneration in general appeared to be high in comparison with other professions, with the possible exception of barristers, the consultants and specialists of the legal profession.[18]

Problems of Hospital Organization

The confusion in medical practice was linked with the confused hospital situation. Voluntary hospitals clustered round medical teaching centers and foci of private practices or were small units scattered throughout the countryside. The large voluntary hospitals, as in the past, were staffed by consultants who, by being linked with the hospitals' expanding specialist departments, were often specialists rather than general physicians and surgeons. The great majority of voluntary hospitals were, however, small, and many, if not most of them, were staffed by GPs who might or might not themselves provide specialist services. Both consultants and GPs, customarily generalists, were simultaneously acquiring specialist skills. Surgery, for example, was being increasingly regarded as a specialist subject, yet no fewer than 2.5 million surgical operations were performed by general practitioners in 1938–39:

17. Spens Report on Consultants, p. 6.

18. A physician in "consulting or superior general practice" in about 1930 was thought to earn at least an average of £2,000 at about age 40. This placed him on the same level as a university graduate solicitor or a top-level executive in industry, and well above the administrative class of the civil service. *Royal Commission on the Civil Service, 1929–30*; Appendix VIII to the *Minutes of Evidence;* statement submitted by the Association of First Division Civil Servants, p. 51. See also Hill, *J. Roy. Statistical Soc.* (1951), p. 30; Spens Report on General Practitioners, p. 20; Spens Report on Consultants, pp. 20–30; P.E.P. *Report*, p. 10.

an average of three per doctor per week.[19] Since the voluntary hospitals were in no way linked, the range and standards of such skills might vary considerably from one to another—for example, from the consultant ear, nose, and throat surgeon in a major teaching center to the GP who performed tonsillectomies in his local cottage hospital.

The role of the hospital was changing under the impact of technical advances. It was no longer a mere hostel for the sick poor, but increasingly a center for scientific work. One result of this was that the hospitals had opened their doors to the middle class and the well-to-do. The number of hospitals and nursing homes rose; hospital prepayment plans sprang up and flourished; and hospital consultants, having to spend more time in hospitals and finding themselves treating an increasing number of middle-class patients (who paid the hospital for its services) began to demand payment for their hospital work.[20] In the meantime, hospital costs rose rapidly, owing to the increase in number of hospital nurses and technicians and the more complex equipment needed in a specialist environment.[21] This added to the financial difficulties of the voluntary hospitals, which had emerged in straitened circumstances from World War I.

A second complicating factor in the hospital scene was the development of the municipal hospital. Under the Local Government Act, 1929, poor-law infirmaries (the old workhouses) began gradually to be appropriated by the health departments of the larger local governments which were already responsible for mental and infectious disease hospitals and tuberculosis sanatoria. By the end of the 1930s, local authorities were responsible for 130,000 beds in general hospitals, some of which were of a standard to rival the neighboring voluntary hospitals.[22] But these too (except in London, where the County Council had created a grouped hospital service) were organized

19. Hill, *J. Roy. Statistical Soc.* (1951), p. 17.

20. The introduction of direct patient billing and the rise of prepayment plans between the wars changed the character of the voluntary hospitals: they were no longer *charitable* institutions. By 1935 less than half their income came from donations and endowments. About one of four of the population was a member of a hospital contributory scheme, and there was an increasing demand for beds for private patients in the hospitals and for single rooms instead of ward accommodation. Nevertheless, private beds remained a small minority. Some voluntary hospitals were precluded by their original charters from providing private beds until Parliament passed the Private Patients Act in 1936. Only 2,400 pay beds of a total of over 18,000 were recorded in London voluntary hospitals in 1938. Patients in beds which were not part of the private pay block were charged for their hospital services, but they were usually not billed by the attending consultants. See P.E.P. *Report*, pp. 16, 234; and *Hospitals Year Book*, 1938, pp. 53, 175–84.

21. Between 1933 and 1937 alone, for example, it was estimated that nursing staff rose by over 12% in voluntary and 18% in municipal hospitals. The first National Register of Medical Auxiliaries, including physiotherapists, radiographers, dispensing opticians, and "biophysical assistants" appeared in 1937. Abel-Smith, *History of the Nursing Profession*, p. 270; PEP *Report*, p. 193.

22. Ministry of Health, Department of Health for Scotland, *A National Health Service*, Cmd. 6502 (London, 1944), "The 1944 White Paper," pp. 55–56.

in relation to their own small service areas. Both voluntary and local public hospitals were insular institutions. Coordination between them was almost nonexistent, and national and even regional planning was unknown. Except for teaching purposes in university centers, they rarely joined forces; nor did either type of hospital plan its services to complement others of its own type nearby.

Voluntary hospitals provided a much greater outpatient service, but the municipal hospitals were rapidly catching up and provided a second considerable pool of employment for consultants; their patients were beginning to rival the voluntary hospitals as teaching material for the aspiring doctor. The *British Medical Journal* commended the local government hospital service not only to those who "seek a secure position with superannuation at the end" but also to "the ambitious who desire experience." [23] Wholetime consultants were employed on a salary. Part-timers, who were often the same consultants who attended at the local voluntary hospital, were also reimbursed. The London County Council, for example, paid consultants according to the number of hospital sessions they attended; fees ranged from £125 a year for one session (half-day) a week.[24] Although this sum was relatively small, it was not unimportant to consultants engaged in building a private practice.

The consultant on the staff of the voluntary hospital was still normally unpaid, especially in the hospitals of greatest prestige. In 1935 it was claimed that only seventy-four hospitals in England and Wales, and only three in London, allocated some proportion of patients' payments to a medical staff fund.[25] In his capacity as honorary physician or surgeon to a voluntary hospital, the consultant had his own block of labeled beds in open hospital wards and, of rising importance, he also had a number of consultative clinics in the outpatient department, at which he saw patients referred to him by general practitioners.

With the exception of professorial units in teaching hospitals, the staffing structure of the large voluntary hospitals was little different from that at the beginning of the century.[26] Below the consultants came the salaried hospital staff of registrar, house physician or house surgeon, and perhaps a quota of

23. *Brit. Med. J. ii* (1937), 504.
24. PEP *Report*, p. 253.
25. Abel-Smith, *The Hospitals*, p. 389.
26. All but four of the medical schools in England, Wales, and Scotland were attached to universities in 1938–39, the twelve London undergraduate schools coming under the umbrella of the University of London. Professorial, or university, medical and surgical units had been developed, largely at the instigation of the Board (Ministry) of Education, from 1909 (when St. Mary's Hospital applied for the first Board grant) to coordinate undergraduate clinical teaching within the hospital. The professorial unit had its own beds and clinics, like any other hospital "firm," but the system encouraged the appointment of whole-time clinicians and teachers of consultant caliber on university salaries. Other consultants on the staff of the teaching hospital were expected to undertake clinical teaching as part of their regular hospital duties.

students. The "firm" system inhibited the development of hierarchical departments in the clinical specialties. There was no movement either within single specialties or across specialties for consultants formally to unite as a team, although they might be called together to work with particular patients.

The firm system had not spread to the municipal hospitals. There the staffing was comparatively simple; at the head was the medical superintendent and below him a hierarchy of salaried assistants. Consultants engaged by local authorities, unlike those in voluntary hospitals, usually had a purely consultative function: they gave advice to the permanent staff on any case, and they did not have a block of beds. The majority of consultants committed only part of their time to hospital work, but there was a trend toward full-time employment in certain specialties. London teaching hospitals employed forty-nine full-time pathologists in 1938, together with eleven full-time anesthesiologists and nine full-time radiologists. In contrast, full-time salaried employment in any type of hospital was rare among consultants in general medicine and surgery.[27]

There were disadvantages in both the voluntary and municipal hospital methods of staffing. The honorary service in the voluntary hospitals was held responsible for the unequal and unsatisfactory geographical distribution of consultants and specialists, who were naturally drawn toward the areas where private practice flourished. Municipal hospital methods resulted in understaffing. The visiting consultant had no continuing charge over patients and therefore little stake in the work of the hospital, and the system of paying low salaries for whole-time specialists and high salaries to medical superintendents had, it was claimed, driven good clinicians, for financial reasons, into administrative posts.[28]

Plans for Hospital Reorganization

The existence of the two kinds of hospital made the question of coordination both more urgent and, because of the voluntary hospitals' innate distrust of local authorities, more difficult. There was no lack of discussion of hospital reform. Rumors had appeared in the press in 1918 of a scheme aimed at "nothing less than the nationalization of the medical profession, involving free medical attendance for all without any element of charity".[29] The Dawson Committee (1920), set up by the new Ministry of Health, recommended a comprehensive health service which would provide for all aspects of medicine, preventive and curative, through a national network of

27. In 1938, there were in London's voluntary and municipal hospitals only 11 general physicians and 9 surgeons on a full-time hospital salary. Gray and Topping, *Hospital Services of London*, pp. 83, 181.

28. Nuffield Provincial Hospitals Trust *The Hospital Surveys: The Domesday Book of the Hospital Services* (London, 1946), pp. 11–13.

29. Abel-Smith, *The Hospitals*, p. 286.

primary (GP) and secondary (specialist) health centers which were to be mutually dependent.[30] The following year the Cave Committee (1921) proposed administrative machinery to coordinate the work and finances of the voluntary hospitals through a central commission and local committees based on county and county–borough areas. But little was done; the problem was deferred from one year to the next.

Sixteen years after the Cave Committee report the Sankey report (1937) recommended regional planning of voluntary hospitals.[31] This suggestion was attractive since it eschewed any question of subordination of the voluntary hospitals to local government: To "surrender control to a Regional Council is not the same thing for a voluntary hospital board as to hand over to the local authority."[32] Distrust of local authorities also inhibited any suggestion that the public hospitals be included in any such grand design, the next logical step in the progress to a national regionalized hospital service. Meanwhile, the hospitals remained badly distributed, uncoordinated, and in many cases chronically short of money, staff, and equipment.

It was calculated from the results of the hospital surveys published during and after World War II that available hospital beds fell short of overall need by about one third, and the deficiencies were far from even. Even more important, however, were deficiencies in specialist staffing. Some counties were without a single gynecologist. The eastern area had no thoracic surgeons, dermatologists, or pediatricians, and only two hospitals had psychiatrists. In the Sheffield and East Midlands area (with a population of four million), pediatrics was a relatively underdeveloped subject; there was no plastic surgery, and there were fewer than six doctors who restricted their work to the administration of anesthetics. Some consultants accepted posts on the staff of a number of small hospitals and spent an inordinate amount of time traveling from one to the other. Outside the radius of the large medical centers, hospital committees had to do the best they could by appointing staff from the general practitioners in the neighborhood.[33] Both voluntary and public hospitals were guilty of allowing surgery to be done by inadequately trained practitioners.

Such findings highlighted the dilemma of medical practice in the late 1930s. The geographical distribution of consultants had probably not radically changed, and may have improved, in the previous quarter century. The difference now was that care by GPs only, which until this time had

30. Ministry of Health, Consultative Council on Medical and Allied Services, *Interim Report on the Future Provision of Medical and Allied Services* (Dawson report) Cmd. 693 (London, 1920).

31. British Hospitals Association, *Report of the Voluntary Hospitals Commission* (Sankey report) (London, 1937).

32. PEP *Report,* p. 263. Lord Sankey himself remarked on regionalization of hospitals that he had "never found such unanimity among witnesses." "Address by the Rt. Hon. Viscount Sankey," reported in the *Hospitals Year Book,* 1937, p. 1.

33. *The Hospital Surveys,* p. 7, and passim; R.M. Titmuss, *Problems of Social Policy* (London, 1950), p. 71.

sufficed for the great majority of the population, was no longer enough—or no longer a practicable system—in the rapidly changing environment of medicine. The nineteenth-century GP with his LSA and MRCS was, in the light of the knowledge of the day, a reasonably competent practitioner. The GP of the 1930s was only too aware of the deficiencies in his technical knowledge; indeed, it was no longer possible to be a competent *general* practitioner. Most GPs undertook midwifery as part of their normal practice but, as the development of postgraduate diplomas indicated only too plainly, certain other aspects of medicine required more skill than were expected of the ordinary GP, or fell outside the duties expected of him. Thus the GP who anesthetized patients for a visiting consultant became a "part-time anesthetist," and the GP who read the X rays, a "part-time radiologist."

Each year the gap between the technical specialist and the ordinary GP grew wider. As it did, the problems of availability and quality of technical care in the many small hospitals became more pressing. Regional hospital planning, by linking and focusing specialist services over a relatively wide area, appeared to doctors and planners alike the obvious eventual solution. "Our hospital system is radically wrong," the president of the Bristol and Bath branch of the BMA had said as early as 1927. "It is wrong because it consists of isolated units without public control." [34] Out of this growing conviction emerged the present regionalized hospital service, established under the National Health Service in 1948.

Perhaps the most significant trend of all in the 1920s and 1930s was the growing commitment of the medical profession to consideration of these issues. This applied not only to the BMA, which was already involved in government negotiations through the National Health Insurance system, but also to the Royal Colleges, which had retained the consultants' primary allegiance. A joint committee of the Royal College of Physicians and Royal College of Surgeons had been formed as early as 1933 to "consider matters of common concern." [35] Three years later an advisory committee was constituted by the Minister of Health, of which the presidents of the two Colleges were members, to maintain contact between the Ministry and the profession as a whole. In the words of Lord Dawson, Chairman of the Dawson Committee and then President of the Royal College of Physicians, by 1938 this latter committee was "taking root and doing good service and training us all to pull together." Increasing specialization thus brought the consultants into the sphere of national policy and planning, even though they were excluded from National Health Insurance.

The opportunity for participating in the coming changes was seized readily. In reply to the question on what the Colleges would do, Lord Dawson had one answer:

34. *Brit. Med. J. ii* (1927), 133 (E.W.H. Groves).
35. Royal College of Physicians of London "Annual Address Delivered to the Royal College of Physicians of London by the President," Viscount Dawson of Penn (Royal College of Physicians, 1933).

Surely they had to seek the co-operation and secure the unity of the scattered forces within the profession with the Colleges leading the way. . . . What is the alternative? Why, the effacement of the Colleges and medicine drifting into the control of bureaucratic government and a lifeless formalism.[36]

This acceptance of leadership was to serve consultants well in the coming negotiations for a National Health Service.

36. Ibid.; and "Annual Address," 1938.

II

Specialism, Generalism, and the National Health Service Act

5

The Design
of a National Health Service

The approach of World War II in 1939 dramatically emphasized the weakness of existing medical facilities and the need for reform, particularly in relation to national and regional planning of hospital and specialist services. Heavy civilian casualties from air raids were expected in the first months of hostilities, and both beds and medical staff would be needed. The existing rapport between the Ministry of Health and the Royal Colleges facilitated such arrangements. The presidents of the Colleges urged doctors to accept the terms of the new Emergency Medical Service (EMS) in 1939,[1] and leading members of the Colleges were influential in ensuring its overall administration and success. From these wartime arrangements of medical services, and from a number of reports issued during the war and immediately after, came a new National Health Service—catalyzed by the disruption of the war years but built on ideas that had crystallized in the 1930s.

Consultants and the Emergency Medical Service

For the first time consultants became actively engaged in national medical policy. Leading consultants advised on the development of a regional blood transfusion service and a national pathology service.[2] Regional hospital officers were appointed to plan, coordinate, and organize services over a geographical area, with the county and county–borough medical officers of health acting as their agents for casualty services in their areas. In London, which became the focus of ten sectors radiating from one or more of the London teaching hospitals, administration was by the Ministry of Health,

1. In a letter written to the *British Medical Journal,* Suppl. *ii* (1939), 231.
2. Sir Philip Panton, a pathologist at the Ministry of Health during the war, reported: "I went to see the Director and pointed out to him that . . . we had made no provision for blood transfusion in the event of air raids on the big provincial cities. I was told to . . . make out a scheme, provided it did not cost appreciably more than £90,000 a year. I made out a scheme for him there and then. . . . I learned that the medical man is in an immensely strong position when advising the administrative side on a vital matter affecting public health and safety, and the corollary that one must be very sure of being right before advising." Panton, *Leaves from a Doctor's Life* (London, 1951), p. 194.

but representatives of the teaching hospitals were appointed officers of the sectors. Outside London, hospital officers were appointed from the voluntary and municipal hospitals. Some of these officers were laymen, but many were distinguished consultants and specialists. For the first time, in many cases, medical staff from the teaching hospitals were assigned under the EMS to public-assistance institutions. At Billericay, for example, according to the biographer of the London Hospital, "Hermon Taylor started prostatectomies on a large scale and got many elderly men back to their homes. At Orsett, William Evans found patients dying of pernicious anaemia who had never been treated with liver extract." [3] The potential of a regional organization as a means of redistributing staff and upgrading facilities was, although in a very limited sphere, at last being realized.

The idea of wide regional planning and of focusing particular services in special centers, instead of dispersing them among different hospitals, was an early and logical outcome of national responsibility for medical services; specialized centers were established at strategic points for particular types of war injury. By the middle of 1940, plans were being executed for centers for orthopedic and fracture surgery, chest and head injuries, plastic and jaw surgery, burns, and neurosis and effort-syndrome centers. Regional consultants and specialists were appointed to inspect and report on the work of these centers. In addition, regional and (later) group advisers in general medicine and surgery were appointed to tour the emergency hospitals to monitor standards and procedures; their duties were to see that patients were transferred to hospitals with special facilities, that consultants were called in, that patients needing special treatment were not unduly detained in the receiving hospitals, and that convalescent homes and rehabilitation hospitals were fully used. These consultants had executive authority in the EMS structure to direct patients to hospitals where the best treatment was available. Contractual arrangements were made with individual authorities for the use of certain of their beds for the emergency service, but the government pledged that there would be "no interference by the Department in the internal administration of any hospital, voluntary or municipal." [4] The basic division between voluntary and municipal hospitals thus remained. But, in addition, hospitals were built directly for the Emergency Service.

It was initially proposed that there be a corps of EMS doctors, from house officer to consultant, who would reinforce the full-time salaried staff of municipal hospitals and would serve in voluntary hospitals on a full-time salary for the duration of the war. They would not be allowed a private practice. The salary offered (£800 to £950) was a pittance in comparison with the prewar incomes of reasonably successful practitioners, but many

3. A. E. Clark-Kennedy, *The London—A Study in the Voluntary Hospital System. Volume Two 1840–1948* (London, 1963), p. 244. Information on the Emergency Medical Service in this chapter is largely derived from R. M. Titmuss, *Problems of Social Policy*, p. 76 and passim.

4. Quoted by Abel-Smith, *The Hospitals*, p. 426.

specialists willingly moved out of London to work in EMS units, thus "sacrificing incomes much greater than those they now received while still bearing the cost of expensive consulting rooms, town flats or houses, and often enormous life insurance premiums." [5] When the expected massive air raids did not immediately materialize, it seemed to many such consultants that their sacrifice had been in vain. Their private practices were evaporating in their absence and they were underemployed in their new locations.

Thus, almost immediately and chiefly to safeguard private practice, both the BMA and the Royal Colleges urged the Ministry to change the EMS regulations. A new advisory committee, chaired by the president of the Royal College of Physicians, was established. It drew up substantial amendments to the Emergency Service, which the Ministry agreed to accept in November 1939—before the war had been in progress for three months. Doctors of consultant or specialist rank were released from whole-time duty to return to private practice, but they also retained a government salary for standby emergency duties (£500 per year), and beds were returned to general use in the London teaching hospitals. The House of Commons Select Committee on National Expenditure later described these terms as "neither in the interests of the country nor in accord with the dignity of the profession." [6] But they shed light on the strength of the medical profession in influencing national policy, and they introduced the Royal Colleges, together with the BMA, to negotiations with the government over conditions of service.[7]

The Emergency Medical Service treated not only wartime civilian casualties but also the armed forces. The Ministry of Health took responsibility under the EMS for the treatment of all wounded arriving from the "Second Front" in 1944. By April 1945, a reserve of 99,000 hospital beds was available to the Emergency Service, representing about a third of all nonmental hospital beds in the country.[8] Although the service at no time covered more than a small proportion of the civilian population, it had an immediate effect on the attitude of the medical profession toward the desirability of reorganizing hospital services, and thus ultimately on the long-term organization of medical care in Britain. The Ministry of Health had assumed, for a section of the hospital services in both voluntary and municipal institutions,

---

5. *Lancet ii* (1939), 947, quoted by Titmuss, p. 197.

6. Quoted by Titmuss, p. 199.

7. On the amendments to the EMS, the president of the Royal College of Physicians observed: "it may fairly be claimed that the Royal Colleges have not been backward in asserting their rightful positions as advisers of the Government in these matters and that it is untrue to say—as I have heard it said—that they have 'abrogated in favour of the British Medical Association.' " Sir Robert Hutchison in his annual presidential address to the Royal College of Physicians, March 18, 1940.

8. At the end of 1948 there were approximately 311,000 beds in teaching hospitals and nonteaching general and special hospitals. It is assumed that the overall number of beds did not vary significantly between 1945 and 1948. See Ministry circular RHB (48) No. 1, and Ministry of Health *Annual Report for 1945*, Cmd. 6710, p. 40.

a national responsibility that was centrally directed, regionally organized, and locally administered. Consultants had accepted payment for their duties in voluntary hospitals; national pathological and public health laboratories had been set up and a national blood transfusion service introduced; the idea of regionally grouped hospitals with specialist centers was accepted; new ancillary services were introduced into hospitals; and hospital standards were raised.[9] Some of the ideals of the 1930s were thus being put into practice under wartime conditions to meet wartime needs.

Plans for Postwar Medical Reform

Both the medical profession and the government continued to agree, in the early years of war, on the need for reform of civilian health services. In 1940 the British Medical Association, in cooperation with the Royal Colleges and the Scottish Medical Corporations, set up the Medical Planning Commission to review the status and future of health services. The report, published in 1942, described once more the sense of isolation of the general practitioner, the rift between the general practitioner and both voluntary and municipal hospital authorities, the need for a unified health plan, and the advantage of cooperative general practice based on health centers. The Planning Commission set out unequivocal aims:

a. To provide a system of medical service directed towards the achievement of positive health, the prevention of disease, and the relief of sickness.

b. To render available to every individual all necessary medical services, both general and specialist, and both domiciliary and institutional.[10]

The various plans and counterproposals for a unified health service during the course of the war indicated a remarkable unanimity in basic philosophy. Apart from debate whether the service should cover the lower 90 per cent of the population (favored by the BMA) or the whole population, discussion centered around the means and not the end.[11] Some kind of national health service seemed inevitable long before the Coalition Government issued the intimation of new legislation in its White Paper of 1944.

Given the existing facilities and tradition there seemed to be two main choices. The National Health Insurance scheme could be extended to include comprehensive medical services, as was suggested by the BMA and others to the Royal Commission of 1926. Alternatively, the existing deficiencies could be met in some other way—for example, through government contracts with hospitals and specialists—or (as was eventually to happen)

9. See Titmuss, pp. 466–84.

10. "Medical Planning Commission, Draft Interim Report," *Brit. Med. J. i* (1942), 743.

11. See A. J. Willcocks, "A Process of Erosion?" *Sociological Review Monograph No. 5* (Keele, 1962).

through nationalization of hospitals and direct employment of specialists. The 1944 White Paper included measures for the abolition of health insurance and for the establishment of a system of government contracts of service with medical practitioners and hospitals.[12] General practitioners, hospitals, and local health services would come under the Ministry of Health. Regional or area planning would be effected by a joint authority, from one or more local governments, which would coordinate the work of voluntary and municipal hospitals and plan comprehensive health services for the whole area. Following the BMA's own recommendations, general practice would be focused partly on health centers in which groups of practitioners would work (possibly remunerated by salary), and partly on individual practice. A central medical board would watch the overall distribution of general practitioners and would be entitled to refuse consent to doctors wishing to engage in public practice in overmanned areas. The consultant's work would include regular and frequent visiting at more than one major hospital, to enable a common consultant staff to be built up as an effective link between hospitals, and he would have both inpatient and outpatient duties. The consultant would also visit general practitioner hospitals, health centers, and clinics. In addition, and this was an important innovation in public medical planning, the consultant would, in case of need, be expected to visit the patient's home at the request of the general practitioner. For these duties the consultant would be remunerated on a whole-time or a part-time basis.

The nub of the White Paper proposals was the joint health authority which, besides having executive responsibility for hospital and specialist services, was to have planning responsibility for all three parts of the service: hospital and specialist, general practitioner, and home care. Voluntary hospitals were to be left as they were, providing the joint health authority with services under contract. Consultants would, however, have a direct relationship with the authority—and this was to prove a major stumbling block. Lord Moran, President of the Royal College of Physicians, while admitting that there were local authorities which were "first rate and most progressive," voiced the consultants' anxieties when he continued: "taking the whole picture of England we know perfectly well that in every discussion in which specialists and consultants have taken part it has been dominated almost entirely by the fear that they will come under local authorities." [13] The concept of the joint planning authority (or area health board), with broad, comprehensive functions, was thereby doomed: not because it was inapplicable but because it was impolitic. The voluntary hospital consultant, however unfairly, was terrified by the vision of himself reduced to the level of the lowest municipal doctor.

As the ideas of this White Paper faded, the concept of hospital regions was taking shape. Regions were now envisaged by the BMA and others as

12. *A National Health Service,* Cmd. 6502 (HMSO, 1944).
13. "Annual Presidential Address" to the Royal College of Physicians of London, April 1946.

"natural hospital areas centred on universities." [14] Since there were relatively few university medical schools, this meant a much larger region than was implied by the joint health authorities suggested in the White Paper. The university-centered region was described in detail in the report of an official committee (the Goodenough report), four months after the White Paper. "The spirit of education," the report stressed, "must permeate the whole service." [15] This was to be done by practical means: all hospitals would be linked directly or indirectly with a medical teaching center. The Goodenough Committee rejected the White Paper's proposal of a common medical staff for teaching and nonteaching hospitals on the grounds that the university teaching staff ought to spend a considerable amount of time with students in the teaching center. Instead, there would be other links in the form of a "series of educational associations with all the major hospitals in a wide area around." These would include associations for the training of house officers in their first year of practice (recommended by the report as a compulsory extra year of training before registration); medical school affiliation for specialists supervising such house officers; the establishment of a joint committee for postgraduate studies, most of which would be undertaken in hospitals outside the medical teaching center; and recognition by the appointment committees in teaching hospitals of medical experience in a nonteaching hospital. Under these proposals the teaching hospital would remain independent of the university; but the teaching center as a whole would be the pivot around which hospitals would revolve. The concept was bold and imaginative, but how well these somewhat tenuous links would work in practice remained to be seen.

The regional idea was carried one final step further in the publication of detailed hospital surveys in 1945 and 1946.[16] The hospital surveys gave substance to new concepts of specialist care within a regional framework. The isolation of specialist hospitals from general hospitals had, in the view of the surveyors—some of whom were consultants—resulted in underdevelopment and neglect of certain ancillary services and aids to diagnosis and treatment. Outside the few teaching hospitals, individual general or special units were not large enough to justify the employment and provision of full specialist facilities. This applied not only to such comparatively rare and expensive specialties as neurosurgery or radiotherapy (which might best be provided in specialized regional units) but to services which had rapidly become essential to the efficiency of a modern general hospital—comprehensive laboratory, X-ray, and other diagnostic services, and continuous coverage of the hospital by fully trained specialists. The obvious solution was provision

14. British Medical Association, *The Doctors and a National Health Service*, undated pamphlet.

15. Ministry of Health, Department of State for Scotland, *Report of the Interdepartmental Committee on Medical Schools* (HMSO, 1944) (Goodenough report), p. 15. The committee consisted of eminent clinicians and teachers.

16. See Nuffield Provincial Hospitals Trust, *The Hospital Surveys*, 1946.

of such facilities on a group basis, through a combined "hospital center" or complex, which would include beds for medicine and surgery, infectious diseases, maternity, tuberculosis, pediatrics, and chronic diseases, all in close proximity. This concept was not controversial. As was remarked at the time, the general hospital center, district, or group would "counteract the centrifugal tendency of the excessive specialism which has lately character-ised medicine in all countries." [17] Thus a two-tier system of hospital organi-zation was envisaged: the hospital district, with a population of 100,000 to 300,000, forming part of a larger region, based on a university town with a medical school, or on a "planning area" within the region.

By 1945, most of the ideas which were to be incorporated in the National Health Service Bill were under general discussion. These included an ex-panded general practitioner service based on health centers; control of the distribution of general practitioners by a central professional committee; university-based hospital regions and multipurpose hospital groups; a paid consultant service based on hospitals; and an implied separation in the administration of the different services. There was still, however, one major question to be resolved; this was the control and administration of hospitals under a new regional plan. As the war drew to its close, the medical pro-fession was anxious to settle future plans. Nearly a fourth of the general practitioners were serving in the armed forces.[18] Continuance of the existing hospital system meant a limitation of posts in both voluntary and municipal hospitals. Returning servicemen found it difficult to get appointments as honorary consultants to voluntary hospitals because the sitting candidates were favored. Individual doctors wanted to know what future they might expect. The BMA had set out its views on several occasions of the desir-ability of an extended organized health plan; GPs had expressed satisfaction with Health Insurance, and never before had the government and the con-sultant branch worked so closely together. The time was thus propitious for change.

The National Health Service Bill

The 1945 election put a Labour Government into power and Aneurin Bevan into the Ministry of Health—a combination that assured the ac-ceptance, first, of a free health service available to the whole population, without an income limit; and second, of nationalization of the hospitals. Bevan introduced his White Paper for a National Health Service in March 1946. Nationalization was perhaps at the time the only viable solution to the hospital reorganization problem. It would have been foolhardy to ask volun-tary hospitals and doctors to work under local authorities, and, although there was a feeling among consultants that they were being persuaded to

17. *Lancet* i (1946), 965; and see Ministry of Health *Annual Report for 1946,* Cmd. 7119 (HMSO, 1947), pp. 63–80.
18. Ministry of Health *Annual Report for 1945,* Cmd. 6710 (HMSO, 1946), p. 56.

allow the voluntary system to die in order to save them from this fate,[19] a number of concessions was made to tempt the powerful teaching hospitals to accept nationalization as an attractive alternative.

The National Health Service Bill arranged for both voluntary and municipal hospitals to be transferred to the Ministry of Health. The endowments of the voluntary hospitals would pass into a new hospital endowment fund, to be set up and supervised by the Ministry. Operation of the hospitals would be entrusted to regional hospital boards, each associated with a university medical school. These boards would be composed of persons appointed by the Minister after consultation with medical and other bodies, and members would be unpaid. Each board would be required to appoint local hospital management committees: "one for each large hospital or related group of hospitals forming a reasonably self-contained hospital service unit." [20] The regional board would undertake, on behalf of the Minister, the general administration and planning of the hospital and specialist services in its region; and the management committees would carry out day-to-day hospital management in the combined hospital groups.

Teaching hospitals—associated with university medical schools—were, however, to be excluded from these arrangements. The great voluntary general and special hospitals would thus escape the fate of being linked on a regional basis with the small hospitals and the municipal institutions. Instead, they were to have direct access to the Ministry of Health. Although the regions were all to be based on a teaching hospital, that hospital was to be excluded from the regional organization, i.e. treated as a region in itself. Teaching hospitals would be nationalized, but each would be administered by a specially constituted board of governors including representatives of the university, the regional board for the area, the local authorities, and, significantly, the senior staff of the hospital. In addition, boards of governors were to retain the endowments of the voluntary teaching hospitals, some of which were very wealthy. Although, as with regional hospitals, they would be generally financed from the government exchequer, these provisions were tempting to the teaching hospitals; moreover, they were exempted from the old idea of a joint local authority. The teaching hospitals were being offered a superior status in the new Health Service and would be able to retain their favored wartime relationship with the Ministry of Health.

Under the National Health Service, consultants and specialists were to be employed by regional hospital boards and boards of governors of the teaching hospitals either on a whole-time or part-time basis, and the part-time specialist would be allowed to continue private practice outside the service. Nor was that all. The Minister was also to be empowered to provide separate accommodations for patients who chose to pay the whole cost and who could be privately treated by part-time specialists within the service. Senior

19. Lord Moran, "Annual Presidential Address" to the Royal College of Physicians of London, April 1946.
20. *National Health Service Bill*, Cmd. 6761 (HMSO, 1946), p. 6.

medical staff would be appointed by the boards to advertised vacancies, according to regulations to be determined by the Minister after consultation with the profession.

Recommendations for the general practitioner services followed the broad lines of the 1944 White Paper. A system of health centers, based on premises technically equipped and staffed at public cost, would be set up for general medical and dental services, for many local health authority clinics, and "sometimes also for out-post clinics of the hospital and specialist services." [21] A national Medical Practices Committee would regulate the succession to old general practices and the opening of new ones. As under National Health Insurance, doctors would be free to practice from their own premises, to join or abstain from the new service, and to continue to see private patients. General practitioners, together with general dental practitioners, would be in contract with a new body, the local executive council (an expanded successor to the existing insurance committee), which would also be responsible for providing a supplementary eye service and for reimbursing those pharmacists who had agreed to supply drugs on a Health Service doctor's prescription. Local government authorities would retain their existing domiciliary services, including midwifery, maternity and child welfare, home nursing and home help, ambulance service, and other preventive and after-care services. Local authorities would also have a duty to provide and to maintain the health centers in which both specialized clinics and general practitioner clinics might be held. But—since their own hospitals would be nationalized—they were to lose all control over hospitals.

Through these separate administrative arrangements for each branch of the service—hospital and specialist, general medical and dental, and local health—the National Health Service Bill created a tripartite organizational structure around traditional patterns of care. The three arms were coordinated only at the Ministry of Health level. In an ideal environment, the whole framework would have been realigned and united, for example, into primary and secondary medical centers, as had been suggested over twenty-five years before in the Dawson report. But, as one writer remarked at the time, "it is understandable that a Minister seeking general acquiescence should avoid or postpone this solution." [22] The Bill, by being built on existing foundations, was realistic, but it naturally contained some of the weaknesses of compromise. By bringing hospitals together under common management and by paying the specialist, thus making him no longer dependent on the general practitioner's good will or referrals for his income, the ties between specialists were to become stronger but those between specialist and general practitioner weaker. The difference in administration of the program for specialists and for general practitioners was to become one of the chief crises of the future service; the division between teaching and nonteaching hospitals was to be another.

21. Ibid., p. 9.
22. *Lancet i* (1946), 422.

In 1946 these problems lay in the future. The honorary unpaid hospital consultant, the medical teacher at the university hospital center, and the ex-serviceman wondering about his future could only be impressed by the conditions outlined for specialist practice. The consultant was to retain opportunities for private office and hospital practice. He was to be employed in a new, and presumably expanded, regional hospital service. The old nepotism for hospital appointment would be lessened, hospitals would receive a necessary infusion of public money, and consultants would be paid for hospital work.

Not surprisingly, consultants were far more receptive to the National Health Service than were general practitioners—they had more to gain and they had more room to maneuver. Specialists were offered a new, state-controlled service, with the principles outlined but with most of the operating details still to be filled in. Their leaders had established a good working partnership with the government in their activities during the war. Consultants had molded the Emergency Medical Service; they had selected London specialists for service in the army; they had created a pathology and blood transfusion service; they had sat on the Goodenough Committee on medical schools on behalf of the government; and they had helped to prepare the hospital surveys. The influence of the presidents of the Royal Colleges in persuading the profession to enter the health service was to be equally profound. Indeed, their actions were to mark a new era in the functions of the Colleges.

The Medical Profession and the Bill

The administrative separation of consultants and general practitioners implicit in the National Health Service Act was underlined in May 1946, before the bill was passed, by the publication of the official report of the Spens Committee on the remuneration of general practitioners.[23] The committee's survey was made against the background of capitation fees paid for patients under National Health Insurance regulations, which remained in force until 1948, and of private practice. The report was noncommittal on the best method of paying the suggested incomes in the new service but seemed to favor the continuation of capitation payment, despite the fact that the system depended solely on the extent of a practice and not at all on its quality or on the experience or age of the practitioner; and although a continuation of the capitation system would further differentiate general practitioners from specialists, who were likely to be paid by salary. Yet at this stage and for long after, the profession seemed well pleased with the system. Through the BMA it gave its "wholehearted support and cooperation" to the Spens report, the general tenor of which had been that general practi-

23. Ministry of Health and Department of Health for Scotland, *Report of the Inter-departmental Committee on Remuneration of General Practitioners*, Cmd. 6810 (HMSO, 1946).

tioners' incomes were too low.[24] The Minister of Health, on the other hand, expressed only qualified approval.

It was at this point that the bogey of salaried medical service was raised. General practitioners, who had regarded the capitation fee system of National Health Insurance as a bulwark against public control of their practice, had a morbid fear of salaried practice. It was now learned that Mr. Bevan hoped to introduce a basic salary (£300 a year) as part of the income of general practitioners, the remainder to be made up of capitation fees and special fees and allowances for certain extra duties. Agreement was shattered. Bevan might see his proposal as a means of helping the practitioner to get started and of assuring all doctors of a basic income, but to the general practitioner, accustomed after thirty-five years of National Health Insurance practice to the principle of capitation, the introduction of a "fixed element" was a move to reduce doctors to the rank of civil servants. They felt, perhaps with some justification, that this was the thin end of a wedge. Consultants did not have the same qualms about salaried service. Some were already under salary as university teachers or as consultants to municipal hospitals. Others, possibly, did not impute a sinister motive to the mechanism of payment for sessions of work done. The part-time paid consultant continued as he had before as an "honorary," but with the added prize of a monthly cheque; emotionally, this was felt to be a fee for consultant duties rather than a part-time salary. Mr. Bevan, later berated for confusing the two terms, was to remark that "members of the medical profession have a terminological sensitiveness which astonishes me." [25] Whatever the semantics, the consultant looked forward to the National Health Service with few qualms—the GP with many.

The imminence of the NHS, with its separate arrangements for each branch of practice, thus had the somewhat remarkable effect not of creating one stalwart profession united against bureaucracy but of reopening the old social division between consultants and general practitioners. Reflecting the increased political authority and interest of the Colleges, the professional negotiating committee set up to deal with the Ministry over the National Health Service included representatives of the Royal Colleges as well as the British Medical Association. Instead of speaking for the whole of the profession, the BMA became further identified with the cause of general practitioners, a source of immediate irritation and of future crisis when the interests of the two groups diverged more seriously. Representing the GPs, the Association held bitter protest meetings against certain provisions in the Bill. Its mood of calm reasonableness evaporated, and it seemed to have forgotten its earlier dicta on the influence of the profession in the National Health Insurance scheme. Meanwhile the Royal Colleges gave impressive and apparently cordial dinners for members of the government. Their aristocratic lineage

24. Quoted in evidence of the BMA to the *Royal Commission on Doctors' and Dentists' Remuneration 1957–1960. Minutes of Evidence,* p. 218.

25. *Lancet i* (1946), 829.

held firm; at times their links with the royal family appeared stronger than those with their brothers in general practice. The Princess Royal visited the Royal College of Surgeons, of which she was an honorary Fellow, to look at their plans for rebuilding, in the month in which the Bill was laid before Parliament, and again later to pay tribute to a survey of anesthesiology before the Bill was enacted. While it was in committee stage and general practitioners' feelings were at their height, the Queen graciously accepted the office of Patron of the Royal College of Obstetricians and Gynaecologists. That same month (June 1946) the Labour Prime Minister, a Hunterian trustee, attended a dinner at the Royal College of Surgeons. Other examples can be enumerated of the interplay of the Royal Colleges with the social "establishment" of England. "The college spirit in medicine," said Eardley Holland, President of the Royal College of Obstetricians and Gynaecologists at a dinner at that college in September 1946, "is precious, is unique, and is peculiarly British, and its flame must never die down." [26] The power of the Colleges, the president emphasized, now depended not on privileges but on cultural and even spiritual qualities; and it was essential that they should achieve unity and harmony. He might have been addressing a group of British subalterns in the outposts of Empire, or the assembled body of an English "public" school. Beside this suave rhetoric, the activities of the BMA appeared rough and naive.

The two senior Colleges held meetings to consider the Bill in May 1946. The president of the Royal College of Surgeons, Sir Alfred Webb-Johnson, agreed that the Bill was "bold and statesmanlike," although many objections were raised by senior fellows. The College promised the Negotiating Committee of the profession its full support in its claims for general practitioners and urged it to press for direct and independent representation of the medical profession on all statutory bodies to be set up to administer the new service. The Surgeons did not agree that state ownership of hospitals was essential to the successful administration of a National Health Service; it viewed "with apprehension" the appropriation of voluntary hospital trust funds, and it was worried about the effect of government monopoly of the hospitals on the specialist's freedom. It was also stressed that fees payable by private patients should be fixed by the medical profession "without interference by outside authorities." [27] But from the Royal Colleges there was no move to veto the Bill or to obstruct it in any way.

The Royal College of Physicians, or at least its leaders, were actively in favor of the Bill. The president, Lord Moran, had himself moved in the House of Lords on April 16 that "This House, while regretting any measures which might impair the efficiency of the general practitioner service, welcome

26. See *Lancet i* (1946), 560; *ii, 35; i, 912; ii, 503.

27. See *Lancet i* (1946), 751; *Brit. Med. J. i* (1946), 855. It is interesting to compare the selective reporting of this meeting by the *Lancet* and the *British Medical Journal*. The *Lancet,* the champion of consultants, was largely in favor of the bill, the *Journal* against it.

proposals for the better coordination of the hospital service of the country." A special meeting of the College in May upheld this view. The College acknowledged "the urgent necessity for reorganisation of the hospital service" and approved the principles of the relevant proposals in the Bill. The Physicians also made no conditions of acceptance; however, they agreed that "much will depend on the regional boards," and they believed it essential to allow hospitals as much independence in administration "as is compatible with the regional plan." [28]

The emergence of the Royal Colleges as leaders of the consultant branch of the medical profession, whereas the BMA spoke primarily for the general practitioner, emphasized the administrative division between the two branches that was built into the National Health Service Bill. Apart from nationalization of the hospitals, however—which was a matter of concern to the hospital boards rather than to the medical profession—there was little that was radical in the actual Bill and much that was familiar. It was, the *Lancet* commented, much less socialistic than was predicted a year earlier.[29] Much of it had resulted from reports originating within the medical profession.

Despite the furore in the BMA, relatively few changes were made in the National Health Service Bill before its enactment in November 1946. Even the Act was, however, only an outline, not a blueprint. It could not be implemented until the proposed machinery was put into effect and until numerous detailed decisions had been made. The real testing period was still to come.

28. *Lancet i* (1946), 632 and 786.
29. *ii* (1946), 719.

6

The Medical Profession
and the Appointed Day

The National Health Service Act provided the framework of a new organization which would come into operation on an "appointed day," which was later disclosed as July 5, 1948. In the meantime, decisive negotiations were to take place between the Ministry of Health and the medical profession. The regulations agreed on in this period, and the concessions obtained, gave substance to the Act. They ensured its final acceptance by medical practitioners and provided new machinery for representing consultant interests.

The Profession Agrees to Negotiate

Immediately after the Act was passed, the medical profession had to decide whether, and how far, it would cooperate with the Ministry in framing the administrative regulations which were necessary before the Act could be put into operation.[1] The BMA decided to conduct a plebiscite among its members to sound out their views. The presidents of the Royal Colleges were already committed in favor of cooperation. At the annual meeting of the Royal College of Surgeons in November 1946, Sir Alfred Webb-Johnson spoke of "important concessions" already made by the Minister as a result of their representations, and at a special meeting of fellows in the same month he added: "I believe considerable concessions may be obtained in the form of regulations."[2] Again, however, the body of surgeons was not so easy to convince. One Fellow urged that the Royal College of Surgeons "shall take no action which is not in accord with the wishes of the main body of the profession"; which, he later elaborated, was meant to assure general practitioners, many of whom were deeply concerned about their future under the new service, "that the surgeons were with them and not against them"—a statement that was greeted with loud applause. The president reminded the assembly that a "considerable majority" of the Council of the College had already voted in favor of negotiation. There were suspicions among both surgeons and physicians that they were being steam-rollered into the health

1. See e.g. *Lancet* leader "Yes or No?" *Lancet ii* (1946), 719.
2. *Brit. Med. J. ii* (1946), 840 and 869–71.

service by their own leaders. Nevertheless, there was comparatively little overt disapproval from consultants; the major complaints were from general practitioners.

The Royal Colleges officially agreed to negotiate independently of the BMA, in January 1947, in a joint letter from the presidents of the three Colleges to the Minister of Health.[3] They pointed out that the form of the service would depend to a great extent upon "what the regulations contained," and that several objections of the profession might be allayed in making the regulations. The letter was conciliatory; the Minister's reply was in the same vein. He assured the Colleges that by entering into negotiation they would not compromise their ultimate stand on whether or not to enter the service, and he assured the profession of further discussion on all the main points at issue. There would be "no interference with the clinical freedom of any doctor—specialist or general practitioner"; specialists would be free to join or not, and to be full-time, part-time, or honorary members of hospital staffs; and consultants would be able to treat patients in private beds in hospitals, "subject to availability." Both letters stressed the need for satisfactory arrangements to be made to encourage specialists to work within the precincts of the hospital.

Already the profession had obtained certain safeguards. As the Parliamentary Secretary to the Minister of Health had said during the parliamentary debates, "no body of public or private employees has ever had the same freedom as the medical profession will have under this Bill." [4] The executive councils would have more medical members on them than had the insurance committees which they would replace; the hospital boards and committees would have medical members on them and would be advised by medical committees; and there would be medical members on the Central Health Services Council (which would advise the Minister) and on the Medical Practices Committee. Moreover, the BMA and other organizations, and the medical press, would still retain their power to influence opinion. "Need we really fear an abashed silence?" questioned the *Lancet*. "Can we not even hope to realise our own kind of service in which neither red tape, nor inefficiency, nor ignorance, nor poverty, nor any other creature, stands between our patient and the best we can give him?" [5]

The profession set up a negotiating committee of thirty-three members, appointed jointly by the BMA (eighteen members), the English and Scottish Royal Colleges (eleven members) and other medical bodies; the proportions indicated their relative importance. The Colleges agreed to negotiate unconditionally. The BMA agreed only if acceptance of the Act was subject to a plebiscite of the profession after this series of discussions was completed, and if the possibility of new legislation was not excluded. With this the

3. Both the letter and the reply were published in *Brit. Med. J.* i (1947), 66–67.
4. See *Hansard*, H. of C. vol. 426 (1946) cols. 392–97. Quoted by Almont Lindsey, *Socialized Medicine in England and Wales* (Chapel Hill, 1962), p. 45.
5. *Lancet* i (1947), 68.

Minister concurred; [6] negotiations began. Neither the general public nor the profession was informed on the progress of the discussions or of their content. In answer to a question in the House of Commons Mr. Bevan stated: "This is essentially a matter for the medical profession in the first instance, and afterwards for the House, if it wishes." [7] But as the months went by, anxiety began to be expressed about what decisions were being made behind drawn curtains. An occasional chink revealed very little except a spirit of resolution. "We have stuck to our principles," reported Dr. Guy Dain to the annual representative meeting of the BMA in 1947; "we have not made concessions or retreated at any point from the position we had taken up." [8] Such remarks did not indicate that the discussions were resulting in acceptable solutions. Would doctors agree to serve in the new health service before the Act was due to be implemented?

During the nine months of discussion between the profession's negotiating team and Ministry officials, the part of the administrative framework that was clearly defined in the National Health Service Act or was subsequently agreed on began to take shape. As early as November 1946 the Ministry of Health sent out to more than two hundred separate bodies its proposals for the boundaries of the new regional hospital areas. These followed the proposals set out in the wartime Goodenough Committee. There were to be fourteen regions in England and Wales, of which four would be based on London; all were centered on university medical schools. The regions varied considerably in size, and populations ranged from 1.5 million to over 4 million.[9] Five of the regional hospital boards were advised to set up subsidiary committees for the more remote areas of their regions; and one of these, Wessex, was to become a fifteenth board in 1959.

By the middle of 1947, members of the regional hospital boards were appointed. Their duties were to review and organize existing resources; to assess the need for new resources; to administer, largely through constituent local hospital management committees, the whole reorganized service; and generally to secure a "proper and sufficient service of all kinds" for all persons in their area.[10] In a large town, it was suggested, a voluntary general hospital, a municipal general hospital, a maternity home, and an isolation hospital might be grouped together, with three or four cottage hospitals in small neighboring towns linked with the central unit and included in the group. Special hospitals were as far as possible grouped with general hospital units, in order to create the equivalent of a single, large, all-purpose general hospital for a district. The regional boards were to guide and control the

6. *Lancet i* (1947), 297; British Medical Association, *The Profession and the National Health Service Act,* Pamphlet, Nov. 1947.

7. *Lancet ii* (1947), 37.

8. *Brit. Med. J. ii* (1947), 178.

9. *Lancet ii* (1946), 804 and *i* (1947), 38. Regional hospital areas were confirmed under Statutory Instrument, 1946, no. 2158.

10. Ministry Circular to Regional Hospital Boards (hereafter RHB) (47), no. 1.

planning of services in their area. Hospital management committees would perform day-to-day administration of the group of hospitals, but they would not be allowed to undertake on their own volition any but minimal building or engineering projects. The board of governors of a group of teaching hospitals, on the other hand, was given power similar to that of a regional hospital board.

The task facing the new boards was immense. The question was not one merely of long-term redistribution of facilities but also of short-term crisis. A recent report had brought out the scarcity of beds for the chronic sick; this problem was to dog the boards in the early years of their existence and, nearly twenty years later, it is still largely unsolved. There was an acute shortage of personnel for nursing services, with many hospitals in dire straits. The distribution of hospital medical staff was out of balance; one survey in Oxford had shown doctor to bed ratios ranging from 1:170 in an old poor-law hospital to 1:10 in a neighboring surgical professorial unit.[11] Finally, the country was faced by an economic crisis, the government was being urged to drop its nationalization programs, and there was a serious possibility that the national situation might damage the development of the whole health service. It was against this background that the new boards, which as yet had no executive authority over the hospitals, took stock of their resources throughout the second half of 1947 and the first half of 1948, consulted with local administrative bodies, and drew up plans that could be put into immediate effect on the day appointed for the Service to begin.

In November 1947, eight months before the appointed day, the curtain between the Negotiating Committee's discussion with the Ministry and the public was finally raised. The auguries were only partly hopeful. While the Ministry had been appointing the new regional hospital boards and executive councils for general medical and dental services, and while these were sketching out the broad lines of the new service, the medical profession had been discussing the same points over and over to the point of deadlock. The profession was not, it was stressed, against a national health service but against certain aspects of this particular Act; and it had become clear that there were some basic differences that could not be settled without high-level decision.

Most of the acute anxiety concerned proposals for general practice, possibly because of the relatively detailed framing of the Act in relation to general practitioners and the vagueness (and therefore the flexibility) still attaching to the proposed condition of the specialist. The two features that had aroused the gravest misgivings were the abolition of the custom of buying and selling the goodwill of general practices, and the proposed establishment, in the Medical Practices Committee, of a machinery of "negative direction" over the movements of general practitioners. The profession also insisted that the remuneration of general practitioners should continue to be

11. *Lancet i* (1947), 105–06; G. E. Gask, *Lancet i* (1947), 336.

by capitation fee and not by salary, and that the right to appeal on disciplinary matters should be allowed from the disciplinary tribunal set up by the Act to the High Court of Justice.[12] Of these, undoubtedly the biggest stumbling block was the question of the sale of practices.

None of these subjects applied to specialists. The sale of their practices was not in question; no machinery was envisaged at this time to redistribute specialists; no statement on their remuneration had been made; and no disciplinary machinery was foreseen. Thus the Negotiating Committee was free on hospital questions to deal with wider issues; it concentrated on private practice. The committee justly claimed that the Act made possible a state monopoly of hospitals. If private nursing homes were also to be incorporated under the Act, the specialist's private patients would occupy beds assigned by the Minister of Health. The committee asked for clarification on this point, adding that "the continuance of independent practice is necessary to the maintenance of a high standard of medical service." It also asked for concessions on certain other aspects of private work and methods of payment. Other points to emerge included strong professional support of the referral system: "There should not be conferred on the patient the right to consult a particular specialist."

Here then, while the general public was eagerly awaiting the National Health Service, was the fruit of months of secret discussion. "Instead of discussing how best the National Health Service can be made to work," said the *Lancet*, "they seem to have spent the past nine months in elaborating the case for its amendment." [13]

The Minister of Health, in a public reply to the profession in December 1947, took a firm line in respect to the general practitioners. He rebutted the idea that the Medical Practices Committee would "direct" doctors; he pointed out that, although goodwill of a general practice would no longer be marketable, partnerships would still be bought and sold; and he refused to allow the profession a final appeal to the courts on questions of discipline, on the ground that it would undermine ultimate ministerial responsibility for the National Health Service.[14]

On the subjects touching hospital and specialist practice, however, he showed himself to be more flexible. The first important statement was that any private nursing home would have "prima facie grounds for exclusion" from the Act. It was also emphasized that all hospitals not required by the service would be "disclaimed," that is, not taken over on the appointed day. Thus specialists would retain accommodations for private patients in hospitals outside the National Health Service; and there would be no control over fee schedules for such patients. Second, the Minister was prepared to accept some of the profession's requests for private beds in public hospitals. Although "reasonable limits" would normally be set on the doctor bills of

12. *Brit. Med. J.* Suppl. *ii* (1947), 141–62; *Lancet ii* (1947), 922.
13. Ibid., p. 913.
14. Published with the original statement.

patients in private beds in NHS hospitals, he was agreeable to allowing a proportion of the available private beds to be used without any prescribed maximum charge. By this move, patients in beds provided at public expense could be liable to no-ceiling medical bills. The action was a deliberate concession to the consultant branch.

Thus the specialists were partly placated, the general practitioners foiled. The *Lancet* reminded the profession that Mr. Bevan had been "consistently conciliatory and reasonable in his pronouncements of the past year." The BMA, which had become more and more the voice of the general practitioner, saw no such indications. "On no single major issue", stated the BMA Council in December 1947, "has the Minister responded to the reasoned arguments of the profession." [15] It was claimed that the Minister of Health had actively wooed the consultant branch of the profession, in order to develop and so trade on the natural rift between the ancient orders: "Those who observed the difference in Mr. Bevan's manner when he addressed himself to the Consultant section of the Negotiating Committee on Dec. 2 and 3 were left in no doubt that he hoped to rule by dividing." [16] A major theme of the new health service was emerging: pre-existing administrative and professional divisions between the historical branches of practice were to be widened, not abolished.

The Last Phase

In January 1948, recommendations were issued on the future development of the regional hospital and specialist services.[17] The regional hospital boards would remunerate specialists in the new service. By making new consultant appointments they would be able to provide extra staff where they were most needed: "Regional planning then becomes possible." The basis of such planning was similar to that emphasized in the Goodenough report; a coordinated system of regional and hospital centers was to be established. Hospital groups would provide all normal specialist services, including as a bare minimum a resident physician, surgeon, obstetrician, and anesthesiologist. Specialty services such as neurosurgery, plastic surgery, and radiotherapy would be provided at regional centers. Except in cottage hospitals, staffed by general practitioners, all patients in hospitals were to be under the direct care of a specialist. The GP would thus not normally be entitled to admit patients to hospitals under his own care. This system was that of the teaching and other large general hospitals where consultants had for long had a monopoly of beds. It was now to be extended to all hospital groups.

The document also set out the suggested policy to be followed by the employing boards in relation to particular specialties. Thus, it was "undesirable that general medicine should be so rigidly sub-divided that all the cardiological or neurological work becomes concentrated in the hands of

15. *Lancet ii* (1947), 914; *i* (1948), 35.
16. *Brit. Med. J. i* (1948), 17.
17. RHB (48), no. 1. *The Development of Specialist Services* (HMSO, 1950), p. 5.

consultants engaged in these subjects"; "The time is hardly ripe for separate genito-urinary work entirely, except perhaps at Regional Centres"; and "Radiology is a separate specialty which should be the sole interest of the practitioner undertaking it." Such policy statements—which emanated from the Ministry of Health's medical department after discussion with consultant bodies—translated prevalent medical opinion into administrative action. Through the kinds of appointments it made, the employing board (regional hospital board or board of governors of a teaching hospital) influenced the subsequent development of specialist practice.[18]

There was, however, still no definition of "consultant" and "specialist" status. The Ministry exhorted the regional boards to ensure that only specialists of a "high degree of competence" be appointed to posts of responsibility, but no interpretation of these terms was provided. Consultant grading was to depend on competitive appointment to a post offered by an employing board. The regional boards, together with the boards of the teaching hospitals, accepted responsibility both for the proportional and geographical distribution of specialists, and—using their own definition of quality—for the minimum standard of consultant practice. Only recently has this method been seriously questioned.

The Ministry circular on specialist planning gave estimates of the number of specialists appropriate to units of population, although it was still not clear how many specialists there were in the country, or how many would enter the service. These planning figures, admittedly tentative, represented an effort by the Ministry to establish yardsticks for future development. However, the estimates (produced by the Ministry itself) proved unattainable, and their failure was to lead to an eclipse of statistically oriented staff planning in England for many years.[19] Furthermore, the specialist estimates failed to take into account any possible developments of general practitioner services, which were excluded from the regional structure. Not only were these not mentioned; they appear not even to have been considered as factors influencing the demand and need for specialist facilities in areas where the existing number of general practitioners was considerably higher or considerably lower than the national average. The two services seemed fated to run in parallel, never in tandem.

18. In 1964, for example, there were only 44 NHS consultants in England and Wales whose appointments were solely in urology, compared with 834 general surgeons; and only 40 cardiologists and 90 neurologists, compared with 777 general physicians. The strong relationship between the Ministry of Health and the Royal Colleges left its mark on all aspects of specialist staffing; it undoubtedly discouraged formal fragmentation into specialties.

19. According to the ratios given there should have been over 1,400 specialist general physicians and geriatricians to the population existing in 1962; only 780 consultants and SHMOs were actually in post. Similarly, the circular's ratios would have produced 235 specialists in physical medicine in 1962; in fact there were only 86. Psychiatry stood almost alone in achieving the desired ratios by 1962. By this time, however, new norms were required, readjusted to changing patterns in medicine.

While the outline of the salaried specialist service was being developed, with few objections from the Royal Colleges, the fear of a salaried GP service reached frenzied proportions. In one of the militant leading articles in the *British Medical Journal* at this time, the Minister was brought to task because he referred at a meeting with the professional Negotiating Committee to the doctors of the new health service as "public servants." [20] A special representative meeting of the BMA resolved in the same month that the National Health Service Act was "so grossly at variance with the essential principles of our profession that it should be rejected absolutely by all practitioners." [21] At the same time the *British Medical Journal* endeavored to stir up activity on the BMA's behalf among the consultant branch. In an editorial, "Consultants and the Act," the *Journal* resurrected the prewar decision of the Royal College presidents to urge entry into the wartime medical service, in which they had assured the profession that it was not the Minister's intention to take over the hospitals. This, in retrospect, was seen to be the thin end of the wedge; it was also an implied criticism of current activities of the presidents of the Colleges.[22] Dr. Charles Hill, Secretary of the BMA, was meanwhile calling for united rejection of the Minister's proposals, primarily because doctors would in his view become whole-time salaried servants of the state and partly because hospitals would become a state monopoly and private practice would be destroyed.[23]

The results of a BMA plebiscite had shown general disapproval of the Act in its current form. The BMA reaffirmed the "whole-hearted desire of the medical profession for a comprehensive health service available to everyone," [24] but it made no move to break the deadlock. Once again, the initiative for compromise came from the Royal College of Physicians. The College suggested an amending act, to prevent a whole-time service from being introduced without further legislation. In almost expected sequence, this was followed by a letter from the president of the Royal College of Surgeons announcing his council's approval of the Physicians' resolution. The president also urged the Minister to modify the proposed method of remuneration of general practitioners in order to "encourage members of the profession to give the service their general support." The president of the Royal College of Obstetricians and Gynaecologists followed suit.[25]

April 7, 1948, saw the climax of this final stage in the drama between the profession and the Minister. On that day the Minister made a conciliatory statement in the House of Commons, following which six BMA delegates met with him to discuss the point at issue. Mr. Bevan agreed to make it statutorily clear that a whole-time service was not his intention, an understanding

20. *ii* (1947), 1037.
21. *Brit. Med. J. i* (1948), 112.
22. Ibid., p. 17.
23. *Lancet i* (1948), 78.
24. Ibid., p. 485.
25. Ibid., pp. 561, 579; *Brit. Med. J. i* (1948), 694.

that was later confirmed in an amendment Act in 1949. He agreed that the basic salary for general practitioners should be optional, except for new practitioners entering the service during their first three years of practice; he assured the profession that every doctor would have complete freedom to publish his views of the service; and he stated that he would set up an expert legal committee to study the effect of partnership agreements among general practitioners.

At the same time, the BMA modified its objections to abolition of the sale of goodwill and to the distribution of GPs through a Medical Practices Committee. In February 1948 it had been hinted in the *Journal* that the right to sell goodwill might no longer be insisted upon if Mr. Bevan gave the profession the alternative of payment by capitation fee only. This the BMA now seemed prepared to ratify.[26] It was now also realized that the National Health Insurance provisions (which were still in effect) would cease to operate on July 5, 1948, *whether or not* the National Health Service Act was brought in on that day, since other forms of social insurance were being implemented at that time. Any delay in introducing the health service could therefore only redound unfavorably on the general practitioner, for he would automatically lose a substantial part of his income. Also, since the implementation of the Health Service Act would reduce the amount of private practice, there would ultimately be less goodwill to sell. The compensation offered to GPs for their goodwill was by no means ungenerous, and the profession's politicians apparently decided it was better to take limited compensation then than see practices lose their commercial value entirely.

The question of the Medical Practices Committee also had an ironic twist. As members of the general public hastened to register with their general practitioners before and after July 5, the uneven distribution of doctors was thrown into prominence. Some doctors found they had very small lists of National Health Service patients. Within the first month of the new service these doctors were rushing to the Medical Practices Committee, asking it to declare their areas "overdoctored" and thus closed to all new applicants. "Negative direction" had begun.

Down to eight weeks before the appointed day, very little was known about the future of consultant practice, and temporary arrangements were made for specialists to work in the Health Service. Regional hospital boards and boards of governors were busy finding out how many medical and dental staff they had; it was planned to undertake detailed reviews in order that long-term contracts might be made before the end of March 1949. Preliminary arrangements were also under way for setting up the new domiciliary specialist service.[27] According to the Ministry of Health, all specialists were to feel they were "members of one team," in whichever hospitals their duties lay. The Ministry suggested there should be opportunities for members of the staffs of hospital centers to do temporary duty in the regional center and

26. *Lancet i* (1948), 251.
27. Ministry of Health Circulars RHB (48), no. 15 and no. 18.

vice versa; that heads of the departments of the teaching hospital and other eminent consultants should visit outlying units; and that professional associations of specialties should be fostered on a regional basis.

One unfortunate result of the compromises made before the Act was, however, the separation of the teaching and nonteaching hospitals: boards of governors of teaching hospitals and regional hospital boards were to be allowed to appoint their specialists independently.[28] Various other factors also made it unlikely that teaching hospitals would endear themselves to nonteaching hospital staff. Teaching hospitals were allowed relatively more private beds than nonteaching hospitals, and to continue to select their cases; they would not be expected to act as district general hospitals with responsibility for accepting cases referred to them. It continued to be more prestigious and lucrative to be attached to a teaching hospital. The old jealousies were not to be removed overnight nor a unified specialist service established.

Who Should Represent the Specialist?

The most important professional question in the few weeks before the Act was implemented was that of an appropriate body to represent the consultant branch in the discussions with the Ministry that remuneration and other urgent matters would require. Apart from the Colleges, consultants as a group were not nationally organized. Those working in municipal hospitals could belong to the Association of Municipal Specialists, but those attached to the voluntary hospitals had no identifiable association. Moreover, the term "specialist" included a wide variety of doctors. It was reasonably easy to recognize a general practitioner—if only by whether or not he did "panel" practice. It was not easy to define a specialist. The medical officer at a mental hospital or tuberculosis sanatorium was more alien to the average teaching hospital consultant than any general practitioner. Specialists were not a homogeneous group.

More than eight of ten consultants were members of the BMA; indeed, their rate of joining was higher than that of general practitioners. The BMA, with its long history of negotiations, would seem the obvious body to represent the specialist in negotiations that would inevitably at times require the numerical strength and political organization that such an association could offer.[29] It already had a local and national structure to represent the GPs, and the BMA Council, in its *Annual Report* published in April 1948, suggested the establishment of a parallel structure for consultants.[30] Regional consultants and specialists committees would be set up, together with an elected Central Consultants and Specialists Committee, closely associated, as was the general practitioners' Negotiating Committee, with the BMA.

28. RHB (48), no. 1, p. 6.

29. The BMA Statistical Department (personal communication) reported 82% of consultants and 78% of general practitioners with National Health Insurance contracts were BMA members in 1947.

30. *Brit. Med. J.* Suppl. *i* (1948), 77

Each regional committee would contain between two and five teaching hospital consultants and between twelve and twenty consultants from hospitals under the regional board, together with five other members. Consultants from the nonteaching hospitals would thus have a clear majority, and the ancient dominance of teaching hospital staff would be destroyed.

But the Royal Colleges were so firmly entrenched in the field of negotiations, and had been so successful, that they were unlikely at this point to withdraw. The BMA's suggestion was not apt to find favor in the eyes of top London and provincial consultants, whom the *Lancet* championed. In its view, the central body proposed by the BMA could have "neither the experience nor the authority" to determine the criteria of the consultant and specialist (which was, by implication, the duty of the Colleges), and it was argued that consultants did not accept wholeheartedly the leadership of the BMA. There seemed to be two other alternatives. One was a joint committee of the Royal Colleges. The second—and this was eventually accepted—was some kind of combined specialist body, containing both Royal College and BMA representatives.

The opposing views were epitomized in the two medical journals, one inclining toward the consultant, the other toward the general practitioner. The *Lancet* came down squarely in favor of the compromise: "Mr. Bevan is offering us plenty of new wine: let us not be afraid to make a new bottle." [31] The *British Medical Journal* stressed the traditional role of the BMA and the inappropriate nature of the Colleges as negotiating bodies. Any new group would "seem to aim at creating antagonism between two important groups of one profession"—a prophecy that was unfortunately to be fulfilled. But the *Lancet*, as champion of the Colleges, was ready with a reply. "For the moment," it said, "it seems as if the BMA's need to represent the specialist is greater than the specialist's need to be represented by the BMA." [32]

Publication of the Spens report on specialist remuneration (June 1948), barely a month before the National Health Service was to be put into effect, emphasized the need for proper negotiating machinery.[33] The Spens recommendations were immediately accepted by the government, but there was no time to make detailed regulations to put them into effect by the appointed day, even if there had been a consultant negotiating body. Specialists entered the new service under their pre-existing arrangements, and the question of professional representation of the specialist was temporarily deferred.

The Spens Committee set out a series of hospital grades, together with recommended salary levels, from house officer up to consultant. There was to be equality of income status among hospitals, whether teaching or nonteaching; but to counteract this leveling tendency, a predominantly profes-

31. *i* (1948), 715.

32. *Brit. Med. J. i* (1948), 985, 1189; *Lancet i* (1948), 991.

33. Ministry of Health and Department of Health for Scotland. *Report of the Interdepartmental Committee on the Remuneration of Consultants and Specialists,* Cmd. 7420 (HMSO, 1948).

sional committee was to be set up to award substantial extra sums to specialists for particular merit or distinction. The immediate reaction of the profession to the Spens Committee pay scales was overall approval, with some reservations, and the distinction award concept had a mixed reception. The *Lancet* called the sums mentioned "substantial," though not extravagant.[34] Lord Moran, President of the Royal College of Physicians (and a member of the Spens Committee), later described the terms as "so generous that they have been attacked in most quarters outside the medical profession." He added that the Chancellor of the Exchequer "is reported to have spoken of inflation when they were presented to him." [35]

The National Health Service Is Implemented

Some 11,000 specialists and other medical practitioners working in hospitals and some 18,000 general medical practitioners entered the National Health Service on July 5, 1948.[36] National Health Insurance provisions ceased; National Health Service rules and regulations took over. About 2,800 of the 3,000 voluntary and local authority hospitals in England and Wales—general, mental, and special, with their associated clinics and departments and all their staff—were officially transferred to the Minister of Health, but, in accordance with the Minister's statement to the Negotiating Committee, about 1,500 nursing homes were left under private management.[37] Apart from a few thousand patients in private beds, patients in the nationalized hospitals overnight became freed from financial responsibility. The fourteen regional hospital boards in England and Wales now had 388 constituent hospital management committees, and there were thirty-six boards of governors of teaching hospital groups independent of the regional hospital boards.

To the general practitioner July 5 came and went with little fuss. Patients had been signing up for some weeks beforehand. In many respects the new service represented little more than the extension of previous "panel" practice to a much greater proportion of the GP's patients. No health centers sprang up overnight. On the contrary, health centers showed signs of disappearing over the horizon, for the Minister of Health, concerned about the more vital need for new housing, had warned local authorities that no general construction of centers should be undertaken. In the following years some experimental centers were set up, but the mood for health centers passed. One early plan for an experimental center in Birmingham was obstructed by a dispute between the local general practitioners and the Minister

34. *i* (1948), 911.

35. Annual presidential address to the Royal College of Physicians of London on Monday, April 11, 1949.

36. The hospital figure is an estimate from BMA data, the GP figure an estimate from the Ministry of Health. Exact figures are not available.

37. Acton Society Trust, *Hospitals and the State, Background and Blueprint* (1955), pp. 17–18.

on whether private patients might be treated at such centers.[38] The enthusiasm for health center practice that had distinguished reports in the 1920s and 1930s was replaced by doubt of their necessity. By the time the Guillebaud Committee reported in 1956, the majority of witnesses were still taking the line that "health centers must for some time remain in the experimental phase," [39] a situation that has continued to the present day.

July 5 came and went with the biggest problem still to come: namely, the relationship between the two branches of the medical profession. The National Health Service Act had set up administrative divisions between them. During the course of the negotiations the case for general practitioners had been considered separately from that of consultant and specialist staff. The 1948 plan for development of consultant services had not even touched on the relationship of the specialist services with general practice. The conflict between the BMA and the Royal Colleges had widened the gap between the two branches of the profession; and the publication of the Spens report forced it farther apart. General practitioners entered the service on terms completely different from those of specialists. Their method of payment was different—by capitation fee instead of by salary. In addition, the question of differential payment between general and specialist practice, which had not arisen when the two branches were not members of the same service, was thrown into prominence. An earlier *Lancet* editorial had suggested that the established consultant in the new service be assured of a rather larger income than that of the general practitioner, although the scales should overlap and there should be exceptional openings for doctors in each category.[40] The two Spens reports, while not overtly considering the relationship of general and consultant practice, created a clear-cut financial advantage in specializing. General practice was already in the doldrums; the decision was not likely to improve the quality of new entrants, especially as the lower grades of hospital staff, from whom consultants were in the future exclusively to be chosen, were now to be paid a reasonable salary.

The BMA continued with its own arrangements for establishing regional consultants and specialists committees, "to protect specialists' interests." Each of these appointed two representatives to a Central Consultants and Specialists Committee, where they were joined by other specialist members; the total committee was an autonomous body, but within the BMA framework. Thus the BMA had created two autonomous structures—one for general practitioners and one for hospital staffs—from local to national level. These existed side by side with the combined core organization of local divisions and branches, whose representatives formed the BMA's national representative body.

As surmised, specialists themselves were not in complete approval of

38. *Lancet i* (1948), 523; *ii*, 419.
39. *Report of the Committee of Enquiry into the Cost of the National Health Service,* Cmd, 9663 (HMSO, 1956), p. 207.
40. *Lancet i* (1948), 293.

democratic regional committees. One consultant wrote that nonteaching consultants had been "well-treated" financially, but stressed that "this does not make them equal in other ways." [41] Signs of conflict between the staff of the two types of hospital were appearing. By the end of July 1948 a compromise seemed possible. Representatives of the Royal Colleges, the Scottish Corporations, and the BMA met at the Royal College of Surgeons to discuss the whole question of representation. The group agreed to suggest to their constituent bodies proposals for a joint committee of the Colleges and Corporations and the BMA. By November the composition of the new Joint Consultants Committee was established. It was to consist of three members each from the Royal College of Physicians and the Royal College of Surgeons, two from the Royal College of Obstetricians and Gynaecologists, one from each of the three Scottish Corporations, and six from the Consultants and Specialists Committee of the BMA.[42]

The Colleges had gained the advantage. Since 1942, as the BMA rightly complained, they had "been inevitably drawn into the more controversial field of medical politics." They were now firmly entrenched. The Joint Committee was "to speak for consultants with one voice," [43] and to negotiate with the Ministry of Health and the Department of Health for Scotland in all matters concerning hospital and specialist practice, save those directly concerning terms and conditions of service. At the same time—and the cause of future crisis—the BMA, whose structure was by now irrevocably confused by the simultaneous existence of sectional and integrated representative machinery, lost its right to speak with equal authority for all categories of doctor.

The medical profession as a whole emerged as a strong force from the negotiations surrounding the Act—especially the barely organized specialist branch. "As a profession," one medical member of a regional board claimed in July 1948, "we are in a more powerful position than ever before." [44] At the center the Minister was advised by the Central Health Services Council, a predominantly medical body. At each layer of administration there was substantial medical representation. The profession had taken a part in the framing of important regulations and had gained some notable concessions —for example, the retention of private practice and the right of part-time service. General practitioners had control over their overall distribution through the Medical Practices Committee; and they had won the right for executive councils to elect their own chairmen. The consultant branch had established a Joint Consultants Committee to negotiate on important policy questions; and, through a distinction awards scheme, a professional committee would allocate large sums of public money to consultants of their choice. The Spens Committee had come out in favor of substantial salaries

41. Ibid., *ii,* 118 (W. A. Bourne).
42. Ibid., p. 239; *Brit. Med. J.* Suppl. *ii* (1948), 173.
43. *Brit. Med. J. ii* (1948), 343; *Lancet ii* (1948), 994.
44. Ibid., p. 26.

for hospital staff. In addition, preliminary regulations on the appointment of specialists, made in June 1948, emphasized appointments committees manned predominantly by professionals, with at least five medical members out of a committee of seven. The review committees set up in November 1948, to enable hospital boards to assess and grade hospital staffs, were entirely specialist bodies.[45] Representatives of the medical profession were acting at all levels as agents of, and advisers to, the public administrative structure.

So far the National Health Service had not inhibited professional freedom; on the contrary, the leaders of the profession had more control over the future of doctors than ever before.

45. Statutory Instrument, 1948, no. 1416, and Ministry of Health Circulars RHB (48), no. 30 and no. 83.

7

The Two Branches:
Postwar Realignments 1948–1950

The structure of the National Health Service showed a clear division between the administration of hospital and specialist services and the general practitioner services. General practitioners had already been organized under a different system from consultants since 1912, when the National Health Insurance scheme came into effect. The real problems of relationships under the new service—although they were emphasized by the NHS structure—were those of professional readjustment. Because of the strains imposed on the old patterns by the demands of specialized medical technology, new definitions and alignments needed to be made: on the content and future of general practice, on the role of the hospital, and on the recognition and limitations of consultant status and specialist skill.

The major effects of specialization were bound to affect the position of the general practitioner, no matter in what social structure or payment system he found himself. The number of specialists was increasing, and the number of hospital junior staff was increasing even faster. The specialist needed to spend more of his time in hospital, less in his office in the community. The main advances in medical science were being made in the teaching hospital centers, not in general practice. Hospital care was becoming more expensive year by year as specialized staff and equipment costs expanded faster than overall price and salary levels. Society itself had become specialist conscious, not only in medicine but in all fields of endeavor. All these results, singly and severally, tended to relegate the general practitioner to the back seat.

Before the NHS, the general practitioner had, however, certain relative advantages. The consultant might have spent a period in general practice, and—still practicing on a fee-for-service basis—was dependent on the goodwill of general practitioners for the referral of private patients; thus it was to his advantage to cultivate good relationships with local practitioners. The income of the general practitioner, although in some cases substantially less than that of the consultant, was considerably better than before National Health Insurance. The financial as well as the social gulf between the two branches had shrunk. Finally, because of the insurance scheme, general practitioners were politically organized, whereas consultants were not. Under the combined impact of increasing specialization, World War II, and the National Health Service Act, many of these advantages were reversed.

The most important single factor was the organization of hospitals and its corollary, the organization of consultants. Almost overnight, consultants were welded from a scattered body with primarily local interests into one group, which was regionally organized and had a national income structure; consultants were able to negotiate with government and to influence national hospital policy. This emergence of the consultant as an administrative and policy-making participant in a national hospital service was to leave an indelible mark on intraprofessional relationships. Consultants were rapidly developing as a cohesive group whose interests were not the same as those of general practitioners.

The Structure of Hospital and Specialist Practice

The grouping and regionalizing of hospitals was intended to annul the detrimental effect of a large number of small, scattered hospital units. The hospital group would function as one large hospital, with a common senior medical staff. Two popular features of each hospital system, voluntary and municipal, were combined: the remuneration of consultants and specialists was to follow the local government pattern, through salaried payments on a sessional basis, but the hospital staffing structure was to follow that of the larger voluntary hospitals. Now all consultants would be in charge of blocks of beds and be assisted by grades of medical staff who were themselves aspirants, through a series of training posts of increased responsibility, to full consultant status. This structure would apply to ex-voluntary and ex-municipal hospitals alike, and to mental, special, and general hospitals.

One of the first tasks of the National Health Service was to survey and assess the position of each member of the medical profession so that each could be incorporated into an appropriate grade. The vital problem here was to grade practitioners in relation to their work in hospitals. Through the new hospital structure, general practitioners could be encouraged or discouraged from undertaking hospital specialist practice. If the number of consultants were limited, and they were given exclusive control of hospital beds (as the Ministry had already indicated was its policy) a high standard of hospital practice might be maintained. On the other hand, if general practitioners were excluded from general hospitals, and thus implicitly from specialist practice, the gap between the two branches would be deliberately restated; acute problems of communication and coordination might result between hospital consultants and GPs who were not attached to hospitals.

The staffing structure set out in the Spens report specified grades of limited tenure and of progressive experience up to the rank of full consultant— senior house officer, junior registrar, and senior registrar.[1] There was no place in this outline for the part-time general practitioner specialist who had

1. Spens Report on Consultants and Specialists, pp. 8–9.

been a common feature of small-town hospitals and the mainstay of rural specialist practice. The first count of specialist staff above the grade of registrar revealed only two thousand specialists employed full time in hospitals in England and Wales in 1948; there were nearly eight times that number of part-time hospital appointments.[2] Specialists attached to teaching and to other large general hospitals were often clearly of consultant status. But there remained several thousand self-styled specialists who might not fit into the Spens definitions. They could not suddenly be jettisoned; indeed, the hospital surveys had described acute shortages of specialists in the very areas in which many were practicing. Some would be eligible for consultant status, but by no means all; and it was not in the interests either of the government or of the leaders of the consultant branch to encourage their mass inclusion into the service at the highest level.

In the course of discussions of the medical profession with the Ministry of Health and the Scottish Health Department in 1948, it was decided that there should be a second specialist grade below the consultant. This grade would accommodate a number of established and experienced specialists "who were not trainees but who had not the training and standing necessary to justify grading them as consultants."[3] These were seen to fall into two groups: local government medical officers, who were largely wholetime employees (e.g. tuberculosis officers), and general practitioners who held posts of some seniority in the hospitals in their districts, with titles such as physician or surgeon, but were not considered to be of consultant quality as measured against teaching hospital staff. The second grade would enable consultant status to be maintained, yet many of those who had felt entitled to call themselves "consultants" by virtue of hospital appointments could be assigned to the junior specialist grade.

The new grade was announced by the Ministry of Health soon after the Spens report was published. Specialists in the new grade were to be termed Senior Hospital Medical Officers (SHMO), and to be of a somewhat lower level than full consultants; SHMOs would, like consultants, have charge of beds and have unrestricted tenure, but their basic salary would be less[4] and they would not be eligible for additional distinction awards. In the absence of recognized criteria for specialists, however, no concrete definition could be fixed on exactly what the difference in level or function would be—a difficulty that was to provoke enormous problems of relative responsibility and status. In 1948, however, the need for a second specialist grade was expected to be temporary. It was widely thought that the general practitioner-

2. There were 1,756 full-time and 13,210 part-time senior staff appointments at nonteaching hospitals; and 313 and 2,367 respectively at university-connected teaching hospitals. But an individual could hold more than one part-time appointment. *Report of the Ministry of Health for the Year Ended 31st March 1949,* Cmd. 7910 (HMSO, 1950), pp. 356–57.

3. *Royal Commission on Doctors' and Dentists' Remuneration* (hereafter *Royal Commission); Minutes of Evidence,* pp. 710–11.

4. £1,300 to £1,750, compared with the consultants' £1,500 to £2,500.

specialist would fall into the SHMO category.[5] As GP specialists retired, their place would be taken by full-fledged consultants: thus the number of SHMOs would decline and eventually disappear.

The agreed staffing structure made it quite clear that specialist status would be contingent on a salaried hospital post, either as a consultant or, at a somewhat lesser level, as a SHMO. There would be no place in the National Health Service for the self-styled specialist—no matter what his ability or training. It would still be possible for the general practitioner to have a part-time hospital appointment as a specialist, in hospital grades of registrar status and above. But, with the decline of private practice under the NHS, it would no longer be possible for him to establish his standing by creating a private specialist practice in the community. The granting of specialist status was to follow the system long held in voluntary and municipal hospitals; it was to be the prerogative not of the specialty associations but of the hospital boards.

The Ministry of Health made no claim to define either consultant or specialist status. Indeed, the official position was that "No general criterion of specialist status can be laid down." Definitions were left to leading consultants in special regional review committees set up for this purpose at the end of 1948. These consisted of two physicians, two surgeons, and one obstetrician-gynecologist from the regional hospital board area, together with two specialists from the branch under review, of whom one was nominated by the regional university. The committees contained no laymen and no general practitioners. They had two major functions: first, to decide how many specialists were required to staff the hospitals for which the board was responsible, and second, to assess existing specialists.[6] In many cases the status of the individual was clear-cut. In borderline cases decisions could be reached only after consideration by the review committee, according to the standards they themselves considered appropriate. Since consultant and SHMO appointments were to be linked with a number of beds and clinics, they would be of limited number and attainable only through a competitive process. Thus, ultimately, consultant or specialist (SHMO) status rested on a personal grading system. This system had long been used by the major voluntary hospitals. The difference was that now the method was universally applied and regionally controlled.

The overriding philosophy of what was and what was not consultant status was soon made clear; the GP specialist was not to be regarded as a consultant. Appeals were allowed from individuals who felt they had been unfairly graded by the committees, but their appeals were heard by the same review committee, this time augmented by two additional consultants, one appointed by the appropriate Royal College and one from another hospital region. The same criteria that had applied in the original decision were used in the appeal. As a result of the review, some 5,300 doctors were graded as

5. *Lancet i* (1949), 963.
6. Ministry of Health Circular RHB (48), no. 83.

consultants in 1949, and another 2,000 were graded as senior hospital medical officers. Many general practitioners who had been doing specialist work were replaced by fully trained specialists; others gave up their general practice and became full-time specialists. Very few men still engaged in general practice were designated as consultants; and even in the new SHMO group, expected by many to be the haven of general practice, only a minority continued as GP specialists. Instead, the SHMO grade was largely used for those who were full-time specialists but of lesser caliber than was agreed befitted consultant status—for example, municipal doctors employed before 1948, many of whom had been working in such special fields as infectious disease and mental illness.[7]

Thus the National Health Service set its seal to a policy of a small number of highly trained and experienced consultants, fed (the necessary corollary) by a relatively large number of general practitioners, and assisted by a junior specialist grade. In 1949 the proportion of consultants to GPs was less than one to three. There was little room for the hybrid. As the *Lancet* remarked, while approving the action of the review committees, there were "unpleasant consequences" for those who did not qualify;[8] but there were broader implications in these decisions than personal inconvenience. Long-term effects had to be considered. There was the unpalatable probability, as the Ministry of Health was aware, of an increasing divorce between general practitioners and the hospitals.[9] Although general practitioners were already excluded from access to beds in major general hospitals, and at the same time consultants were already becoming more firmly based on hospitals, these trends were accelerated by the process of review. More definite functional boundaries were set up between the two branches: general practice was based on the office and the home, specialist practice on the hospital.

There was a danger in such geographical limitation of recreating two professions, or at least two demarcated branches of a single profession. Viewed historically, the wheel had come full circle. The inheritors of the teaching hospitals and of the Royal Colleges were once more in control of key hospitals; the general practitioners were once more on the outside. Only now the move had been substantially complete, embracing 90 per cent of all hospitals

7. Many graded as senior hospital medical officer thought they had been unfairly treated, either because of their qualifications or because they suspected the grade was a device to reduce expenditure on specialist services. The BMA championed the SHMO until the grade was closed to new entrants in 1964. But there were other cases where GPs abandoned general practice for appointments as consultants. According to the Central Medical War Committee, there were at the end of World War II only 3,550 recognized part-time "consultants or specialists" in England and Wales, including those in the armed services, out of a grand total of over 45,000 doctors; and the BMA's own figures for 1947 give 4,000 consultants and specialists for Great Britain. The grading would therefore signify a marked *increase* in consultant appointments. (Data kindly supplied by Statistics Branch, BMA.)

8. *i* (1949), 963.

9. *Report of the Ministry of Health for the year ended 31st March 1950*, Part I, Cmd. 8342, p. 17.

in the country, and it had been made in a situation not of private enterprise but of government service.

The Effect of the NHS Structure on the General Practitioner

Both consultant and general practitioner status were arbitrarily defined. The consultant was someone appointed to a hospital consultant post and paid by the hospital board; the GP was someone recognized and paid by the local executive council, a totally different branch of the National Health Service. Doctors were defined by their titles rather than by the actual work they did, and they were separated by the referral system.

The new system guaranteed to raise the general standards of hospital medicine. But it left general practice with problems of its own: the same problems that existed before World War II, but thrown into prominence by the new administrative structure. Because of the referral system, general practice had a function, patients being expected to see their GPs no matter what their problem, and only in special circumstances being referred to consultants. But it did not have a well-defined specialty. The growth of specialties in the previous decade had emphasized unique or expert skills which were brought to bear on a single focus of interest; it was fashionable to be narrow, it was unfashionable to be broad. The GP could claim no exclusive skill. Within the Royal Colleges the new elites of neurosurgeons, plastic surgeons, and thoracic surgeons, or cardiologists and endocrinologists, were forming their own specialized subgroups, their own professional identities, their own sense of being exclusive, esoteric groups. The general practitioner, lacking a scientific label, could not expect to rival them in glamor.

The prewar insecurity of the general practitioner had already been intensified—on both sides of the Atlantic—by the impetus the war gave to the development of specialties. In England it was feared that this tendency would be accelerated by the National Health Service because, "if hospital work were adequately paid, it will be much easier to specialize and so to avoid the 'drudgery of general practice', and to obtain a larger income than can be obtained in family work." There was no financial inducement for the general practitioner to rise above a certain level of mediocrity. On the contrary, it was claimed, the more time and trouble the GP, compensated on a capitation basis, gave to his individual cases, the fewer potential patients could be accepted on his list and the lower his income.[10] The pay scales agreed for the National Health Service clearly favored specialist over general practice. On the average, consultants had always earned more than general practitioners. But the financial advantage, it was feared, would encourage many doctors to enter specialist practice.[11]

Even more significant was the assumption that, given a free choice, the young doctor would prefer to specialize. This argument had been used by the

10. *Brit. Med. J. i* (1948), 809 (W. Edwards). For an analysis of the relative status shifts in medical practice between generalists and specialists, See R. M. Titmuss, *Essays on the Welfare State* (London, 1958), Chap. 10.

11. *Lancet i* (1948), 911.

Spens Committee concerning general practitioners in 1946. Unless the financial expectations in general practice were substantially improved, the committee claimed, the great majority of the abler men would seek to become specialists, "in view of the fact that as specialists they have an equal outlet for their interests in medicine, can more easily keep close contact with hospitals and with medical progress and will have a less arduous life." [12] Young men were reported to be champing at the bit for specialist appointments. "Shall we perhaps," said Sir Lionel Whitby in 1947, voicing the fears of many members of the profession, "like a Gilbertian navy, be all admirals and suffer from a galaxy of specialists with none to do the field work, the work in the home?" [13]

The introduction of better pay conditions for junior hospital staff, coupled with the expectations of a substantial salary if and when consultant status were achieved, gave to the able student an effective choice of careers. In addition, the development of state aid to higher education widened choice of career at the medical student level. Under grants from public monies, the longer training of the medical course was no longer prohibitively more expensive than other university courses; and by 1956, two of three medical students were receiving some kind of government grant or scholarship.[14] Given a choice reasonably free from financial pressure, the GP's motives for entering that branch of practice took on a new light. Lord Moran was to claim, in a now famous statement, that general practitioners were those who fell off the career ladder. He discounted the possibility that general practice might be a vocation: "If a man's vocation was obviously trying to help the community, would he not have more opportunities as a consultant?" [15] By implication, GPs were less able than consultants, a view long held by some consultants but rarely publicly stated.

Thus the general practitioner was attacked simultaneously from a number of points. He was excluded from larger hospitals (but not from cottage hospitals in rural areas). He lacked specialist status. It was assumed that he was of lesser intellectual caliber than the specialist. He had no technological expertise. He had no Royal College. He had no health centers, except for one or two lone experiments. He had fought against salaried service only to see hospital staffs reaping its benefits: holidays with pay, sickness and study leave, distinction awards, free secretarial services, and an advantageous pension plan. To the further chagrin of many, general practice was also ill organized and often inefficient.

The final blow to the GP's dignity fell with the publication of an article by an Australian visitor in 1950.[16] Dr. Collings surveyed three different areas of general practice: industrial, urban-residential, and rural. The report did

12. Spens Report on General Practitioners, p. 5.
13. *Lancet i* (1947), 895.
14. R. K. Kelsall, "Applications for Admission to University," quoted in *Royal Commission; Minutes of Evidence*, p. 767.
15. *Minutes of Evidence*, Questions 1020–22, 1030.
16. Joseph S. Collings, *Lancet i* (1950), 555–85.

not give a heartening picture of general practice. It was worst, Dr. Collings alleged, in close proximity to the large hospitals and the clinical centers, and improved in scope and quality almost in proportion to the distance away from the centers. This meant that general practice was worst where there was the greatest and most urgent demand for good medical service—in areas of dense population. Surgeries and equipment, organization, and staffing of many practices were rated unsatisfactory. In some cases, especially in industrial areas, the working conditions were "so bad as to override the abilities and skills of the individual doctor." Many doctors were isolated from hospital facilities and working in situations which made useless much of their "elaborate and expensive training" and nullified the disciplines taught in the hospital and medical school. Some conditions of general practice were "bad enough to change a good doctor to a bad one within a very short time." Rural practice represented "the last outpost of family doctoring," and in some respects it gained more from medical knowledge and techniques than did urban practice. The overall state of general practice, Dr. Collings felt, was bad and still deteriorating; the National Health Service had caused an increased load to be heaped on the general practitioner and at some points had caused "serious strain or near breakdown."

These comments, which were widely read and were to be long remembered, caused a sensation. Many disputed the evidence adduced for the conclusions. The *British Medical Journal* judged the picture offered as "inexact and unfair." [17] As the *Lancet* noted, Dr. Collings had looked at only fifty-five practices, which statistically was a very small sample, not even selected at random; too much emphasis had been laid on unimportant details like filing cabinets and examining couches, and it was easily arguable that a wrong impression had been gained from a few hours observation under artificial conditions. But it welcomed the report as a major challenge and made a plea for a constructive rather than defensive reaction to it.[18] Whatever its defects as research material, the paper had a salutary effect on general practice by galvanizing GPs to undertake some self-diagnosis; they began to emerge from the lethargy into which general practice had fallen.

It prompted a number of other surveys which did not produce such disparaging conclusions. Lord Taylor's *Good General Practice,* based on observations made in 1951–52 of ninety-four general practitioners in thirty practices, became the most celebrated normative study on the subject. Another inquiry was undertaken by Dr. S. J. Hadfield, then Assistant Secretary of the British Medical Association. This survey, the only one of the three based on random selection of practitioners, produced findings entirely opposite to Dr. Collings'. In addition, the BMA set up a council to conduct a postal survey among 13,000 general practitioners, and the Ministry of Health began to examine the subject through a special committee of the Central Health Services Council.

17. *i* (1950), 709.
18. *i* (1950), 547–49.

Further encouragement was also given to an already existing idea of founding a separate professional institution specially designed for the needs of general practice—a body that would endow the GP with the kind of status given to consultants by the Royal Colleges and would enable general practitioners to reorganize themselves as one professional body. Since the institution of the Conjoint Board in 1884, few general practitioners had taken the basic diploma of the Society of Apothecaries; that society had ceased long since to represent the interests of general practitioners. No comparable body had taken its place. GPs were generally recognized only at the lowest and least influential level of the Royal College hierarchy, through the basic LRCP and MRCS diplomas. The BMA represented the general practitioner in negotiations and in matters of general interest, but it did not impose educational requirements. Moreover, after its great efforts to modify the National Health Service Act, the BMA seemed to have lost its grip. It had not come out of the conflict unsullied. Already there was doubt whether all the noise had really been necessary. "Will posterity regard today's disputants as champions of noble if conflicting causes, or as something rather more closely resembling Tweedledum and Tweedledee?" questioned one far-sighted correspondent in 1948.[19] Sir Robert Platt, sometime president of the Royal College of Physicians, later offered a considered answer: "it seems inconceivable that the same concessions could not have been won by peaceful negotiations as between men of honour." [20]

The BMA was by no means idle, but its effort was directed at general policy reports, rather than specific efforts to raise the GP's status. In 1948 it had published a report on the undergraduate medical curriculum, with recommendations for change; and in the same year a report on health centers was issued.[21] This report laid stress on the central position of the general practitioner as the "only possible co-ordinating center for all that is done for his patient by specialists, nurses and others." The report spoke of the need for intellectual stimulus in general practice, and warned that many doctors were working too much in isolation. It recommended assimilation of general practice with preventive clinic work (run by the local health authorities), the grouping of doctors into family practice units, improved working conditions and ancillary help, the provision of additional general practitioner beds in hospitals, and easy access to hospital diagnostic facilities. And it concluded that the most satisfactory form of practice "at present and in the immediate future" was partnership practice from a common surgery, from which, ultimately, the logical future development would be the provision of specially designed health centers.

19. *Lancet i* (1948), 189.
20. *Doctor and Patient—Ethics, Morale, Government* (Nuffield Provincial Hospitals Trust, 1963), p. 56.
21. *The Training of a Doctor*, Report of the Medical Curriculum Committee of the British Medical Association (London, 1948); *Interim Report by the Council of the Association on Health Centres* (BMA, July 1948).

Two years later (1950) an impressive committee of the BMA, under Professor Sir Henry Cohen, issued a report more specifically concerned with general practice as a career and with the need for continuous education.[22] This committee made a number of concrete recommendations. It proposed a three-year career program for the GP, including one year as a trainee assistant in general practice, a recommendation that was put into action as the present paid-traineeship program by the Ministry of Health before the publication of the report, but was to have only a limited impact on the career structure in general practice. Of greater long-term significance was a recommendation that the GP be enabled to attend hospitals as a "clinical assistant." The stated purpose of the clinical assistantship was to keep the GP in touch with hospital work and with the progress in diagnosis and treatment, in order to develop any special interest he might have in particular aspects of general practice and to maintain contact with the medical staff of hospitals. This too was taken up by the Ministry of Health; it resulted in the part-time hospital grade of clinical assistant, specifically for general practitioners, broadly corresponding to the level of hospital registrar.

The Cohen Committee, as others, endorsed the wide spectrum of general practice. It saw general practice as a special branch of medical practice dealing with the "whole man," and it deprecated the "traditional distinction in status and prestige between general practice on the one hand and any and every specialty on the other." But although it provided an important and practical boost to the long-term development of general practice, it did not offer the immediate incentive many general practitioners felt they should have—nor did it offer professional leadership. Less than a third of the investigating committee were general practitioners; the majority were consultants or university teachers. The report proposed methods of relinking the GP to the expanding hospital service. It did not provide the symbol of regeneration that the GP desperately required. The Royal Colleges had shown their strength as policy makers in the National Health Service; later, GPs were to turn to the College system for their own salvation. Meanwhile the old problems remained, and new ones were established.

The division of the medical profession between consultants and general practitioners had been sharpened by the grading undertaken by the consultant review committees. All NHS hospitals were now assured of salaried specialist staff of recognized consultant caliber (that is, recognized by the review committees and by the appointments committees set up to appoint to new posts), assisted by the second (and presumably temporary) specialist grade of SHMO. General practitioners, employed under local executive councils, were reconfirmed as domiciliary or family doctors whose work was almost entirely apart from the hospital. The most singular aspect of medical practice between 1948 and 1950 was the ready acceptance of this division.

The immediate needs were twofold if, as a number of reports had stated,

22. *General Practice and the Training of the General Practitioner,* The Report of a Committee of the Association (London, 1950).

the GP was in fact to be the cornerstone of medical practice under the National Health Service. First, the status of general practice, which was at a low ebb, had to be raised. Second, to avoid an increasing divergence between the two branches, new means had to be found to link GPs with the reorganized hospital service. The health center program—whereby consultants would visit GP centers—did not offer a solution as a means of communication between the two branches, since few were developed. As hospitals were reorganized and expanded, consultants devoted more of their time to salaried hospital work. The only immediate answer seemed to be the encouragement of schemes such as the clinical assistantship, by which general practitioners might be more firmly attached to individual hospitals.

8

Specialism and the Royal Colleges in the 1940s

The emergence of the Royal Colleges (and particularly the two older ones) as policy-making bodies within the National Health Service obscured but in no way replaced their primary role as educational institutions. Indeed, the war had come at a critical stage in postgraduate educational development, for it interrupted the process of fragmentation of specialties into new professional groups, each with its own status and its own control over specialty standards. The specialist caste system did not only affect the role of the general practitioner; it also had a profound impact on the traditionally generalist cultures of the older Royal Colleges. The Colleges, assailed by the demands of growing specialty groups, had to come to some decision on their future organization both as educational and as representative bodies in the NHS structure.

The Colleges, the University of London, and the Special Hospitals

The Royal College of Obstetricians and Gynaecologists had been founded as a specialist college. The Royal Colleges of Physicians and Surgeons were still primarily generalist; that is, their membership included eminent practitioners in all spheres of medical practice from pathology to cardiology or psychiatry, and in all the surgical specialties, including anesthesiology. But each had only one postgraduate diploma: the MRCP for physicians, the FRCS for surgeons. Each college had now to decide whether it could retain this diploma for the whole spectrum of medicine or surgery, when general medicine and general surgery themselves were declining as fields of practice; and whether, if it did, it could still claim to represent the majority of consultants no matter what their specialty. The first was a question of technical content. The second question concerned the intangibles of specialty status, of influence, and of the numerical balance of rapidly growing specialist fields —matters that would be of increasing importance in the National Health Service where the consultant staffing pattern would change quickly under the program of expansion. Finally, the Colleges needed to reconsider their responsibilities vis à vis the universities, which were now at the hub of a regionalized hospital system.

If consultants remained as a small elite, recognized through appointment to a hospital, there would be less need to define specialist status by examination; on the other hand, there would be greater need to have benchmarks by which training and experience could be assessed by the new appointments committees. In the United States, where there was no comparable consultant branch, sixteen separate specialty boards had been set up by 1940 to certify specialist competence. But in England, it was not clear whether "specialty" referred to an examination (as did, for example, membership in the College of Obstetricians and Gynaecologists), to a personal working bias toward a particular area, or to appointment to a hospital post. Each pertained in part. Now more concrete efforts had to be made to realign specialist training around the special hospitals, the Royal Colleges, or the universities—or some combination of all three.

The 1944 Goodenough report had recommended, on the advice of the Royal Colleges, the development through university affiliation of the postgraduate schools attached to the major London special hospitals, and the concentration of specialist diplomas within the Royal Colleges.[1] University-based hospital regions were established by the National Health Service Act. By this time, following the Goodenough Committee's recommendations, the reorganization of postgraduate medical schools in London was well under way.

The major London special hospitals, such as Moorfields Eye Hospital and the Hospital for Sick Children, Great Ormond Street, had provided postgraduate teaching facilities for many years. But until 1935 there had been no formal postgraduate link with the University of London as there was, for example, between the University and the London undergraduate medical schools. In 1935 the British Postgraduate Medical School had been opened as an independent school of London University; it was attached to the Hammersmith Hospital (which had evolved from an old workhouse infirmary) instead of to one of the existing voluntary hospitals. It was thought at the time that this school might provide a national focal point for postgraduate education; but there was reluctance on the part of the voluntary special hospitals in London to accept any encroachment on their independence as teaching institutions, particularly by an institution with such an unfashionable heritage. Another solution therefore had to be found. The obvious one, which was put into effect ten years later, was the establishment of another body, attached to the University, which would coordinate the work of the Hammersmith school, the school of psychiatry at the Maudsley Hospital (which had been a school of the University of London since 1924), and the major voluntary special hospitals in the city (which encompassed twelve separate specialty groups). Accordingly, following the recommendation of

1. It was recommended that the award of all postgraduate medical diplomas other than those in public health, clinical pathology, bacteriology, and tropical medicine (which would remain with the universities) should be undertaken solely by the Royal Colleges. Goodenough report, 1944, Chap. 19, 20.

the Goodenough Committee and predating the National Health Service Act, the British Postgraduate Medical Federation was established by London University in 1945. The federation received a Royal Charter in 1947 and in the same year became a school of London University.

In July 1948, when the National Health Service came into effect, twelve constituent institutes had been set up within the British Postgraduate Medical Federation; and the establishment of the remaining three was in progress by the end of 1951. The institutes included two general schools—the Postgraduate School of Hammersmith and the Institute of Basic Medical Sciences of the Royal College of Surgeons—and thirteen specialty schools.[2] Their associated hospitals, taken over by the Minister of Health in 1948, were recognized as postgraduate teaching hospitals. Hammersmith Hospital and each of the thirteen specialty hospitals, or group of hospitals in the same specialty, had its own board of governors, directly responsible to the Ministry of Health. They thus had the same relationship to the Ministry as the undergraduate teaching hospitals. These arrangements were peculiar to London; outside London the special hospitals were incorporated with undergraduate teaching hospitals or into nonteaching hospital groups.

The establishment of the British Postgraduate Medical Federation marked an extension of the University's role in providing specialist education, training, and research at the same time that the undergraduate schools were being given a central position in the regional hospital service. But unlike the undergraduate schools, the institutes were not exclusive training facilities. A period attached to one of the institutes would stand the prospective consultant in good stead before an appointments committee, but it was not *necessary* for consultant status. The institutes did not become involved in determining the levels of competence of specific grades in the hospital service. Indeed, as part of the University of London, they were outside the NHS. Nor were they primarily concerned with preparation for university degrees or diplomas; in most cases, there was no appropriate degree to give. Instead, the institutes remained free to mount such courses and training programs as each thought fit. Moreover, the universities were not responsible for the most important basic higher diplomas of medical practice, specifically, the MRCP and the FRCS.

2. The specialist institutes, which became integral departments of the University, are the Institutes of Cancer Research (1951), Cardiology (1954), Child Health (1949), Dental Surgery (1951), Dermatology (1959,) Diseases of the Chest (1955), Laryngology and Otology (1949), Neurology (1950), Obstetrics and Gynaecology (1949), Ophthalmology (1949), Orthopaedics (1951), Psychiatry (1924), Urology (1957). Thus many of the nineteenth-century special hospitals were linked through their schools to London University. St. Peter's Hospital for the Stone, for example, was associated with the Institute of Urology; Moorfields Eye Hospital with the Institute of Ophthalmology; St. John's Hospital for Diseases of the Skin with the Institute of Dermatology; and the National Hospital for Nervous Diseases with the Institute of Neurology. *Handbook for the Session 1962–63,* University of London, British Postgraduate Medical Federation.

The Royal Colleges, on the other hand, although responsible for these diplomas, had no way of enforcing the specialist training of those who held the MRCP or FRCS. Since these were designed as general diplomas, they were taken by candidates perhaps two or three years after registration. The aspiring specialist still had several rungs to climb before he reached consultant status, but the Royal Colleges ceased to have any formal means of controlling standards in this vital training period. The standards of the forty existing specialty diplomas given by the universities and the Conjoint Boards were too low for specialist trainees. Although their standards varied, they were generally lower than those required by the Royal Colleges for the MRCP and FRCS. It was claimed that many of the diplomas encouraged "ill-grounded and immature specialization." At the same time, the benefits of specialist diplomas held by the nonspecialist—the reverse side of the coin —were dubious. Such diplomas, it was feared, would give rise to "misconceptions in the minds of the public or of appointing authorities." [3] They had sufficed for the 1920s and 1930s, but political, professional and scientific changes had made a reworking of the system essential.

There was a general consensus that specialist status should be determined by "some suitable central machinery," [4] and that this should be provided by the Royal Colleges. But there was also support for the continuance of the MRCP and FRCS as *generalist* postgraduate diplomas. The two were not incompatible. Specialist diplomas might, for example, have been developed as subspecialties of the MRCP or FRCS. Alternatively, new colleges or diplomas might have been set up for specialties that did not clearly fall into either general category, such an anesthesiology or psychiatry. A third possibility was for appointments committees to ignore the possession of diplomas and to concentrate on training and experience; and a fourth would be to bring the Colleges together as one institution or academy with oversight of all the specialty branches. Each of these was a possible development in 1948.

The Royal Colleges were thus being pressed for change by a number of external and internal forces: the expanding role of the university, the need to define a specialist and to enforce recommended specialty training, and the delayed demands of groups of specialists for their own examinations inside or outside the College structure. Last but not least were the increased, and increasing, policy-making activities of the Colleges within the National Health Service. "The influence of the College," said Lord Moran of the Royal College of Physicians in 1945, "can be measured by its prestige." [5] This prestige undoubtedly encouraged some specialty groups to seek their solutions within the College framework. As one ophthalmologist had said before the National Health Service Bill was enacted, the members of the specialties felt a desire to "present a united front to the Minister of Health

3. Goodenough report, pp. 231, 233.
4. Ibid., p. 212.
5. Presidential address to the Royal College of Physicians, 1945.

when the time comes." [6] At the same time the assertion of authority by the Colleges led to demands for increased representation of specialty interests in the college organization.

The acceptance by the Colleges of the mantle of spokesman for consultants in National Health Service negotiations implied that they were equally representative of all groups of specialist practice. In fact, they were not. Radiologists had their own independent faculty. Other specialists were not as strongly represented within the Colleges as were the specialties of general medicine and surgery. If the Royal Colleges were to continue as spokesmen for all branches, internal pressures from specialty groups would be likely to increase as their number and their influence expanded. In the immediate postwar years this was particularly true of anesthesiology, dentistry, ophthalmology, and otolaryngology, all traditionally contained within the Royal College of Surgeons. If special arrangements were not made for these groups, there was danger that they would be encouraged to set up new colleges outside its jurisdiction. At the same time there were problems in establishing, as a precedent, new examinations for these groups within the College structure. The Royal College of Physicians was not to feel the similar irresistible pressures from pathology, psychiatry, and pediatrics until the 1960s. It was therefore not surprising that the two Colleges in the immediate postwar period should reach different organizational conclusions.

Development of Faculties within the Royal College of Surgeons

A special meeting was held at the Royal College of Surgeons in May 1944 to consider the co-option of additional members to the College Council. This had as its aim representation on the College Council of certain special branches of practice. The Council was traditionally elected by the whole body of fellows, that is, those who had passed the FRCS examination. It was now proposed to co-opt additional Council members after consultation with certain branches of practice. The Royal College of Surgeons had begun to consider the special plight of anesthesiologists, ophthalmologists, and ear-nose-throat surgeons in 1939. Apart from general medicine and general surgery, and the two specialties that had already formed their own organizations (obstetrics and radiology), these were the largest specialty groupings at that time; the figures are given in Table 1. They might therefore be assumed to feel entitled to special arrangements. The specialty societies invited to suggest names were the Council of British Ophthalmologists, the Association of Otolaryngologists, the Faculty of Radiologists, and the Association of Anaesthetists. Dental surgery was added to the list later, and finally, in May 1946, the Council invited the College of Obstetricians and Gynaecologists to

6. This comment was provoked by the announcement of the formation of an independent Faculty of Ophthalmologists in February 1945. Unlike the Faculty of Radiologists, however, this body set up no examinations and remained a specialist association rather than a complement to the other colleges and faculties. *Brit. Med. J. i* (1945), 311 (C. R. Duncan Leeds).

TABLE 1. *Distribution of Specialists by Specialty; England and Wales, 1938–1964*

	1938–39*		1949		1959		1964	
	No.	%	No.	%	No.	%	No.	%
Total	1,620	100	5,316	100	7,031	100	7,973	100
General surgery and related specialties	375	23.1	1,126	21.2	1,308	18.6	1,400	17.6
Gynecology & obstetrics	137	8.5	370	7.0	439	6.2	485	6.1
Ear-nose-throat	156	9.6	276	5.2	304	4.3	312	3.9
Ophthalmology	244	15.1	295	5.5	299	4.3	306	3.8
Orthopedics	67	4.1	227	4.3	329	4.7	394	4.9
Anesthesiology	76	4.7	459	8.6	791	11.3	906	11.4
General medicine & related specialties	291	18.0	1,217	22.9	1,577	22.4	1,764	22.1
Dermatology	51	3.1	114	2.1	140	2.0	145	1.8
Psychiatry	38	2.3	405	7.6	637	9.1	799	10.0
Pathology	64	4.0	454	8.5	629	8.9	810	10.2
Radiology & radiotherapy	121	7.5	373	7.0	578	8.2	652	8.2

* England, Wales, and Scotland.

The 1938–39 data are drawn from a retrospective study of incomes made by Bradford Hill for the Spens report on consultants and specialists. They do not include all specialists practicing in 1938–39, merely those who were alive and who replied to a questionnaire in 1947. It is not known how far these figures stray from the actual situation.

The 1949–64 figures refer to the number of consultants employed under the National Health Service. "General surgery and related specialties" include urology, neurosurgery, plastic and thoracic surgery, and hospital dentistry and orthodontics. "General medicine and related specialties" include chest diseases, neurology, cardiology, pediatrics, geriatrics, physical medicine, infectious diseases, venereology, and social medicine. Comparable percentages for these subgroups are not available for 1938–39.

Source: *Report of Interdepartmental Committee on Remuneration of Consultants and Specialists* (Spens report), pp. 22 and 25; and Annual Reports of the Ministry of Health.

nominate one of their members to attend its meetings as an additional co-opted member.

In addition, and in reply to a demand that had been raised by the Society of Members of the College for some fifty years "as they were by far the more numerous and contribute more to the College funds than any others," it was decided to include general practitioner representation on the College Council as a gesture of cooperation.[7] In fact, the efforts of members for representation had become feebler—and perhaps less justified—as the number of fellows increased to thousands, and surgery became more clearly differentiated from general practice; and it was not now intended to provide specific training arrangements for general practitioners within the College. All these arrangements were confirmed by amendments to the College Charter in 1947. By widening the sphere of representation on its College Council, the Royal College of Surgeons emphasized the broad approach to the surgical spectrum that was to be its postwar keynote.

Reconstructing the College Council might provide a broader base for national negotiation but to four major specialty groups (ophthalmologists, otolaryngologists, dental surgeons, and anesthesiologists) this was not enough. It did not answer their growing demands for a separate training structure, which had developed as the specialty fields expanded their own esoteric techniques. Ophthalmologists no longer considered themselves general surgeons with a special interest in eye surgery; they wanted a fellowship examination in ophthalmology alone. This request gained the agreement of the Council in July 1943. A similar request was made by the British Association of Otolaryngologists on behalf of its members in 1945. The FRCS in ophthalmology and the FRCS in otolaryngology were instituted in 1947.[8] Ophthalmologists and otolaryngologists continued to take the College's primary examination in the basic medical sciences, but they were no longer examined in general surgery in their final. Since the fellowship in ophthalmology or otolaryngology was intended to be comparable in standard to the usual final examination for the general FRCS, there was no distinction in regard to status or privilege between fellows admitted under either system.

The third specialty to request special arrangements was dental surgery, for which the Royal College of Surgeons already awarded a basic license (LDS, RCS). Dental surgery had developed as a highly complex branch of jaw and facial surgery during World War II, and became recognized as a medical as well as a dental specialty. But even before the war there had been suggestions for a postgraduate grade of dentistry within the Royal College of Surgeons. The old division between dentistry and medicine was no longer applicable to hospital dentistry, and the small body of hospital or consultant dental surgeons wanted due recognition of their expertise. "We need more dental doctors. . . . We cannot expect to get them unless we give this medical specialty the honour which is its due and the partnership which, on theoretical and practical grounds, it deserves." [9] In 1945 the Council of the Royal College of Surgeons duly confirmed its previous intention to grant a special

7. *Brit. Med. J. ii* (1944), 19 (Alfred Webb-Johnson); Cope, *History of the RCS*, p. 211. *Brit. Med. J. ii* (1944), 256 (Percy B. Spurgin, President, Society of Members, RCS).

8. Cope, p. 214.

9. *Brit. Med. J. ii* (1943), 590 (L. Michaelis).

Fellowship in Dental Surgery as a higher diploma. In the following year, a further and rather different request was made, which was accepted by the College: to form a semiautonomous Faculty of Dental Surgery within the Royal College of Surgeons. It was decided that the board of the faculty was to be comprised of the president and two vice-presidents of the Royal College of Surgeons, with eighteen fellows and three licentiates in dental surgery elected by the faculty itself. A Fellowship in Dental Surgery (FDS, RCS) was created by the charter of 1947, with the intention of making the standard as high in dental surgery as in general surgery, but the examination was made the responsibility of the faculty. The College was authorized to confer the fellowship without examination on not more than 250 dental surgeons during the three years after the granting of the charter. The first fellows of the faculty were nominated and the first dean of the faculty elected in July 1947.[10] Dental surgery thus received somewhat different treatment from ophthalmology and otolaryngology, which effectively were treated as alternatives to the general FRCS and which had no College faculty.

The fourth and final specialty to be given special treatment by the Royal College of Surgeons was anesthesiology. The scientific advances in anesthetics, made in the interwar period, had not been reflected in improved teaching or higher status. By the end of World War II, anesthesiologists were in short supply, although GP anesthetists were relatively common. If anesthesiology were a specialty, it was argued, it ought to be confined to practitioners with special qualifications. "Until the medical profession as a whole regards it in this light," said a correspondent in 1944, "the present unsatisfactory position will continue. Surgeons themselves were partially responsible for the present anomalous state of affairs by permitting general practitioners to anaesthetize their own cases." [11] In November 1947 the Association of Anaesthetists requested a faculty of anesthetists within the College, similar to that already set up for dental surgeons. The request was approved. It was recommended, and agreed, that all holders of the Diploma of Anaesthetics granted by the Conjoint Board should be eligible to be members of the new faculty, and other duly qualified practitioners could join on the recommendation of the faculty board, which was similar in structure to that of the Faculty of Dental Surgeons. The first meeting of the board was held in March 1948. It was decided to offer a special fellowship in anesthetics (FFA, RCS). The fellowship was awarded until 1952 by election to medical practitioners who had made distinguished contributions to anesthesiology, and after that by examination. The faculty grew quickly, and within six months from its foundation it had seven hundred members.[12]

Thus by 1948 the Royal College of Surgeons had made special arrange-

10. Cope, p. 213; *Annals of the Royal College of Surgeons of England 47*(1), 61, July-Dec. 1947; *Brit. Med. J. ii* (1947), 353.

11. *Brit. Med. J. i* (1944), 233 (M. Dawkins).

12. The faculty board was composed of the president and two vice-presidents of the Royal College of Surgeons with 21 diplomates in anesthesiology of the College. Cope, p. 213.

ments for four specialty groups. Anesthesiology and dental surgery were given semiautonomous faculties with responsibility for their own postgraduate examinations (FFA and FDS). Ophthalmologists and otolaryngologists were kept within the FRCS framework, continuing to sit for the common primary examination, but with a specialty-tailored final examination. At this point fragmentation ceased. Other surgical specialists remained largely content with their own specialty association or set up particular bodies with limited functions. For example, a Joint Committee for Post-Graduate Orthopaedic Training was formed in 1948 under the aegis, among others, of the Royal College of Surgeons, the British Orthopaedics Association, and the Institute of Orthopaedics. Orthopedics, neurosurgery, plastic surgery, and urology, which were all developing rapidly as scientific areas of medical practice, made no move for independent examinations. They were already status specialties, able to exert influence within the Royal College of Surgeons. Indeed, given the consultant appointment machinery, there was little to be gained from a separate examining structure. Consultants were chosen by committees of their peers—they were not self-selected—and the committees were likely to favor the man with a broad rather than an over-specialized training record. Moreover, because the total number of consultants was small relative to the number of medical practitioners, the number of consultants in the new specialties was sometimes minute. In 1949, for example, there were only thirty-one consultant neurosurgeons working in the National Health Service, which was a virtual monopoly, in the whole of England and Wales; there were twenty-seven consultant plastic surgeons, and forty-four thoracic surgeons.[13] The needs of these groups could be well served by their small exclusive specialist societies or through the appropriate section of the Royal Society of Medicine. These surgeons continued to take the general FRCS examination (the primary, which examined in the basic medical sciences, and the final, in general surgery) before embarking on apprenticeship in the registrar and senior registrar grades in their chosen surgical field.

Postwar Committees of the Royal College of Physicians

The Royal College of Physicians was also undergoing a period of up-heaval. The equation of membership in the College with success in a professional examination provoked problems of organization and representation equally difficult to those experienced by the Royal College of Surgeons. But unlike the Surgeons, specialty groups within the Royal College of Physicians were less demanding of specialist examinations, less vociferous, or less concerned about their relative status. Thus, whereas the Surgeons provided arrangements for splinter groups, the Physicians, in the immediate postwar period, did not. Instead, activities in the College at the end of the war included pressure by members for representation in the government of the

13. *Report of the Ministry of Health for 1961, Part I,* Cmnd. 1754, p. 160.

College and extensive committee work among all the chief subspecialties of general medicine.

The three-tier organization of the College gave governing powers not to the members but to the elected fellows, who together formed the Comitia. The Comitia in turn nominated the officers and council. Thus, whereas the surgeon holding the FRCS could vote for, and be a member of his College Council, the physician of similar professional status had no vote. Indeed, a college bye-law stated that members "shall not be entitled to attend or vote at General Meetings of the Corporation and shall have such share only in the Government as is provided in the Bye-Laws." [14] The body of fellows of the Royal College of Physicians was, and is, self-perpetuating, new fellows being nominated from the members according to a subjective assessment of their relative professional eminence. With the growing involvement of the College in public policy, the question of representation acquired additional importance.

Members complained of their impotence with regard to control of the College in 1946. "Our College," wrote three correspondents, "instead of remaining a mere academic institution should become a dynamic force, capable of exercising a profound influence for good on various medical, social and educational problems confronting us and pressing urgently for solution." [15] The first step, it was suggested, was the creation of facilities for active participation by members in the management of the College. Further protests came from Dr. Ffrangcon Roberts, writing from Cambridge. He reported in 1946 that he had resigned his MRCP because he had not been considered for a fellowship and felt he must be "socially undesirable" to the College; furthermore, he claimed he had had poor return from his association with it. "The College, beyond granting me a licence to practice (for which it was handsomely remunerated) six months earlier than I could have obtained it from my University, has not contributed one iota to my education." [16] A defense against such charges was put by the registrar of the Royal College of Physicians, who pointed out that its president had called a meeting of members in January 1946 which was attended by a group of three hundred. It was decided that there should be an organization of members of the College, with provision for meetings and the election of two representative members to serve on the Council.[17] Nevertheless, the Royal College of Physicians remained a much more oligarchic organization than the Royal College of Surgeons, and the real seat of authority remained with the Comitia of Fellows. It was this system that was later to provoke adverse and bitter criticism and complaints of inadequate representation on the Comitia from psychiatrists and pathologists, whose interests, among others, the College served.

14. Royal College of Physicians of London, Bye-Law 111.
15. *Brit. Med. J. ii* 1946), 476 (C. Anderson et al.).
16. Ibid., p. 591 (F. Roberts).
17. Ibid., p. 591 (H. E. A. Boldero).

In the 1940s the question of specialty representation among the Physicians had less urgency than it had among the Surgeons because the growth of the specialties of general medicine had been somewhat different. Whereas surgical specialties such as ophthalmology were focused on small areas with advanced technical skills, developments in the medical specialties tended to be broader. Developing specialties like geriatrics, pediatrics, and psychiatry had vital links not only with general medicine but with general practice and with a variety of paramedical social services. Pediatrics, for example, was not so much a specialty as general medicine applied to a limited section of the population. It was thus "holistic," and to some critics more easily justifiable as an area of practice than were specialties relating to single conditions, organs, functions, or techniques. The holistic approach permeated the extensive committee work undertaken at this time by specialist subcommittees of the Royal College of Physicians. The committee on neurology, for example, did not favor the creation of a special diploma in neurology; it was felt that the consultant status of the neurologist was secured by a higher diploma in general medicine (the MRCP). The *British Medical Journal* agreed; the neurologist was a "consultant rather than a specialist": a man with the breadth to generalize and advise on the nature, origins, and outcome of an illness and the disposal of a sick person (albeit from a neurologist's viewpoint), rather than the peddler of a particular type of treatment.[18]

The recommendations of the College reports thus followed the strong conviction expressed in the Goodenough report, that consultant practice should be based on the general surgeon and general physician with special interests, rather than on specialties per se. Not only undergraduate but also much of the postgraduate education was to be primarily general in interest. The MRCP, an examination in general medicine which required no specified training or experience and which included no choice of special subject, was at least in theory an ideal examination for the general physician—and thus by implication for all those in the medical subspecialties—as was the FRCS for the general surgeon.

But even as these sentiments were being expressed, certain medical subspecialties were rapidly rising in numbers and status. The Royal College of Surgeons had recognized some branches of surgery as being distinct from general surgery, at the request of particular specialty associations. It was only a matter of time before the Royal College of Physicians would be faced with similar pressures: to decide, in effect, whether *general* medicine, including almost all the nonsurgical specialties, was still a viable concept or whether it should be sectioned into internal medicine and its subspecialties, with special arrangements for the relatively large and influential groups in pediatrics, pathology, and psychiatry. Each of these was being recognized as a distinct kind of practice; each had a relatively large number of adherents; and each was soon to burgeon into a number of subspecialties of its own. In the 1940s and 1950s the Physicians were able to stand firm, and to offer

18. *ii* (1945), 292.

exclusively the general MRCP; but the question of division was becoming more urgent.

Symbolic of the rise of pediatrics during and after World War II was the increase in the importance of the role of the British Paediatric Association (BPA).[19] By the end of the war it had become usual for a hospital, about to make an appointment to a new pediatric department, to seek the association's advice, and the BPA thus played a part in planning pediatric services within the National Health Service. In November 1945 the BPA was for the first time asked to advise on the foundation of a university department of pediatrics and child health, and in 1946 an observer appointed by the Ministry of Health began to attend BPA meetings. Everywhere, new children's hospitals and departments in general hospitals were started, and chairs in all universities were almost simultaneously instituted.

The Paediatric Committee set up by the Royal College of Physicians suggested in its report (1945) that pediatrics be regarded as a major clinical subject.[20] Among its detailed proposals for both undergraduate and postgraduate education, it proposed a period of not less than one third of that devoted to clinical medicine to be set aside for clinical pediatrics, that from the departments of psychiatry, radiology, and pathology a member of staff should interest himself particularly in the problems of childhood, and that questions of pediatrics should be included in the undergraduate final examinations. It was implied that pediatrics should embrace all aspects of child health and would have a much wider social content than general medicine. Pediatrics appeared to be developing as an *alternative* to, rather than a subspecialty of, general medicine. The development raised questions of redefining the scope of "general medicine." Was it to remain the sum of all the nonsurgical specialties except radiology—which already had its own faculty —or was it, as was becoming increasingly the case in the practice of general medicine, to be limited to "internal" medicine?

The same question was particularly relevant to psychiatry and pathology, both much larger specialties than pediatrics. Moreover, whereas the consultant pediatrician continued to be a member or fellow of the Royal College of Physicians or hold an approved higher degree in general medicine rather than a pediatric diploma, outside the teaching hospitals pathologists and psychiatrists normally held the special diploma given by the Conjoint Board or one of the universities rather than the MRCP. There was already a tendency to regard psychiatry as a distinct and separate branch of medicine. "Psychiatry is the other half of medicine," said the president of the Royal Medico-Psychological Association in 1946, "and not just another specialty."[21] The reports of the Royal College of Physicians on psychiatry concentrated on reforming the standard of the Diploma in Psychological Medicine (DPM). The aim was to allow for the diversity of experience now

19. The material on pediatrics is drawn from Cameron, *The British Paediatric Association*.

20. *Brit. Med. J. i* (1945), 705.

21. *Lancet ii* (1946), 160 (D. K. Henderson).

necessary for the psychiatrist, and to prevent the tendency for psychiatry to split into a series of specialties with little in common.[22] Thus the emphasis was on relating the components of psychiatry to general psychiatry rather than relating psychiatry as a whole to general medicine.

Pathology also had a growing claim as a distinct branch of medicine. Before World War II, pathology, like psychiatry, had been a low-status specialty. The pathologist had a double stigma: he was usually employed on a salary, and he had no hospital beds. It had been the widespread custom to regard as ineligible for appointment to the medical staff committee of a hospital any salaried (even part-time) person. The pathologist, whose work gave him little scope for private practice, was often excluded from a share in hospital affairs on equal terms with his clinical colleagues, because he was thought to have a vested interest. "This unwarranted prejudice," wrote one complainant as late as 1960, "has left its mark on staff relations to this day."[23] The war had had a great effect on pathologists, whose specialty was recognized by the government; emergency arrangements for blood transfusion, the Emergency Public Health Laboratory Service, and the pathological laboratories of the Emergency Medical Service remained under the National Health Service. Pathologists were rising in status, and at the same time pathology as a subject was becoming more highly specialized. These trends were to continue in the early years of the National Health Service and to force the issue of the separate organization of pathology.

Pediatrics, psychiatry, and pathology became organizationally distinct from internal medicine in the 1960s. Other new and smaller specialties of general medicine with equally valid cases for separate treatment, particularly geriatrics and endocrinology, did not press their claims. Geriatrics, consonant with the higher proportion of old people in the population, expanded after World War II. People over 65 years were expected to represent 11.5 per cent of the total population by 1951.[24] This large increase among the old, and the special nature of their illnesses and of the care they needed, presented problems for administration. A BMA report on the care of the aged sick (1947) postulated the provision of a geriatric department in each district hospital,[25] a goal that has not yet been attained. The new specialty developed its own particular skills, but most of the early geriatricians were general physicians or general practitioners who, through interest or force of circumstance—for example, appointment to a group of NHS hospitals which included a large "chronic sick" institution—came into daily contact with the problems of the elderly. The British Geriatrics Society was organized, but there was no university or Conjoint Board diploma.[26]

22. *Brit. Med. J. i* (1945), 302.

23. D. F. Cappell, *Lancet, ii* (1960), 864.

24. Dudley Committee's reports on the design of dwellings, 1944, quoted in *Brit. Med. J. i* (1946), 617.

25. *Brit. Med. J. ii* (1947), 870.

26. Geriatrics, some insisted, "should be regarded more as an outlook than as a specialty," *Brit. Med. J. ii* (1948), 401 (T. H. Howell); *i* (1952), 650 (M. C. Binnie).

Endocrinology dated back to the discovery in 1902 of secretin, the first of the hormones, but as a specialty it attained no organization until World War II. The first number of the *Journal of Endocrinology* was published in June 1939, the Section of Endocrinology of the Royal Society of Medicine was founded in 1946, and in the same year the Society for Endocrinology held its inaugural meeting. Endocrinology was a wide specialty in that it had no anatomical boundaries, but its scientific content was such that it could not easily be encompassed by a general physician. By 1946, two hospitals had appointed endocrinologists, as such, to their honorary staffs, and a professorship in London University was planned. But the specialty seemed unlikely to attain the numbers that would lead to separate recognition.[27] As with neurology and cardiology, practitioners in this field were a relatively small elite.

Taken as a whole, the specialties arising from general medicine in the 1940s represented at least as wide a range as those arising from general surgery. Indeed it could be argued that the anesthesiologist had more in common with the ophthalmologist, or the dental surgeon had more in common with the otolaryngologist (all of whom had to pass special College examinations) than the psychiatrist had with the pathologist, or the endocrinologist with the pediatrician. The Royal College of Surgeons was faced with more intensive, and thus narrower, specialties. The Royal College of Physicians, however, was confronted with a number of specialties which were different aspects of virtually the whole spectrum of medicine. Traditionally, medical practice had been neatly divided between the two Colleges. Obstetricians and radiologists, by founding separate examining bodies, had set a precedent whose influence might be profound; they had implied that their two branches were clearly and equally distinguishable from general medicine and general surgery. The basic question of the logical division of specialties remained. How many branches of medicine should there be? If anesthesiologists had a separate faculty, why not psychiatry or pathology?

An Academy of Medicine?

This question might have been more easily resolved had the Royal Colleges combined; and, indeed, serious proposals for a combined Academy of Medicine were made by the Royal College of Surgeons in 1945. Part of its own building had been destroyed in the air raids of 1941 and the College owned a large site in Lincoln's Inn Fields. The possibility of including all three Royal Colleges on the site inspired the new president, Sir Alfred Webb-Johnson (created a baron in 1948). With the Council's agreement, several adjacent houses were purchased, and a proposition was put to the other two Royal Colleges for joint development. The decision rested with the Royal College of Physicians, whose officers had for some time been contemplating rebuilding, for the Royal College of Obstetricians and Gynaecologists declared that it was not willing to move unless all three colleges were housed together. The Joint Committee of the three Royal Colleges, formed in Janu-

27. *Lancet i* (1946), 820.

ary 1942, decided unanimously that a single site for the Colleges was more important than the qualities of any particular site.[28] The scheme was beginning to take on a substance of reality. A building committee was set up and an architect engaged. The Royal College of Surgeons pledged funds to the extent of £100,000 to provide the opportunity for the three Colleges to meet on one site; physical union had become a concrete possibility. But so far all the enthusiasm had emanated from the Surgeons, who had both the land and the desire to proceed. They even had an artist's sketch of the proposed building—in the center, an imposing portico for the Royal College of Surgeons, and on each side, a lesser entrance for each of the other two Colleges.[29]

When it came to the point, the Royal College of Physicians were not so enthusiastic as some of their remarks had suggested, and in October 1945 wrote to the Royal College of Surgeons that they had concluded their interests were best served by remaining in their present premises. After an abortive exchange of letters between the presidents of the two Colleges, a last bid to save the proposal, accompanied by a large financial inducement, was made by the Surgeons in February 1946.[30] But the Physicians were not to be tempted. They remained firm in isolation, partly perhaps for fear of appearing a victim of annexation by the restless and enthusiastic Webb-Johnson. By August 1946 final deadlock was reached, by which time the main outline of the plans for rebuilding had been provisionally designed.[31] The space had therefore to be put to other uses.

Many rumors surround the reasons for the final decision, one of which, with variations, concerns the Physicians' reluctance, as the oldest College, to be placed on one corner of the site while the Surgeons sat grandly in the middle. But both the organization and the outlook of the Colleges were very different. The energy exhibited by the Surgeons in reconstructing and expanding their college after the war—and their notable success as fund raisers—set them apart from the Physicians, whose mood was more conservative. Sir Robert Platt, himself a president of the Royal College of Physicians, was later to remark:

> Surgeons, I suspect see themselves in a setting of glamour, conquering disease by the bold strokes of sheer technical skill. Physicians quietly

28. *Brit. Med. J. i* (1945), 92.

29. *Lancet ii* (1944), 605.

30. The Royal College of Surgeons appealed to common interest and the need for a "single authoritative voice." Lord Moran replied that new responsibilities that would inevitably fall on the three Royal Colleges in connection with the NHS would give them a unity of purpose "which will not be dependent on geography." *Brit. Med. J. ii* (1945), 789, 827. A further donation of £100,000 was made to the Royal College of Surgeons in February 1946, on condition that it offer all sites and property to the east of the college which were not required for its own extension as a free gift to the Royal College of Physicians, the offer to remain open for one year. *Brit. Med. J. i* (1946), 376.

31. Cope, p. 209.

remember that they were educated gentlemen, centuries ago, when surgeons and apothecaries were tradesmen. They see themselves as the traditional thinkers of the profession.[32]

Nor was the Royal College of Obstetricians and Gynaecologists apparently saddened by the news of failure. A spokesman for that College said that there was never serious thought of joining the others, merely of building on the same site: "The Colleges are not bricks and mortar." [33]

With the failure of physical union went the recommendation of the Goodenough Committee that the Colleges be responsible jointly for all postgraduate clinical diplomas and also the broader question of an Academy of Medicine. Although some expressed an opinion that "The mere propinquity of the three Royal Colleges has little to do with and could have little influence on the establishment of an Academy of Medicine," [34] no academy was formed. Physicians continued to be attached to one building, Surgeons to another, and Obstetricians to a third. Both Physicians and Obstetricians were soon to rebuild on sites removed from each other and from the Surgeons.

Each College continued to go its own way. The Royal College of Surgeons continued the expansion that was embodied in its charter of 1947 and in the successful fund-raising activities undertaken by its president. Instead of providing space for the other Colleges, the acquisition of the adjacent sites permitted development of its own premises to accommodate eight departments for research and teaching. Research laboratories had existed at the College since 1928, but an endowment in 1941 made possible the creation of a research professorship in applied physiology. Chairs of anatomy and pathology followed in 1942, although the College had at this time no formal connection with a university. Postgraduate courses in all three subjects were inaugurated in 1945, and the growth of departments in the same fields soon followed, as did the establishment of the further chairs and departments of pharmacology, ophthalmology, anesthesiology, and biochemistry.[35]

Compared with this spate of activity, the Royal College of Physicians remained much as before. It did no routine teaching, it set up no special departments, and its only examination was for the MRCP. The College continued to discuss in a series of further reports the relationships of the general and special aspects of medicine and the relationship of the MRCP to each stage of training. In 1949, the Comitia officially confirmed that examination for the MRCP should be based on general medicine, on a level

32. Nuffield Trust, *Doctor and Patient,* p. 83.

33. Miss A. Holloway, Secretary to the Royal College of Obstetricians and Gynaecologists (personal interview).

34. *Brit. Med. J. i* (1945), 161 (J. H. Parsons). But see *The Times,* January 10. 1945 (Sir Stewart Duke-Elder), for a strong case for a comprehensive academy on a central site.

35. Royal College of Surgeons (personal communication).

higher than that required for the basic medical degree,[36] and that it would be taken early in training, normally about two years after the basic qualification. It was thus not to be recognized as being in any way the hallmark of consultant status—as it was in fact sometimes being used in appointments to NHS hospitals. The College rejected a suggestion that it should prescribe training and experience for candidates to the examination, nor did it wish to accredit training posts. The candidate would continue to stand before the examiners with nothing to recommend him but his performance on that day. In contrast to the FRCS and MRCOG, both of which included primary and final examinations, it was decided that the MRCP examination should be a "single whole." The introduction of a separate primary examination was considered but rejected; the committee saw little relevance in introducing a primary test in anatomy and physiology ("it would probably promote cramming rather than the desired broadening of fundamental knowledge"). Instead, there would be a limitation on the frequency of entry for the examination.

These recommendations were intended to liberalize the examination—to make it a reasonable test of general knowledge, competence, and judgment rather than a rigid examination of basic skills. Unfortunately, the attitude of many candidates was not receptive to such a test, for with the advent of the National Health Service the possession of the MRCP or FRCS had become vitally important: it was the only outward sign of consultant potential. Since consultants would be appointed on the basis of merit alone from candidates who might not be known personally to the appointments committees, these diplomas became a hurdle to be overcome. At the same time, the scope of general medicine and general surgery had become so wide that many felt success in the diplomas was a question of luck. A candidate working in cardiology, psychiatry, or pathology might, for example, be asked to discuss a dermatological case. By the postwar years, the eminent examiners for the MRCP tended themselves to specialize, and had to be restrained from wandering too far into their own fields. Not surprisingly, the attitude of mind of candidates had thus become "morbid rather than natural." The test for the MRCP was dreaded even more than the FRCS. No longer was it the leisured, relaxed examination, followed by a cup of tea, of prewar days. The new candidates were nervous and often ill-prepared senior house officers and registrars, staking once, twice, or many times their future prospects on the consultant career ladder on one examination extending over the broad and formidable field of medicine.

The argument surrounding the MRCP and to a lesser extent the FRCS was generalism versus specialism. The evils of specialization were clearly

36. As a nice reflection on the cultural heritage of the Royal College of Physicians it was agreed that translations from French and German should be retained in the examination: "Besides providing evidence of general education, they enable examiners to give credit to candidates who will be able to expand their knowledge of medicine by reading in these languages." *Lancet ii* (1949), 252–55.

seen by leading clinicians. Textbooks had become "accretions of monographs written by different authors in which the principles of medicine which should pervade all undergraduate teaching are obscured or lost." [37] The population of teaching hospitals was becoming more specialized, so that the student often saw only the rarer forms of disease. Moreover, generalists were alarmed at the predatory tendencies of certain specialists in relating pathological conditions to their particular fields. All these factors bolstered the concept of a firm, general postgraduate experience on which the MRCP and the general FRCS were founded, but which had been largely abandoned by the radiologists, anesthesiologists, dental surgeons, ophthalmologists, otolaryngologists, and obstetricians, although many obstetricians were taking the general FRCS as well as the MRCOG.

At the same time, however, medical knowledge was advancing so fast that true general medicine or general surgery was becoming impossible. One surgeon wrote in 1946: "Those who do not believe in specialists and prefer 'a good general surgeon' forget how much there is to know nowadays." [38] By confirming their chief postgraduate diplomas as general examinations, the Colleges left themselves no way of imposing their recommendations on subsequent specialist training except through indirect influence on consultant appointments committees. There was still no one body responsible for the finished product; there was still a conglomeration of diplomas at all possible levels; there was still no place within the Royal College structure for the postgraduate training of the GP; and there were dangers of further organizational fragmentation.

Finally, there was no clear division of responsibility for postgraduate training. The specialist institutes developed in London around the special hospitals and within the British Postgraduate Medical Federation of London University. The undergraduate medical schools in the hospital regions appointed postgraduate deans to supervise courses within the regional framework. The Royal Colleges maintained their position as the professional leaders of medicine but had few or no direct links with training in the hospitals. No long-term solution had yet been found to the interrelationships of the Colleges with the university medical schools. The possibility of union of the Royal Colleges had come to nothing, and the two older Colleges were clearly set on different courses of development. At the center of all discussion were the MRCP and FRCS, which had been the hallmark of consultant status since their institution in the mid-nineteenth century. Now, like the LRCP and MRCS before them, they had been overtaken by the advances in medical sciences; they were no longer signs of consultant competence, just as consultant medicine was no longer generalized but specialized.

The National Health Service began in this rapidly changing professional environment. It did not initiate the problems that the profession and the

37. See *Proceedings of the Royal Society of Medicine,* March 22, 1949, pp. 1035–39.
38. *Lancet i* (1946), 978 ("Specialist-Surgeon").

Ministry of Health had ultimately to face—the split between consultants and general practitioners, increased specialization within the hospitals and in the professional bodies, and the need to redefine the purpose of postgraduate diplomas; these problems already existed. But they were emphasized by the creation of a national service. Some trends, such as the buildup of consultant time spent in hospitals, the exclusion of general practitioners from the larger hospitals, and the increase of consultants in the less popular but increasingly important specialties of anesthesiology, pathology, and psychiatry, were accelerated by the new administrative machinery. Other questions, such as the hospital staffing structure and the GP's problems, became more noticeable because there was comprehensive national responsibility for providing health services.

The structure of the health service, based as it was on the professional patterns of the past, tended to inhibit change. The distinction between consultant and general practice long antedated modern medical specialization. The hospital staffing structure had been developed by the voluntary hospitals in the eighteenth century. The role of the general practitioner was crystallized in the demarcation disputes between GPs and consultants at the turn of the century and reinforced under the National Health Insurance Act of 1911. The higher professional status of the consultant and the lower status of the general practitioner were centuries old, as was the wariness between the Royal College of Physicians and the Royal College of Surgeons. None of these patterns was ideal for mid-twentieth century medicine. Each had been bent as far as possible to accommodate the needs of specialization and then of a National Health Service. Not surprisingly, new tensions were to arise, as the demands of technology once more outstripped the established structures of medical practice.

III

Emerging Problems:
The National Health Service
1948–1961

9

Determination of Incomes

The National Health Service was absorbed surprisingly quickly into British life. The then Minister of Health (Derek Walker-Smith) looked back with pride in 1959 on three years of Labour and eight years of Conservative administration of comprehensive medical services: "The task of taking over nearly 3000 hospitals, most of them old and of differing size, capacity, standards and traditions was no small one." [1] The change in government in 1951 had made little difference to the basic policy of the service. Certain charges were introduced to patients as an economy measure by the Labour Government in 1951—originally for dentures and optical appliances—and these were increased and extended to include prescription charges under successive Conservative administrations; but even under the increases in 1961 (when Enoch Powell was Minister), payments made by patients using the service represented under 7 per cent of the NHS budget.[2] For the most part the ideal of a comprehensive, free medical service was fulfilled, even though the development of facilities was hindered by national financial stringency.

The structure of the service, founded as it was on pre-existing organizational patterns, undoubtedly facilitated this adjustment. Within the prestigious teaching hospitals, nationalization made little apparent change. The honorary consultant, although now paid, continued to work within the same staffing structure. Ex-municipal hospitals and rural ex-voluntary hospitals were subject to the greatest change, but the change was for the better in terms of patient care and staffing ratios, and few complaints were heard. The GP continued to regard himself as an independent practitioner, treating patients for a capitation fee as he had under National Health Insurance. The machinery of regional hospital planning and national regulation of the distribution of general practitioners were accepted with little question.

Under the strain of increasing specialization, however, the inadequacies of the NHS structure—particularly the divorce between hospitals and general practice—soon became apparent. Acute problems of hospital medical

1. *Report of the Ministry of Health for 1958*, p. iii.
2. The abolition of charges became part of the Labour Party's platform while in opposition. Prescription charges were ended in February 1965. Ibid. for 1964, p. 65.

staffing arose, pre-existing problems in general practice were thrown into prominence and, despite their supposedly educational focus, hospital regions failed to stimulate medical training programs. Finally, there was the question, in some ways the most important, of determining doctors' incomes. In each of these areas pressures were built up through the 1950s, and by the 1960s revision was urgent.

Income and the Divided Professional Structure

Where the state is a monopoly employer and the employee is a monopoly profession, pay negotiations may, if not subtly directed, degenerate into a trial of strength between two forces. If a National Health Service dismisses a practitioner, his alternative means of support are few. If the profession decides to withdraw—as general practitioners have threatened to do on more than one occasion—the health service will collapse. The two parties are thus interdependent, and income levels largely result from the relative pressure each can exert. The determination of income scales under the NHS was, however, complicated by the vital third factor of the division of the medical profession into hospital medical staff and general practitioners. This dichotomy added a disturbing dimension to pay negotiations, for it bore seeds of dissent within the profession.

The traditional income gap between consultants and GPs had narrowed between the two world wars under National Health Insurance. Under the National Health Service, the Ministry of Health took over responsibility for the income of both branches. It thus acquired the unenviable responsibility for deciding how much each ought in future to be paid in relation to the other; income determination would formalize their professional and social distinction. Whatever the system for deciding the national income scale of each branch—through special committees, negotiations, or arbitration—it was more than likely to lead to collision. Consultants wished to maintain a reasonably wide income differential between themselves and general practitioners; they were relatively few in number and wanted to emphasize the enhanced skills and status that set them above the mass; GPs, on the other hand, were naturally in favor of reducing the differential. They had been slowly doing so since 1815, the year of the Apothecaries Act, which turned the apothecary into a professional medical practitioner.

The first determinations of income policy in the National Health Service were made by the Spens committees of 1946 and 1948, which set out suggested scales and methods of remuneration for general medical practitioners and for consultants and specialists. Each committee was independently staffed; their conclusions appeared to have been arrived at independently, and they were inevitably based on the prewar incomes of each branch rather than on the desirable future relativity between general and consultant practice. Figures in the Spens reports indicated that the consultant might expect to earn almost twice as much as a GP. They recommended a median net income (after practice expenses) for a general practitioner aged 40 to 50 years of £1,300; a whole-time specialist was to receive a salary of at least £2,500 at about age 40.[3]

But there were numerous difficulties in interpreting and comparing these figures: general training took less time than specialized training; entrance to general practice was relatively easy, but appointment as a consultant was uniformly difficult; consultants had become accustomed to earning considerably more than general practitioners. Direct comparison of national average incomes had not previously been feasible and had never been used as a gauge by one branch to assess its own income in terms of the other. There were no adequate measurements of relative responsibility or value. Each branch tended to think of itself in absolute terms, and because of the compartmentalism of the NHS structure, they were encouraged to continue along their separate ways. Thus specialists had their own terms of service and their own negotiating machinery, while GPs continued to have a separate organization.

In the debate over the National Health Service Bill, the then Minister of Health (Mr. Bevan) had indicated that future terms of service and remuneration would be subject to consultation and negotiation with the profession.[4] The joint negotiating machinery set up to determine NHS incomes followed the principles of the Whitley Councils which were already familiar in industry and employed in the various parts of the public health service. Nine functional councils were set up for NHS employees, each to deal with certain categories of staff, together with a general council for matters of intergroup interest. Each council consisted of representatives of employees (the staff side) and employers (management), and it was decided that decisions made by the councils should apply to appropriate staff in the whole of Great Britain. One of the functional (or Whitley) councils, divided into three committees, considered medical remuneration.[5] Committee A was intended to negotiate income between the government and general practitioners; but because of the pre-existing relationship between the BMA and the government under National Health Insurance, it was in fact ignored. Committee B, set up to deal with the terms and conditions of service of hospital medical

3. *Spens Report on General Practitioners*, p. 12; *Spens Report on Consultants and Specialists*, pp. 10–11. Subsequent calculations on the Spens Committee figures showed that the average net income for general practitioners over all age groups and from all sources would be £1,111, in terms of the 1939 value of money. *Royal Commission; Report*, p. 11.

4. See *Report of the Ministry of Health for the Year Ended 31st March 1949*, Cmd. 7910, pp. 302–03.

5. Whitley committees were named for Mr. J. H. Whitley, speaker of the House of Commons in 1916, and chairman of a government committee on the relations between employers and employees. The principles of joint negotiation set out in the Whitley Committee reports were applied to government industrial establishments after World War I and were later extended to local government and the civil service. For an account of the setting up of the NHS Whitley machinery, see H. A. Clegg and T. E. Chester, *Wage Policy and the Health Service* (Oxford, 1957), Chap. 1, 2.

and dental staff, was, in contrast, an active participant. Its staff side included the newly established Joint Consultants Committee; the employers were represented by the hospital boards and the Ministry of Health. Committee C negotiated for medical staff in the public health service, including medical officers on the staff of local health authorities.

Unfortunately, the whole Whitley machinery had an inauspicious beginning because of mounting concern over the cost of the health service. Salary claims on behalf of a number of groups in the NHS were deferred or rejected in the first two years of the service because of the general financial situation, and an economic review of medical and other hospital staffs in 1951 did not augur for a brighter prospect in the immediate future. The disadvantages to a profession of being tied to a politically dependent service became apparent. The Ministry of Health as the employer and source of income could not itself commit government funds in addition to those already granted for the National Health Service by the Treasury. Meanwhile, general practitioners were submitting proposals for substantial increases in their remuneration and for changes in their terms of payment.

The GP "Pool" System and the Danckwerts Award

The general practitioner had expressed a desire to continue to be paid a basic capitation fee for each patient registered with him, together with a number of other payments for special services not covered in the general capitation fee. There were two ways in which the capitation fee could be calculated. The first was through a realistic appraisal related to what the GP might otherwise earn as a fee in private practice. The second was to use the capitation system purely as a means of securing reasonably equable incomes among general practitioners with practices of different sizes, in relation to an agreed average income rather than to an agreed individual fee. In other words, either a specific sum could be named as a reasonable payment for total general medical responsibility for one person for one year, and the GP would receive such a total for each person in his NHS "list"; or it could be agreed centrally what the average GP ought to earn, irrespective of the value of services given, and the capitation fee would be calculated backward from this amount. The first method was advantageous to the profession when the population was increasing more rapidly than the number of doctors; the more people on his NHS list, the higher the doctor's total income. The second, being tied to a "fair wage" concept, was desirable when the number of doctors was rising faster than the population.

At the beginning of the National Health Service reimbursement to GPs was calculated according to the first method. A central fund (or pool) was set up; it was based on a capitation fee of 18 shillings, multiplied by the 95 per cent of the population who were expected to take part in the new service.[6] But this system provoked almost immediate outcries from GPs. Despite

6. *Report of the Ministry of Health for 1949*, p. 264.

their desire for independence, they were not in favor of the all-out competition implied in this method. Moreover, there was concern that more doctors were being produced by the medical schools than could easily be absorbed into general practice. "Do the prospects in medicine really justify the present intake of students?" asked the *Lancet* in 1951. The evidence seemed to suggest that England and Wales had "an annual surplus approaching 200 doctors." [7] Under the population system, the greater the number of GPs to a given population, the smaller would be their average income from capitation fees. Thus the profession was interested in tying the size of the central pool to the number of doctors, and the Ministry of Health, with an eye fixed on cost, was not. This difference of opinion reached a deadlock and led to submitting the whole question of general practitioner payment to arbitration by Mr. Justice Danckwerts in 1951.

The Danckwerts proposals were accepted by the Conservative Government in 1952. It was now agreed that the total pool should be dependent on a nationally agreed income for the average doctor; thus the size of the pool would increase as the number of doctors increased. General practitioners had come into the NHS in 1948 with a net average income about 60 per cent above that recommended by the Spens report which was couched in 1939 values. [8] Justice Danckwerts decided that a more appropriate "betterment" or conversion factor was 100 per cent, and GP incomes were increased proportionally to an average net of £2,222. This was, however, to include income from all sources. The individual GP might have a list of some 2,500 potential patients for whom he would receive capitation fees and also (a post-Danckwerts innovation to encourage moderate list sizes) extra "loading" fees for patients 501 to 1,500 on his list. He might also engage in NHS maternity work, collect rural mileage payments, do some private practice, work part time for the local health authority (for example, by undertaking an antenatal clinic) or for a local hospital, and perform other paid duties. If the central pool was to reflect the average income of the GP, it had to be manipulated to include them all.

Estimation of the pool thus became a series of calculations out of which the capitation fee emerged as no more than an artifact. First, an average net income for general practitioners was agreed by negotiation between the Ministry and the profession's General Medical Services Committee. This figure was multiplied by the number of doctors. Next, an agreed amount of practice expenses was added. In 1954–55 this gave a global pool of £70.5 million. Then deductions were made in respect of income earned by GPs outside their commitments to general medical practice, including at this time private practice, and for pension contributions made by the government. This gave a figure for the "central pool"—£57.2 million in 1954–55. [9] The

7. *Lancet i* (1951), ii, 331–32.

8. That is, 60% above the agreed figure of £1,111. *Royal Commission; Report,* p. 12.

9. British Medical Association to *Royal Commission; Minutes of Evidence,* p. 254.

money was then distributed according to previously agreed amounts for each item: for capitation and extra loading fees, initial practice allowances to enable doctors to establish themselves in agreed new locations, supplementary annual payments for additional services not covered by the basic capitation fee, mileage payments, and fees for certain additional procedures. If any money was left in the pool at the end of these disbursements, it was paid to GPs on a pro rata basis as extra amounts for capitation fees and loadings. Equally, however, the central pool could suffer a loss and have to carry a deficit to the following year. Thus the individual practitioner's income might vary from year to year for the same work done.

This complex scheme had come a long way from the basic concept of a capitation fee, but it was a logical extension of the capitation method chosen. There was, however, a built-in disadvantage in the pool system. The more that doctors earned outside their general medical practice, the more was deducted from the global pool, and thus the smaller the amount available in the central pool for distribution as capitation and other fees. It followed that the GP who agreed to work as a clinical assistant in the hospital service for half a day a week—for which he received extra income from the hospital board—was ultimately reducing the income of his colleague down the line who relied solely on capitation fees.

Significantly, the deficiencies in the system were not to be denounced until, in the late 1950s, the population began to rise faster than the number of general practitioners. Meanwhile, despite its anomalies, the pool system continued to be favored by the BMA, which recorded its "firm conviction that any departure from the pool method of payment would be a breach of the undertaking given by the Government to the profession when it entered the Service." [10] The stigma of salaried service was still in evidence. The pool system at least allowed the local GP to earn his income from various different sources. But it gave him no incentive to provide the best service to his general medical patients or to invest in good equipment. The amount allowed for expenses was calculated from a stratified sample of income tax returns made available by the Inland Revenue Service. This sum (about a third of the gross income of GPs) was applied to the global pool and distributed to doctors on a proportional basis, not in relation to the actual money spent by each. This meant that the man who improved his premises received the same expense allowance as the man who did not—another disincentive. Finally, as the pool system became more complex, it became increasingly difficult for the GP to understand fully how each part of his income was derived.

It is debatable whether the revised pool system was different in effect from a salary graduated according to list size. If so, it was without any of the advantages of a salary which are, notably, an increased instead of a decreased income with age when the work load has declined, and the provision of paid staff coverage for vacations, periods of sickness, and other leave. Nevertheless, the capitation ritual followed by this system, because of its

10. Ibid., p. 238.

indirect method of payment and because of its *appearance* as income for work done independently by independent practitioners, was hallowed by GPs as a symbol of their freedom from bureaucracy: "It is traditional and historical, and everyone is familiar with it." [11]

There were also certain sectional advantages on both sides from having a different payment mechanism for GPs and hospital doctors. Each group, in the pay negotiations of the first decade and more of the NHS, tended to play itself off against the other, with direct relativities between the two being impossible to establish except in terms of the two Spens reports. These formed a useful kind of reference which each party could use to its own advantage. After the relatively large income raise given to GPs by the Danckwerts award in 1952, consultants quickly lodged a claim of their own in similar terms.[12] The Minister of Health, however, was chary of automatically linking rises in income to the cost of living. The Spens figures had been evolved from income patterns existing in 1939. It was by no means certain that these same patterns ought to be applied in postwar Britain when professional incomes as a whole were increasing less rapidly than other incomes. There was every incentive for the profession to refer to Spens at every opportunity, but there was every incentive for the Ministry to make no promises of income raises in terms of general economic development. While consultants asked for a post-Danckwerts increase because of the "reduced value of money," the Ministry of Health was careful—while allowing consultants what the Joint Consultants Committee called a "modest increase"— to relate this amount to the need to safeguard consultant recruitment and to help restore the balance between the pay of the two branches.[13] From April 1954 the consultant basic scale was increased to the equivalent of 40 per cent above the Spens figures at the bottom of the age scale and 24 per cent at the top—the new scale being £2,100 to £3,100. Distinction awards, which provided additional income to one of three consultants, remained unchanged. Even so, in terms of the Spens reports, the difference between GP and consultant incomes had been considerably reduced.[14]

11. Sir John Hawton, speaking for the Ministry of Health, ibid., Question 3607.

12. Consultants had entered the service on a basic salary scale about 12% above that recommended in the Spens report, or about 20% above if the new superannuation provisions were also included. The 1948 basic scale was £1,700 to £2,750; but with the government's contribution for superannuation it reached £1,836 to £2,970. *Royal Commission; Written Evidence, Vol. 1,* p. 24. Additional distinction awards remained as suggested in the Spens report. It was recommended that 4% of consultants have a distinction award of £2,500 per annum, 10% have £1,500, and 20% have £500. Thus one of three was expected to earn more than the basic scale, and the actual average income difference between consultants and GPs was greater than comparison with the basic scale alone would imply. Spens Report on Consultants and Specialists, p. 11.

13. Evidence of Joint Consultants Committee in *Royal Commission; Minutes of Evidence,* p. 63.

14. Taking the average net income of GPs and the top of the consultant basic scale, the ratio was less than one to two in the Spens reports (£1,111 and £2,500), and more than two to three in 1954 (£2,222 and £3,100).

The new figures had been arrived at through different mechanisms and for different stated reasons. They could be interpreted in various ways: as a comparative victory for the General Medical Services Committee in forcing the question of GP pay to a state of crisis; as a comparative lack of pressure exerted by the Joint Consultants Committee working through the Whitley negotiating machinery; as an error in the original Spens relativities; or as a mark of the increasing status of the general practitioner. Possibly each of these factors played a part. The Danckwerts award had been a notable achievement for general practitioners. By forcing Parliament to produce the extra money to cover the award through supplementary estimates, it also relieved the Ministry of Health of the unpleasant necessity of refusing income raises because of its straitened health budget. The advantage of having income decisions for major pressure groups made by a nonparticipant was thus apparent to both sides.

The Royal Commission on Doctors' and Dentists' Remuneration

In 1956 the income situation reached a second crisis which again could not be contained within normal negotiating machinery. The General Medical Services Committee and the Joint Consultants Committee set up their own joint negotiating committee to cover both GPs and hospital medical staff, and in June of that year they submitted directly to the Minister and the Secretary of State for Scotland a claim for an across-the-board increase of at least 24 per cent, thus bypassing the Whitley machinery.[15] Later the British Dental Association submitted a claim for the same increase for all NHS dental practitioners and specialists. The medical profession again based its claim on rises in the cost of living since the Spens reports; again the Ministry rejected the request. The medical and dental professions were unified as perhaps never before, and the Ministry of Health was caught once again in the impossible position of being limited by budgetary consideration while faced by the need to maintain good relations with the profession. Joint negotiations for determining broad income levels through the Whitley machinery (for hospital and dental staff) and between the Ministry and the General Medical Services Committee (for GPs) had broken down. In future these committees would be limited to the detailed application of income scales.

The previous income crisis had been resolved by arbitration. This had proved only a short-term solution. It had not determined whether medical incomes should be tied to some kind of gauge, such as the BMA claimed was implied in the Spens Committee reports. If not, then some other foundation for income policy was required, and this could be decided only after full-scale inquiry. The government's solution was the appointment of a Royal Commission early in 1957. Meanwhile, consultants, GPs, and dentists received an interim pay increase of 5 per cent, and junior staff an in-

15. *Report of the Ministry of Health for 1956,* Cmnd. 293, p. 117.

crease of 10 per cent. The antagonism of the medical profession was not allayed by these announcements. The Commissioners began their work, in their own words, "against a background of controversy." [16] The BMA saw the Royal Commission as a delaying tactic. In a strategy that was to be repeated in the equally bitter pay disputes of 1964–65, it proclaimed that resignations would be sought from practitioners, to be held as a threat of withdrawal from the National Health Service if an immediate income settlement were not made.

The efficacy of such action depended on solid support from the whole profession; but GP and consultant interests were not unified. Once again a Royal College president moved independently of the BMA, on an inner circle of public influence. After certain assurances from the Prime Minister and the Royal Commission's chairman (Sir Harry Pilkington), Sir Russell Brain, President of the Royal College of Physicians and Chairman of the profession's Joint Negotiating Committee, rejected the BMA's policy of noncooperation. The BMA was thrown into confusion. Reluctantly, in June 1957, its representative body agreed to give evidence to the Commission and indefinitely to postpone withdrawal of services. The BMA had revealed an essential weakness. It had been neither constructive nor successful in its policy, and thus had satisfied neither its progressive nor its militant members; and it could not count on consultant support.

The Royal Commission reported in 1960; it did not vindicate the BMA's position. The career earnings of consultants in 1955–56 were greater than the career earnings of any of the other professions surveyed, which included accountants, lawyers, architects, university teachers, and university graduates in industry. Although other professions could claim a higher proportion of really large incomes, consultants had the advantage in terms of the majority of their members. Taking the median income of the professions in the age group 30 to 65 years, consultants ranked first, followed by general dental and medical practitioners. Nevertheless, after studying the evidence, the Commission concluded that incomes of both doctors and dentists ought to be raised. Accepting the Commission's advice in every detail, the government agreed to an increase in medical incomes under the NHS by approximately 21 per cent.[17] The award was to be backdated to January 1960 and to apply for approximately three years. The profession appeared reasonably satisfied with this conclusion and agreed to accept the Commission's recommendations as a "package deal." The immediate problem of income levels was thereby settled.

The package included changes in the structure of the GP income pool. Private practice, group practice loans, and government pension contribu-

16. *Royal Commission; Report,* Cmnd. 939 (HMSO, 1960), p. 1.

17. According to the figures collected by the Royal Commission, the average "career earnings" for all NHS doctors in 1955 between the ages of 30 and 65 were £84,000. The Commission recommended an average of about £102,000, an increase of 21.4%. *Royal Commission; Report,* pp. 40, 151.

tions were now to be excluded from the global figure, but two other benefits previously omitted were now included: inducement payments to encourage GPs to work in certain areas, and money earned by GPs after retirement age. Thus, as an additional confusion in an already confused situation, the final approved net average income for general practitioners was not directly comparable to the average income which had existed previously.[18] Two matters were left open in the case of general practitioner pay. The Royal Commission, arguing in favor of a greater spread of incomes, had recommended that £500,000 a year from the central pool be set aside for distribution to GPs as extra pay, unrelated to the capitation scheme and somewhat like the distinction awards system for consultants. Thus some GPs would receive additional awards each year for recognized merit. One suggestion was that 1,000 GPs (out of the total of 21,000) might receive an extra £500 a year as a straight salary benefit, on top of normal income; but this was rejected by the profession. The Ministry of Health had also insisted that £1 million of the increase in the pool money after the package deal be reserved to develop "methods of making the best possible general medical service available to the public." [19] Thus not all of the GP's income under the Commission's award was to be paid in the form of capitation fees. Because the pool was finite, being determined by the agreed average net income and the number of GPs, each new invention or improvement in general practitioner pay took another slice out of the cake. Consultant pay continued to be simple—a straight salary together with certain allowable expenses; general practitioner pay became more complex at each pay award.

For long-term and periodic income reviews the Royal Commission recommended a small "Standing Review Body" which would continue the Commission's work on a permanent basis; it would therefore be formally outside the National Health Service. The Review Body would have some of the characteristics of existing income machinery for senior civil servants—a parallel the BMA did not altogether relish:

> The comparison often made with the Coleraine Committee carries with it the suggestion that the doctor is more and more being looked upon

18. GPs were to receive an average net income after expenses of £2,425 from official sources, which corresponded to a previous income of £1,975; an increase of 22.8%. The new basic scale for consultants was £2,550 to £3,900. This represented an increase between 21% and 26% over the levels agreed in 1954, although there had been two interim increases. In addition, the amounts of distinction awards were also increased.

19. The merit system was rejected by the profession in 1962 but continued to be raised for discussion. For the second proposal, it was recommended that £750,000 should be applied as extra "loading" fees for Patients 1,001 to 1,500 on a doctor's list; but that £250,000 should be reserved as a postgraduate education fund for general practitioners. The sum was to come out of the global pool—and thus out of the total earnings of GPs; consultants, on the other hand, as salaried employees, had their postgraduate training paid outside the amount allocated for their income. See *Brit. Med. J.* Suppl. *ii* (1960), 84, and *Brit. Med. J. i* (1962), 1125.

as a public or civil servant, working in a health "service" rather than as a professional man in direct contact with his patient.[20]

In future, the BMA proclaimed, the virtues of self-reliance, independence, and responsibility, together with the freedom to act without the intervention of a third party, would "find their most fruitful soil in the private practice of medicine, which it has always been the policy of the BMA to safeguard and foster." Nevertheless, the BMA accepted the Review Body with good grace. Indeed, it was difficult to think of an alternative.

The creation of review machinery could be seen as a successful attempt by the medical profession to overcome some of the penalties of being state servants. In terms of income determination, the wheel had come full circle; for the Standing Review Body was performing a function similar to that of the original Spens committees. From the point of view of the Ministry of Health, the Review Body removed from the Ministry's jurisdiction the vital but unpleasant decisions regarding the level of professional remuneration for the most powerful and important group in the health service. No doubt the Ministry was relieved at this arrangement. High-level discussion with the profession might now concentrate exclusively on planning and policy.

To the profession the Review Body posed one immediate problem. Up to this point GPs and consultants had negotiated separately; each branch had presented its claims in terms of the income of the other. The Royal Commission had heard evidence from all interested parties. The Review Body of its very nature was unlikely to make enormous changes in income policy, since all relevant questions had been discussed exhaustively in the Commission's own evidence. At least its first pronouncement would concern general income levels—the pricing of doctors' services—rather than major changes in the relative income or income structure of each branch of the profession.

The Royal Commission had declined to enter the arena of internal differences in income between consultants and GPs, merely observing that "the broad relationship between the earnings of those in the hospital service and of those in general practice should be maintained unchanged." According to the figures of existing incomes from all sources (including consultants' distinction awards and private practice), the average (median) consultant earned £3,130 in 1955–56 and the average GP £2,160—a ratio of about three to two. Since the Royal Commission clearly superseded the Spens reports, it might appear that this magic ratio, arrived at fortuitously, could continue indefinitely and that every increase in pay to one branch would be accompanied by a parallel increase to the other. A new era of difficulty was about to begin.

One question raised in 1948 had been the potential for conflict between the two branches if the British Medical Association represented both in pay negotiations with the National Health Service. This argument had been used

20. *Brit. Med. J. i* (1962), 101.

in support of the Joint Consultants Committee, which included representatives of the Royal Colleges. General practitioners continued to be represented by the General Medical Services Committee, which was for all intents and purposes a BMA committee. The divided administrative structure, with its implications of separate income negotiations, had stimulated this division of professional interest groups. As a result, the basic relativity appropriate to generalist and specialist practice in an increasingly specialized environment tended to be overwhelmed by sectional interests. One result of the new call for unity was to be a crisis within the BMA.

10

Problems of Hospital Medical Staffing

The different methods of pay negotiations underlined the administrative division of the medical profession into general practitioners and hospital staff. There was virtually no career structure in general practice; the young doctor left hospital after one, two, or more years of experience, usually to become an assistant in an established practice in which he hoped before long to become a partner. In hospital practice there was, however, a well-defined model, prescribed under the Spens Committee report of 1948 and based on conditions pertaining in the major voluntary hospitals in the prewar period. This pattern was subject, in the first years of the National Health Service, to the strains not only of an evolving national staffing structure but also of increasing medical specialization. Not surprisingly, problems soon developed at all levels of hospital staffing, and there was an increasing need for a new staffing policy.

The Spens Training Ladder: Immediate Problems

The Ministry memorandum on the development of specialist services (1948) had recommended consultant charge of inpatient beds and outpatient sessions, as had been customary in the old voluntary hospitals.[1] The Spens report envisaged a training ladder of about seven years. This would include one year as a "preregistration" house officer in medicine and surgery before the doctor's name was admitted to the medical register; one further year in a training post as a senior house officer; next a junior registrar post for about two years (at the age of 26 or 27); and eventually a senior registrar or chief assistant post for about three years before attaining consultant status.[2]

The structure was based on traditional teaching patterns rather than on strictly service needs. Little thought was given to modifying the traditional teaching hospital structure for the new comprehensive hospital service; it was merely standardized and transposed to all hospitals. The development of the grade of Senior Hospital Medical Officer (SHMO) as a second junior specialist grade somewhat modified this ladder; and at the same time the

1. Ministry of Health Circular RHB (48), no. 1.
2. Spens Report on Consultants and Specialists, pp. 8–9.

further tenure grade of Junior Hospital Medical Officer (JHMO) was added at about the registrar level. There were thus seven separate hospital grades, each with its own salary level. Each moreover was an established "post"; that is, even the consultant grade appointment was allowable only to an already established vacancy. In the junior positions there were house officers and senior house officers; above them were registrars with limited tenure and JHMOs in permanent posts; and above them were senior registrars, who were consultant trainees, and the two permanent specialist grades of consultant and SHMO. General practitioners might return as part-time clinical assistants to consultants, but these posts again were outside the career ladder for consultant status.

The assumption of responsibility for hospital staff by the Ministry of Health had long-term planning implications that were not at first apparent. Inequalities and inconsistencies there may have been before but, because there was no central responsibility, these were not nationally evident. Even if they had been, there was no action that could be taken nationally to rectify them, since each hospital had been responsible only to itself. Now the Ministry of Health oversaw the total national position and had ultimate control of the number of doctors in each staff grade. Any failures in the staffing structure could thus be laid at the Ministry's door. This was the negative aspect. The positive aspects were the potential opportunity for redeploying specialist services with optimum effect—in terms of geography, specialty distribution, and the balance between general and specialist practice—and the creation of a streamlined educational and training structure.

If the opportunity to redistribute practitioners were to be realized, two conditions had to be met: first that there were adequate planning norms, and second, that the Ministry of Health was in a position to effect any necessary reform. Unfortunately, neither of these assumptions was true in 1948. The National Health Service came into effect at a time of intense social and scientific change. There were no norms capable of sustaining a national medical staffing structure. Indeed, there was a singular dearth of information on the number and characteristics of doctors already working. The BMA did not have a large research and statistics department; and, although it claimed to hold records of all doctors, these were not initially transferred to the Ministry for its own use. Not until 1955 was a statistician appointed to develop a central statistical unit at the Ministry of Health, and it was only in 1958 that detailed descriptions of senior medical staff were requested from the employing boards for punch-card analysis. Policy over the whole of the period 1950–58, eight years of growing hospital staffing difficulties, was handicapped by the lack of readily available data.

The training ladder structure assumed that the individual would start at the bottom as a recruit and end at the top as a fully trained professional. He learned by doing, each grade giving him extra skills and extra responsibility. The internal balance of the system was thus important for its success. If there were more than one or two juniors (for example, one house officer and one registrar) to each consultant or in each "firm" headed by two consultants, the individual tuition that was the essence of apprenticeship was weakened. It was also important that the structure should be so balanced that each promising junior would have a reasonable chance of moving up to the next grade and ultimately, if he wished, to a consultant post. This balance was particularly important under a national system in which the staffing structure was open to public and professional criticism and national trends might for the first time be discerned. It was important in the National Health Service for a further reason: the new hospital service would provide a career structure of its own, and the previous flexibility between junior hospital posts and general practice would concurrently be reduced.

But even at the time of the Spens report (1948), the balance between categories of medical staff in hospitals was being subjected to service demands quite different from those of the training ladder. These were the demands of increasing specialization, both of senior staff and of departments, in teaching and nonteaching hospitals alike. First, the more sophisticated the specialty, the greater was the need for specialized residents. The registrar in general medicine could no longer easily double as registrar in cardiology, psychiatry, or physical medicine. As a result, as the specialties fragmented, the supporting grades also had to diversify and expand in numbers. Second, the role of both the consultant and his junior staff was changing. In the 1930s the senior registrar was the consultant's apprentice. By the 1950s, hospital junior medical staff were required to fulfill necessary technical procedures. The patient was no longer admitted to nursing care while awaiting the weekly visit of the great man. Instead, the junior doctor sprang immediately into action, armed with modern therapeutic drugs and with access to refined pathological and radiological diagnostic facilities. By the time the consultant arrived, all necessary preliminaries were completed. Because of this, hospital care became more effective, the average length of stay was reduced, and the number of inpatients seen in any period rapidly increased. But this in its turn stimulated the demand for an even larger number of junior medical staff to act as ever-more efficient aides to the consultant staff.

A third effect of specialization was that the consultant himself was drawn more intimately into hospital work. Hospital patients were given more medical attention; more procedures required expert help (for example, X rays or laboratory tests) or expensive equipment. The old consultant fields—general medicine, general surgery, and obstetrics—were increasing less rapidly than other specialties that were more explicitly technical. By 1949, 17 per cent of consultants were pathologists or anesthesiologists, and a further 7 per cent were in radiology or radiotherapy. These specialists were virtually tied to hospital work. Other specialists were able to continue flourishing private practices from their consulting rooms in town, but even they were becoming more dependent on hospital facilities, and their practice was hospital rather than office based. For these reasons, realignments in the internal medical staffing structure of the hospital were needed, irrespective of the hospital's new place in a free national service.

The creation of the National Health Service at this particular point of time exaggerated such changes through the introduction of salaried specialist service and by the consequent reduction of private practice; through a more attractive payment system for junior hospital staff (enhanced by government scholarships for those leaving the armed services); through the optimistic picture of future consultant opportunities painted in the Ministry's 1948 circular on the development of specialist services; through the attitude of the consultant review committees and the low state of general practice; and through the expansion of ex-municipal hospital staffs to approach the staffing levels of the ex-voluntary hospitals. The Spens training ladder was doomed to failure from its beginning.

It was not unnaturally expected by young doctors that there would be room at the top for most of those who elected the training ladder. Initial experience bore this out. In the first full year of the service (1949–50), the number of consultants in England and Wales was increased by almost 9 per cent and, in the first three years taken together, consultant numbers rose by a fifth. In some of the nonteaching hospital groups the expansion of medical staff was immediate and dramatic. A typical illustration is provided in Ipswich, an industrial and market town of about 120,000 population.[3] A hospital management committee was set up under the East Anglia Regional Hospital Board to organize local general hospitals. It took over, besides a number of small GP units, two hospitals, each of about 300 beds. One, originally founded as a poor-law hospital, was run by the local authority; the other was a voluntary hospital. In 1947—the year before the Health Service Act came into operation—the two hospitals had a total of fourteen consultants, of whom three (two pathologists and one radiologist) were whole time. There were three full-time doctors in the middle grades (one resident medical officer, one resident surgical officer, and one medical superintendent), and five house officers. Anesthetizing and dental work were undertaken by general practitioners who came in as required. By the end of 1949 the number of consultants had jumped from fourteen to twenty-three, of whom six were full time. These included a number of specialists not previously designated: pediatrics, geriatrics, anesthesiology, dental surgery, and orthodontics. The number of SHMOs, senior registrars, and registrars—the equivalent of the old middle grades—increased from three in 1947 to fourteen in 1949; and in the latter year were spread over nine different specialties. House officer posts increased from five to fourteen in the same period. Thus, in a mere two years the consultant complement was raised by 60 per cent, while the other grades were expanded by 250 per cent. Excluding general practitioners, the total number of medical staff had risen from twenty-two to fifty-one. By far the greatest expansion in this group, as

3. Personal communication from Mr. John Williams, Group Secretary, Ipswich Group Hospital Management Committee

elsewhere, was in the middle grades. Most of the staff were now occupying posts designated by the Spens Committee as part of the consultant training ladder; under the Spens plan, they could reasonably hope to rise to consultant status. The position in Ipswich was no isolated case. This pattern of expansion was being repeated all over the country. In prewar terms, the ranks of the middle grades were becoming excessively swollen. Figures from the BMA indicate that before World War II there were more consultants and specialists than other grades of hospital staffs.[4] After the war the situation was reversed.

It was at this time the deliberate policy of the Ministry of Health to delegate as far as possible planning and policy decisions to the regional hospital boards and boards of governors. The boards had before them the 1948 document on planning consultant services, prepared by the Ministry; and they had requests for additional senior staff coming to them from their medical advisers and from their constituent hospital management committees. There was no national control of medical posts, just as there was no national control of administrative, nursing, or technical staff. Each board decided, on the basis of the money it had available to it, how many staff, in which categories, it required. Staff posts were thus made on the basis of immediate need instead of a long-term, balanced career structure, and one region did not know what the next region was doing. The Spens report did not appear until the middle of 1948—too late for all the ultimate planning ramifications to be considered before the first influx of staff had been appointed. Thus the Minister had a plan but no control of the numbers in post, while the boards had control of numbers but no long-term national plan.[5] All these factors together increased the number of young men and women on the consultant training ladder faster than the consultant posts became available. Ultimately, either the number of posts for consultants and SHMOs would have to be increased or the training period in hospital would have to be lengthened.

Too Many Senior Registrars

The short era of rapid expansion immediately before and after July 1948 soon gave way to one of financial restraint. Public alarm began to be ex-

4. According to BMA figures the number of "consultants and specialists" in Great Britain rose from about 3,000 to 4,000 between 1937 and 1947; the number of staff employed in hospitals in other grades rose from 2,400 to 8,200 in the same period. BMA Statistics Branch (personal communication).

5. In the latter part of the war the proportions needed in the various hospital grades were purportedly "all very carefully worked out before the service started" by the Ministry, and postwar training grants were geared to these predictions. One eminent consultant (Sir James Paterson Ross) ascribed some difficulties in the senior registrar grade to a retirement age for NHS consultants of 65 years, whereas in the prewar voluntary hospitals (the basis of the calculations) it had been age 60. *Royal Commission; Minutes of Evidence,* Questions 4197–99.

pressed at the "excessive" cost of the health service in comparison with original estimates. The worsening of general economic conditions caused the Chancellor of the Exchequer, in March 1950, to impose a ceiling on the amount of money available from the Treasury to the Health Service. A national review of staffs (medical, nursing, and other) was decided on in the latter part of 1950 as a basis for staffing control, and this review was conducted by small teams of experts during the next two years.

In this atmosphere of retrenchment it was forcefully revealed that there were in 1950 over 2,800 registrars and senior registrars in the hospital service. Registrars were expected to remain in that grade for only two years, senior registrars for three. This would imply, if all aspired to consultant status, a complete turnover of 2,800 every five years. But consultant status was limited to the number of available posts, which at the time was only 5,600. If consultant status was to be reached by age 35, the average tenure of consultant posts was some thirty years; the turnover of consultants was therefore relatively slow. Even allowing for continued expansion in the number of consultant posts, it was clear that all those on the training ladder could not be absorbed; and these totals excluded those 2,000 doctors who had originally been graded senior hospital medical officers and could also legitimately aspire to consultant status. According to the Ministry's calculations for the near future a total of only 600 senior registrars and some 1,100 registrars would be needed. It followed that some 800 senior registrars and 300 registrars were redundant.

At this point of crisis (October 1950) the Ministry of Health endeavored to impose central control. The SHMO grade was originally intended to be temporary. Advantages were now claimed for establishing permanent and expanded arrangements for this grade, to provide doctors with a career post of limited scope, of lower responsibility, and requiring less than a consultant's skill, at least in some specialties and in some hospitals.[6] Although the original concept of the SHMO as the GP-specialist was not entirely excluded, the emphasis was now on a permanent hospital staffing grade for all specialties in which a lesser or limited level of skill could be incorporated and which would absorb some of the excess of senior registrars.

The Ministry further recommended discontinuing the appointment of existing senior registrars in their third and subsequent years, termination of second- and third-year registrars, and annual review of the performance of

6. The skill and experience of SHMOs were not thought adequate for general medicine, general surgery, or obstetrics and gynecology; nor for highly technical fields such as neuro, plastic and thoracic surgery. In other specialties a limited field of work was suggested: certain aspects of chronic illness, chest diseases, geriatrics, psychiatry, and infectious diseases, together with certain types of outpatient work (antenatal clinics, child welfare, refraction sessions, venereal disease). SHMO status was thought appropriate in the "service" specialties— anesthesiology, pathology, and radiology. The groups divided themselves neatly into specialties that were fashionable (and thus well staffed with consultants and senior registrars) and those that were relatively unfashionable career choices. See RHB (50), no. 96.

registrars and senior registrars in post.[7] The young specialist could no longer put up his plate in the community and built up a private practice, for there was little market for his services. Since there was no way of becoming a recognized specialist except by being appointed to a consultant or SHMO post, this meant that senior registrars would be forced to emigrate; or to go into general practice, almost certainly with the attitude that it was an inferior calling; or to go into a different field of medicine, possibly ill-equipped to do so because of having worked for several years in another specialty.

The profession's reaction to the Ministry proposals for registrars was one of violent indignation, followed by immediate and effective lobbying to reverse the decision. Under the pressure, the Ministry was forced to modify aspects of the original memorandum. In 1951 the registrar grade was redesignated as a staffing and not a training grade, and tenure of a senior registrar post was increased from three to four years in 1952. Concessions were also made in 1954 for retaining "time-expired" senior registrars on a year-to-year basis while they looked for jobs. The medical profession, largely through the efforts of the Joint Consultants Committee, had won a major battle on behalf of senior registrars. But the Spens training ladder had broken down and the concessions made to the profession, although they reduced individual misery, did not solve the basic issues. The imbalance, although gradually reduced, was to continue for many years. In 1958, all except 220 of the 1,000 senior registrars were 33 years old or over, and 92 were over age 42; the Spens report had envisaged appointment to a consultant post at the age of 32. For one attractive consultant post in obstetrics, the Royal College declared in 1958, thirty to fifty qualified applicants might be expected.[8] With each successive year the chance that "time-expired" senior registrars could gain a consultant post was reduced, and they were becoming less and less able to survive a possible transfer into another branch of practice.

The senior registrar problem, although perhaps the most urgent, was only one of the problems of hospital medical staffing as a whole. There were two others that were equally vexing: the future of the SHMO grade, and the continuous demand for increases in supporting staff at junior levels. These matters were also discussed by the profession and the Ministry of Health in the early 1950s; but, as with the senior registrar dilemma, there were no clear solutions.

The SHMO grade provided a body of salaried specialists who were not generally considered of consultant status or who were not expected to do consultant work. Since there was no definition of consultant status or consultant work, the SHMO's exact role was somewhat obscure. With the ex-

7. RHB (50), no. 106. The background and outcome of the senior registrar question is described in detail by Harry Eckstein, *Pressure Group Politics*, pp. 113–25.
8. Ministry of Health, Department of Health for Scotland. Report of the Joint Working Party, *Medical Staffing Structure in the Hospital Service* (Platt report) (HMSO, 1961), p. 68. *Royal Commission; Minutes of Evidence*, Question 4363.

pansion of numbers and the broadening of the concept of the grade to include new posts, new definitions of responsibility were needed. The British Medical Association, looking back in 1958, considered that SHMOs had been exploited, because many had both the training and responsibilities of full consultants, and the grade carried "an unwarranted stigma of professional inferiority"—a carry-over from the initial grading process. The BMA spoke of great dissatisfaction regarding status, prospects, and remuneration for this grade. The number of SHMOs, instead of declining, was rising almost as rapidly as the number of consultants (Table 2), and the unfortunate older SHMO had to face the permanent prospect of subconsultant status with its "attendant frustration and intense dissatisfaction." Cases were quoted of SHMOs outnumbering consultants in particular areas or particular specialties, and it was stressed that the SHMO was eligible for career earnings of £34,000 less than his consultant colleagues.[9] More than once it was suggested that the Ministry was employing SHMOs as consultants but refusing to pay them the rate for the job.

The strain on both SHMO and senior registrar posts could have been eased if the consultant grade had been enlarged to include both senior and junior specialists, or if the SHMO grade had been redesigned as an essential part of the consultant career ladder. In a sense, therefore, the vital problem was, as before the war, the definition of consultant—a question still unresolved despite the activities of the medical review committees. The existence of a relatively small body of consultants was thought to ensure high standards and enhance status. But it was not clear whether enhanced status was due to the competitive system or to significantly better performance; it might, for example, have been possible to double the number of consultants within a reasonably short period without jeopardizing the standard of consultant care. Certainly, the excess of senior registrars in the early 1950s indicated an untapped pool of potential consultant talent, and there may have been a number of SHMOs who could legitimately aspire to consultant rank, even though they had not been redesignated as consultants in the series of SHMO reviews that followed the initial grading process.

The number of consultants was limited by extraneous forces. Consultants themselves had two built-in and long-held disincentives to expand their rank. First, since hospital beds were a status symbol, the incumbent was loath to share his allocation of beds with new appointees. The bed-block system, hallowed by tradition if not always justified, was thus a barrier to change, and there was little call for additional consultants except in clearly overworked and understaffed specialties. As a result, instead of automatic standardization of beds per consultant in particular fields, existing differences tended to remain. Consultants were also disinclined to share their private practices with expanded ranks. In 1955, one third (32 per cent) of consultants were on whole-time contracts; the remaining two thirds were free to undertake private work. Part-time SHMOs were also entitled to private prac-

9. Ibid., p. 1238 and Appendix, p. 14.

TABLE 2. *Estimated Numbers of Medical and Dental Staff by Grades; England and Wales, 1949–1956*

Grade	1949	1956	Percentage Change 1949–56	
Consultants				
Medical	4,959	6,490	+ 30.9	+ 29.8
Dental	232	249	+ 7.3	
Senior hospital medical				
officers	1,860	2,314	+ 24.4	+ 26.2
Senior hospital dental				
officers	159	234	+ 47.2	
Senior registrars *				
Medical	1,390	1,020	− 26.6	− 24.6
Dental	24	46	+ 91.7	
Registrars *				
Medical	1,462	2,438	+ 66.8	+ 68.3
Dental	16	50	+212.5	
Junior hospital medical				
officers	401	592	+ 47.6	+ 47.6
Junior hospital dental				
officers	1			
Senior house officers *				
(junior registrars)				+148.5
Medical	780	1,932	+147.7	
Dental	4	16	+300.0	
House Officers *	2,633	2,681		+ 1.8
Total				
Medical	13,485	17,467	+ 29.5	
Dental	436	595	+ 36.5	
Medical and dental	13,921	18,062		+ 29.7

* Grades of limited tenure.

Notes: The figures from registrars down exclude a few part-time and honorary staff whose number is unknown. General practitioners working part-time in the hospital service are not included.

Source: Evidence of H.M. Treasury and the Health Departments to the Royal Commission on Doctors' and Dentists' Remuneration, 1957–1960, *Evidence*, p. 708.

tice, but were limited by the referral system; GPs as a whole were more likely to refer patients to specialists of consultant status than to those who had been graded SHMO by consultant appointments and review committees.

The Joint Consultants Committee described appointment to consultant status in 1958 as being "dependent upon the possession of appropriate qualifications and ability." But if this were so it could not be equally true, as was simultaneously being claimed by the BMA, that SHMOs were undertaking consultant work. "First you emphasize," said a perplexed critic, "that a consultant grading is something very personal; then you deal with a post that is a consultant post and a status that is a consultant status." [10] Two conflicting forces were in operation. The consultant elite was concerned to retain the consultant as a high-quality, well-educated, and comparatively rare product—therefore small in numbers. But hospital medicine required a greater number of expert specialists than the consultant branch alone could provide. Meanwhile hospital morale suffered because some 2,500 SHMOs felt they had been dealt with unjustly. Was the SHMO a specialist but not a consultant, or was he a kind of junior or assistant consultant? And how could each term be assessed?

Problems in Junior Hospital Staffing

Despite apparent shortages, consultants constituted the largest single hospital grade, containing well over one third of all hospital doctors. If it were expanded to include the SHMOs and the surplus senior registrars, over half the hospital doctors would be consultants; and the cherished "firm" system —which relied on a consultant and his apprentices—would have to be modified. But already the firm system was changing because of the increased demand for junior medical staff. As indicated in Table 2, the numbers of registrars and senior house officers increased far more rapidly in the first seven years of the service than the more senior or the most junior grades of staff. Clearly, a much greater proportion of young doctors was staying in hospital jobs for a longer period before entering general practice, or these middle grades were being expanded by doctors from abroad, or both factors were in effect.

The great expansion in the number of middle-grade posts in the early 1950s had a further effect on the organization of medical practice. There was a buyer's market in middle-grade posts; the practitioner had great freedom of choice and more opportunties to choose the specialty he preferred and to work in the hospitals with the highest reputation or situated in the most desirable areas. The individual might decide to apply for a registrar post at Hospital A, and, if he were unsuccessful, he might choose to go into general practice rather than go to Hospital B. This inevitably affected the geographical distribution of hospital staffs. Many hospitals by the late 1950s, particularly the nonteaching hospitals, were finding it difficult to get registrars at all, and even to fill their senior registrar posts. The senior registrar at the teaching hospital stood a better chance of being appointed to a consultant vacancy than his opposite number at the nonteaching hospital. In a situation of extreme competition for consultant posts, the man who accepted a

10. Ibid., Question 5033.

post as senior registrar outside a teaching hospital might feel he had taken on a greater risk than the situation merited. New entrants did not want to get their fingers burned as had their predecessors.

Thus, although there were too many senior registrars for the available number of consultant posts, and there were more than twice as many doctors in the grades of registrar, JHMO, and SHO in 1959 as there were in 1949, for about the same number of hospital beds, [11] some regional hospital boards were becoming desperate by the late 1950s for both senior registrars and registrars, especially in such specialties as radiology and psychiatry. Dr. T. Rowland Hill, of the Joint Consultants Committee, expressed the difficulty succinctly in 1958: "If you take a man today who is a senior registrar in general surgery doing advanced surgery, if he had taken up mental hospital work he would long ago have been a consultant." [12] Registrar posts were proving increasingly difficult to fill, especially with graduates of British universities or of British nationality. Sixty per cent of registrars in posts in the Sheffield region in 1957, and more than four out of five applicants for such posts, were of foreign nationality. The situation was worsened by an increasingly rapid turnover of registrars, both of those from abroad who had come to England for a higher diploma (for example the FRCS) and needed specified experience in registrar posts, and from British nationals who decided, on reaching a registrar post, to enter general practice. In Sheffield, between 1955 and 1958, the average registrar in ophthalmology, general surgery, or thoracic surgery remained in post for less than one year.[13] In some hospitals, one foreign registrar with English-language difficulties rapidly followed another.

Despite junior staff increases, the supply could not keep pace with the demand for juniors to perform technical procedures and give continuous hospital coverage. There appeared to be a shortage of consultants, a surplus of senior registrars, and a growing—in some cases desperate—shortage of registrars. There was still no national policy to dovetail the numbers and training of general practitioners with those of specialists. Indeed, the Joint Consultants Committee, which spoke for consultants on matters of hospital policy, thought it impracticable that the relative numbers of general practitioners and consultants should be determined in an "arbitrary manner." [14] Furthermore, it denied that the appropriate numbers in each field were necessarily interdependent. The committee appeared not even to have considered whether there would be a continuing trend toward more consultants and relatively fewer general practitioners.

11. Table 2 gives an estimated number of 2,664 medical and dental staff in the grades of registrar, JHMO, and SHO in 1949. In 1959 there were the whole-time equivalent of 5,801 doctors in these grades. By 1964 the number had risen to 7,429. Ministry of Health, *Annual Report for 1959,* p. 221; ibid. for 1964, p. 144.

12. *Royal Commission; Minutes of Evidence,* Question 351.

13. Ibid., pp. 1112–14.

14. Ibid., p. 1109.

Staffing Reappraisal: The Platt Committee

By 1959, at the end of ten full years of the National Health Service, the hospital staffing structure was in turmoil. The consultant training ladder suggested by the Spens report had shown itself unable to adapt satisfactorily to the new conditions imposed by specialization and by the National Health Service: a greater proportion of specialist time spent in hospitals, greater demands for specialist assistance at both senior and junior levels, the problem of balance between different grades, and the interrelation of teaching and service functions. These were in part problems of balance, of function, and of changed scientific expectations. It was evident that there was first a need for more detailed information on hospital staffs, and second, for a national staffing policy. The Ministry of Health was drawn in on both counts. Despite its reluctance, it was being forced by circumstance to assume greater central control.

In 1958 a joint working party was set up by the Minister of Health to reappraise the hospital staffing problem. The committee, chaired by Sir Robert Platt, President of the Royal College of Physicians, consisted of eleven members drawn from the English and Scottish health departments, the Joint Consultants Committee, the Royal Scottish Medical Corporations (Colleges), and the Central Consultants and Specialists Committee of the British Medical Association. The committee's first concern was the continued problem of too many senior registrars in medicine, surgery, and obstetrics and gynecology. However, it was immediately obvious that it would have to consider the total staffing pattern, and in fact the conclusions related chiefly to the two permanent specialist grades—consultant and Senior Hospital Medical Officer. For on the future of these grades hinged the future of the "firm" system of hospital staffing, the numerical balance between senior and junior staff, and the relative desirability of careers in general and specialist practice. If the consultant grade were considerably expanded, it might absorb some of the SHMOs, and that grade could be abolished. On the other hand, it might be desirable to retain a second specialist grade but incorporate it into the normal career structure so that the candidate would move to consultant status via the SHMO appointment. There were many possibilities. All had implications both for other hospital grades and for parallel developments in general practice, which was almost entirely divorced from the hospital career pattern.

The Platt report, *Medical Staffing Structure in the Hospital Service,* was published in 1961. First and foremost, the report was strongly in favor of continuing the existing system of full consultant responsibility for patients, and for the "firm" system of hospital staffing; a firm of two whole-time or maximum part-time consultants in acute medicine or surgery, working in a nonteaching hospital and with adequate supporting staff (a registrar and two housemen) might, it was thought, take responsibility for sixty to eighty inpatients, with the associated outpatient and emergency duties.[15]

15. Platt report, pp. 18–19.

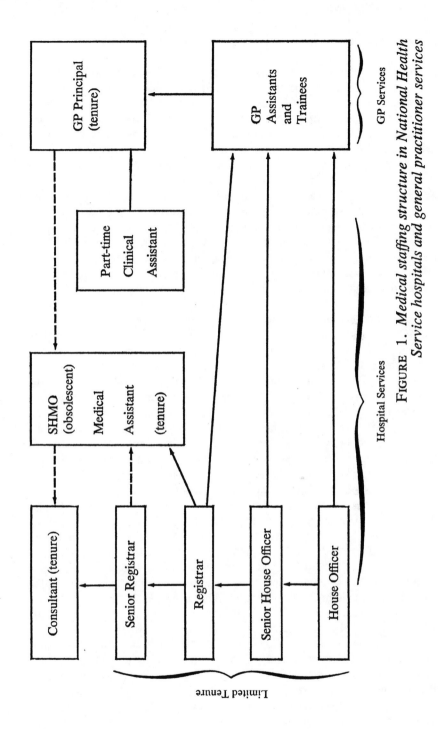

FIGURE 1. *Medical staffing structure in National Health Service hospitals and general practitioner services*

Simple calculations on these figures indicated that there were too few consultant posts, a fact that the committee fully endorsed. From a glut of senior registrars in the early 1950s, the situation had now moved to a supposed shortage of consultants—not necessarily of those of consultant quality but of those holding consultant posts. Exactly how many more were needed had to await the results of a thorough and detailed staff survey, to be undertaken at the report's instigation, for such planning data had not been routinely assembled either by the Ministry of Health or by the regional or teaching hospital boards. Special regional review committees (the Platt review committees) were once more to be established, this time to make a comprehensive survey of short-term senior staffing needs. In addition, permanent joint advisory committees of the university and the teaching and nonteaching hospitals were to be set up in each hospital region to organize and supervise the senior registrar program in their areas, particularly in relation to rotating senior registrars between the teaching and nonteaching hospitals.

The second major recommendation of the Platt report concerned the SHMO. It was agreed that there was a continuing need for a second permanent specialist grade at an assistant level. But the committee was anxious to free this grade from the old stigma of SHMO status and at the same time to widen its scope so that a more flexible use might be made of it and to link it more closely with the overall staffing structure of both general and hospital practice. The new grade would be called "medical assistant"; the SHMO grade would be abolished. Medical assistants would act as assistant radiologists, child welfare clinicians, ophthalmic refractionists, or nonoperating orthopedists—as did SHMOs—and the new grade would also lie outside the main promotion ladder. A major potential of the new medical assistant grade might be to prepare general practitioners for consultant posts.

The suggested structure (Figure 1) was promptly accepted by the Ministry of Health. However, the details of the new grade had yet to be agreed, by negotiation between the Ministry and the profession, on such matters as the future of those then in the SHMO grade and on the appropriate pay scales for medical assistants. Until these negotiations were completed, and until the Platt review committees presented their planning figures, the major part of the Platt Committee's report could not be implemented.

The Platt report represented the crossroads in hospital staffing policy. In 1961 the National Health Service was thirteen years old. The hospital staffing structure had radically changed since 1948, partly because the hospital itself had changed rapidly in this period and partly as a result of the nationalized hospital system. The period of consolidation and acceptance of the National Health Service was over. The Platt report by implication emphasized the need for further information and greater, more efficient use of medical manpower—not only in hospitals but also in relation to general practice. There were two immediate needs: first, for planning data based on the existing situation; second, for an end to the accepted convention of considering hospital problems as if general practice did not exist.

11

Changes in General Practice: The Question of Status

While the problems of hospital staffing were becoming increasingly acute and battles were raging over the question of income determination, general practitioners were being faced with their own problems. Perhaps the most important was their status; for if the GP's status relative to consultants was once determined and accepted, many of the other problems—the content and structure of general practice, the income differential between the two branches, the GP's place in the total manpower situation, and his relationship to the hospital—might be more easily determined.

The College of General Practitioners

It was essential, said one writer among many in 1948, that, if the best features of family practice were to be preserved, there should be a "potentiality both of prestige and financial reward in general practice. There should be some criterion by which a general practitioner can be recognized as outstanding, much as a physician gains prestige from his honorary appointments or his Fellowship [FRCP]." [1] Financial reward, as set up under the system accepted by the general practitioner, did not appear to meet this criterion. The capitation system of payment (described in Chapter 9) did not allow for differing standards of care, only for its overall quantity as judged in the number of patients registered with each doctor. The two Spens reports on doctors' remuneration (on general practitioners, in 1946, and on consultants in 1948) had put a damper on general practitioners' financial expectations relative to those of the consultant. There remained to the GP the same possibility that a number of specialists had already seized on—of improving his status through better postgraduate education programs, which would lead to a diploma that would be a symbol of the well-trained and exceptional general practitioner.

The question of a special diploma for general practitioner had been raised during World War II.[2] A new diploma would have two advantages. First, it would give a quality measurement to general practitioners; it would enable

1. *Brit. Med. J. i* (1948), 809 (W. Edwards).
2. See e.g. Frank Gray, *Brit. Med. J.* Suppl. *i* (1944), 121–22.

the better qualified or more assiduous to be distinguished from the mass, and some recognition of higher quality might eventually be incorporated into the capitation fee system. Second, and of increasing importance, it was recognized that a professional focus for general practice might be provided by a diploma from a College of General Practitioners.

The need for organized representation became more urgent when it was realized that general practice might become academically isolated and politically weakened under the National Health Service, as hospital and specialist services were developed. All agreed on the essential role and the vital function of general practitioners, but there was no ready identification of this role; GPs were, as one correspondent later remarked,

> without headquarters, without academic leadership of their own, without much influence over undergraduate or postgraduate teaching, and without the status of their specialist colleagues. . . . General practitioners had muddled along, and time and time again they had found themselves left behind, left out, edged out and even pushed out—as from certain cottage hospitals. . . . They had never organized themselves, and they had no one of the standing of the executive of the Royal Colleges to put forward their claims when big decisions had to be made.[3]

A plea for a Royal College of General Practitioners was made in 1949 by Dr. P. K. Murphy, who claimed that never had the interest of GPs been so "mismanaged or neglected" as in recent years: "Influence, status, material prosperity, it is complained, are waning." [4] Memoranda on the subject of a College were produced in September 1951 by Dr. F. M. Rose and Dr. J. H. Hunt before the General Practice Review Committee of the BMA. The reception was "by no means unfavorable," but the committee agreed that much further discussion on the subject was needed. Rose and Hunt published joint letters in the medical journals asking for comments for and against the proposal; the response was enthusiastic. Of those who wrote to the journals, or privately, the proportion in favor was over fifty to one. As a result, a steering committee was formed by the two doctors; it was chaired by a former Minister of Health, the Rt. Hon. Henry Willink.[5]

Opposition to a new College rallied around two main points: the financial difficulty of founding such a large-scale venture, and the fear that the movement would encourage further fragmentation of medicine. The first might well be overcome. The second was, however, largely a bogey. Divisions in medicine had begun long before. Consultant physicians, consultant surgeons, and consultant obstetricians—employed under the NHS on the

3. *Report of the College of General Practitioners*, 1953.
4. *Brit. Med. J.* Suppl. *i* (1949), 124.
5. John H. Hunt, *Brit. Med. J.* Suppl. *i* (1952), 335; see also *Brit. Med. J.* *ii* (1951), 908, 1582.

same terms to work in the same hospitals—had more in common than had any of the three with general practitioners, who were performing a different kind of medical role. Yet the Royal Colleges had missed the opportunity to combine on one site, and thus to represent all aspects of medicine. Neither the MRCP nor the FRCS was directly applicable to general practice, although some GPs held one or the other of these diplomas. Obstetricians had shown the advantage to a specialty's educational standards and professional status of founding a prestigious college of their own. Why should general practitioners be content with less?

By the end of 1952, there seemed no alternative to the founding of a separate College. The General Practice Steering Committee, in a unanimous report (November 1952), declared that the evidence was overwhelming for the foundation as soon as possible of an academic body with broad educational aims, to represent general practitioners in Great Britain.[6] The report said no complaint was lodged against the Royal Colleges or the BMA, but there is "a time in any family when the children grow up and want to manage their own affairs." Indeed, with medicine split into thirty different specialties, it was questionable that the Royal Colleges would have time and interest in the future to deal adequately with the academic problems of the 20,000 general practitioners in Great Britain. The Steering Committee had decided against a triple faculty for GPs under the aegis of the three Royal Colleges; it found that correspondents disliked the term "faculty" for its implication of inferiority. A separate College would enable general practitioners to cooperate on equal terms with bodies bearing an analogous relationship to other branches of the profession. "We accept the view," said the *Lancet* "that GPs are as much entitled to a college as are physicians and surgeons." [7]

The primary or overt purpose in founding a new college was educational. Medical students were passing their examinations (declared the Steering Committee) without ever having met or spoken to a GP, and without having seen one at work. The educational difficulties posed by specialization, which were already apparent before World War II, had become acute. At the same time a period of work in general practice for the aspiring consultant had become rare. Specialists spent all their time, from student to consultant, in the hospital environment and knew little of the problems and techniques of general practice: yet at the same time the emphasis of medicine was turning back to community and environmental influences on health and disease. Part of the policy for the new College would be to encourage closer contact between medical students and general practitioners. For postgraduate teaching in general practice, the College might collect information on the specific needs of GPs, help young practitioners to follow a special bent by increasing their knowledge in a particular field, and encourage the doctor to continue his education throughout his career. One of the criteria for membership of

6. *Brit. Med. J. ii* (1952), 1321, and as supplement to the *Practitioner*, Jan. 1953.
7. *i* (1952), 139.

the College might, it was thought, be so many hours of postgraduate instruction every few years—a suggestion that was later put into effect. Furthermore, the College might act as a center for general practitioners to discuss difficulties in their work, and it could sponsor special lectures and an exchange of visits with colleagues overseas; it could encourage and give practical guidance in research and assist the publication of good original work. Since family doctors were widely scattered, one of the early duties of the proposed College would be to establish regional subdivisions or faculties to facilitate communication throughout the country. The educational potential was enormous, and the correspondence columns of the medical journals were filled with enthusiastic suggestions.

It was envisaged that the new College would complement, and not replace, the functions of the BMA. General practitioners were determined to assert their position within the profession, rather than to create a bargaining power; they required more than anything a lustrous figurehead. One of the founder members wrote that the College would not be directly concerned with remuneration or terms and conditions of service.[8] But although the proponents of a new College eschewed questions of pay, they were concerned with other material aspects of the GP's status. One stated aim was to restore, or to establish, hospital beds for the general practitioner. The new College would also press for direct access for all general practitioners to laboratory and X-ray facilities so that they could do as much diagnostic work as possible from their own premises, and to ensure that they play their full part in development of health centers and clinics. A College provided a symbol for the resurgence of the general practitioners. This was of particular importance, for, as the Steering Committee remarked, "If a doctor is discouraged, there is no branch of medicine in which he can deteriorate more rapidly."

Thus, from the germ of an idea of a diploma in general practice, the concept of an academic center had grown; a center, moreover, that would improve general practice and would have a much wider educational role in relation to general practice than the Royal Colleges provided for the specialist. On whether admission to the College should be by examination, as was the case with the Royal Colleges, there was no immediate decision, although some felt that this would be a logical outcome.

The College of General Practitioners was founded in November 1952. Foundation membership opened on 1 January 1953, and during the first three weeks 1,007 members and 142 associates enrolled, most of whom came from the British Isles. By 12 February, 1,600 general practitioners had joined the College, and before it was six months old it had 2,000 members, none of whom, although there were admission requirements, had to take a formal examination. Practitioners applying for membership had to have passed their basic medical examinations from a university or from a

8. *Brit. Med. J.* Suppl. *ii* (1951), 175 (F. M. Rose).

College Conjoint Board not less than seven years earlier and to have engaged in general practice for at least five years; for associate status in the College, three years' practice experience was required. Each applicant was to be sponsored by two members, submit evidence of his practice, experience, and academic and administrative achievements, and, if necessary, be interviewed by the board of censors of the College.

The College went from strength to strength. At the end of its first decade (December 1962) it had 6,200 members and associates, thirty-seven regional faculties, of which fifteen were overseas, and three regional councils (Scotland, New Zealand, South Africa). During its first ten years the College focused largely on special training programs through the *Journal of the College of General Practitioners,* scientific meetings, and building up a library of tapes for circulation (Medical Recording Service) by Drs. John and Valerie Graves.[9] The College also set up evening discussions and courses, and organized a number of fellowships to enable general practitioners to attend a minimum of two weeks' postgraduate study at their old teaching hospital or at any other hospital, clinic, health center, or general practice of their choice in the United Kingdom. Collaboration with the General Register Office produced volumes of morbidity statistics in general practice. Such studies disclosed the potential and willingness among general practitioners for research.

The GP already had a function; he was now asserting his value as a member of a distinct professional group. Through these activities the College aimed to raise the professional standing and expand the role of the general practitioner. But he still did not have a recognized specialty. The GP might be regarded as a respectable participant in epidemiological research. This, however, was an activity additional to the traditional general practice duties of diagnosis, prognosis, treatment, and prevention of disease, by continuing contact with individual patients. The basic administrative problems of general practice remained. These included, besides a basic definition of general practice, imperative questions of its organization and the relative numbers of GPs ideally required in the total medical staffing situation. From these the College stood largely aloof.

9. A questionnaire sent out from the College in 1954–55 revealed the educational isolation of many general practitioners. After five years in a busy practice, the GP hardly had time to read any journals; and even when he did, the advances in medicine had been so swift that the journals were no longer intelligible. Some claimed that all they wanted to know was how to handle the new drugs and "I can get this from the drug firms." The tape circuit system of the College was started in 1957 in an effort to fill the gap. It brought GPs together in a stimulating atmosphere. Two thirds of the recipients of tapes in 1964 (a circuit taking five to six months to complete), invited up to ten persons to listen with them. The tapes covered the major specialties and included such titles as "The Acutely Ill Baby," "Dirty Air and Disease," "Squint," "Facing Facts about Toxemia," and "Sex Problems in General Practice." Some 8,000 tapes were being sent out every year all over the world. (Dr. Valerie Graves, personal communication.)

The General Practitioner and the Hospital

Although the changing role of the general practitioner was due to scientific rather than social forces, it was given extra impetus by the National Health Service. With free hospital treatment assured to all, a previously unfulfilled demand for consultative and specialist care emerged, which coincided with a period of increased technological efficiency in hospitals. Some of the effects of specialist utilization are shown in Table 3. Patients registered for NHS services with general practitioners rose from about 42.2 million in 1949 to 47.8 million in 1964—an increase of about 13 per cent. The number of patients moving through hospital inpatient services increased, in contrast, by 61 per cent in the same period. The new domiciliary specialist service (whereby consultants and SHMOs were able to visit the patient's home at the GP's request) expanded quickly. Outpatient attendances also immediately began to rise, although the number of visits made by each patient remained the same.[10] The hospital was confirmed as the consultative unit; the organization of general practice remained uncertain.

TABLE 3. *Hospital Patients and Patients Registered with General Practitioners, National Health Service; England and Wales, 1949–1964*

	Average Daily Number of Occupied Beds	Inpatients Discharged or Died During Year	New Outpatients at Consultant Clinics	Domiciliary Specialist Visits	Number of Names on GP Lists
	Number of units in thousands, to nearest thousand				
1949	397.6	2,936.6	6,148	132.4	42,200
1950	402.6	3,085.5	6,193	169.0	42,900
1951	406.8	3,259.2	6,299	175.5	43,100
1952	416.1	3,414.4	6,606	186.6	42,200
1953	424.1	3,543.5	6,731	208.4	42,400
1954	427.6	3,630.3	6,767	227.3	42,900
1955	426.0	3,652.0	6,787	241.7	43,500
1956	423.8	3,739.2	6,888	272.4	44,100
1957	420.2	3,793.6	6,927	294.3	44,700
1958	417.6	3,889.2	6,968	294.3	44,632
1959	412.6	4,000.3	7,109	310.1	45,059
1960	410.3	4,136.1	7,123	unknown	45,579
1961	404.4	4,269.0	7,216	307.1	46,264
1962	403.0	4,391.3	7,215	316.0	46,820
1963	404.0	4,575.7	7,383	323.6	47,325
1964	400.3	4,724.7	7,505	323.6	47,820

10. Ministry of Health, *Annual Report for 1949*, p. 119.

Proportional change; 1949 = 100

1949	100	100	100	100	100
1950	101	105	101	128	102
1951	102	111	102	133	102
1952	105	116	107	141	100
1953	107	121	109	157	100
1954	108	124	110	172	102
1955	107	124	110	183	103
1956	107	127	112	206	105
1957	106	129	113	222	106
1958	105	132	113	222	106
1959	104	136	116	234	107
1960	103	141	116	unknown	108
1961	102	145	117	232	110
1962	101	150	117	239	111
1963	102	156	120	244	112
1964	101	161	122	244	113

The figures include all NHS hospitals, general, special, and convalescent, and teaching and nonteaching hospitals. The number of names on GP lists is inflated for such reasons as dual registrations of the same patient. A more accurate assessment of the population is given in Table 8.

Source: Ministry of Health, Statistics Division and Annual Reports.

The general practitioner was caught between two stools. The expanding role of the hospital, allied with the enthusiasm for specialist practice, threatened his traditional function as an all-purpose doctor; the old single-handed practice in domestic surroundings was clearly obsolescent. At the same time, financial stringency had impeded the proposed health-center program, which would have encouraged GPs to work in groups. By the end of 1959 there were only twenty-three health centers in the whole of England, Wales, and Scotland, and not all of these were health centers in the accepted sense of the phrase.[11] They ranged from the elaborate opulence of Woodberry Down—a combined general practitioner and public health center set up for the sum of £198,000—to GP teaching units, GP diagnostic centers, or merely buildings that were specially erected for GPs working in partnership and had little or none of the additional services a health center might suggest. Their facilities varied enormously, their purpose was various, and they served no common population unit. Furthermore, both Ministry and profession were becoming doubtful about the purpose a health center should

11. See Medical Practitioners' Union, *Health Centre Report* (Oct. 1960).

serve. The 1920 Dawson report, when the health center's pattern was first strongly proposed, had been written in a very different medical environment, when the function of general practice was unquestioned and hospitals were mainly institutions providing beds for the treatment of the sick. By the 1950s, hospitals were centers for diagnosis as well as for highly specialized treatment procedures. Were health centers still necessary?

A second major difficulty in health-center development concerned the relationship between general practitioners and the local health authorities who were charged under the Act with providing the centers. Many general practitioners regarded any effort by local government with suspicion if not actual hostility. From many sides came complaints of bad relationships, poor liaison, and lack of consultation; in one case the general practitioners sent a deputation to complain about a local authority to the Ministry of Health. Even in relatively happy centers, there was reportedly a deep-seated distrust of the authority's motives: "It was for many G.P.s an effort to give up surgery premises under their own control to become tenants of the L.H.A. and matters were not helped by the slow rate of progress." [12] In the absence of health centers, the most practicable alternatives for general practice were the encouragement, first, of groups of general practitioners to work together out of common surgeries; and second, of new links between general practitioners and the newly streamlined hospital service.

The Ministry of Health had suggested in 1950 that general practitioners be employed in hospitals as part-time "clinical assistants" to consultants. One primary motive behind this suggestion was to alleviate the growing demand for junior and middle-grade medical staff in hospitals. Appointment as a clinical assistant did not imply full staff status for the GP nor did it allow him to admit his own patients to beds in hospital; typically, he assisted the consultant in the outpatient department by assuming delegated responsibility for particular outpatient sessions. Clinical assistantships appealed to a large number of GPs with special interests or with a desire to be more closely connected with a local general hospital. By 1964 more than 4,400 GPs were part-time clinical assistants, representing one out of every five practitioners. Their overall contribution in terms of hospital staffing was, however, relatively small, representing the equivalent of only 827 full-time hospital staff (Table 4). Furthermore, many clinical assistants were drawn to specialties that were already reasonably staffed; over one third assisted consultants in general medicine, general surgery, and obstetrics and gynecology. It seemed unlikely that the clinical assistant would take over middle-grade hospital work although, because of the peculiarities of the GP payment system (whereby hospital income gained by GPs was deducted from the global income pool), it was not clear how many other practitioners were inhibited from accepting hospital posts as a matter of principle.[13]

12. Ibid., pp. 21–22.

13. A GP who was a clinical assistant received income from the hospital in addition to his capitation fees. But the amount of hospital income—as part of the total

TABLE 4. *Employment of General Practitioners in Hospitals*

	Working in GP Units	Clinical Assistants and Others	
	Number	Number	Whole-time Equivalent
1953	2,908	3,700	480
1955	2,968	3,971	548
1957	3,105	4,187	582
1959	3,200	4,486	634
1961	2,318	4,064	685
1963	2,180	4,288	773
1964	2,174	4,462	827

This table also includes general dental practitioners.

Source: *Digest of Health Service Statistics*, 1962, Table 73, and Ministry of Health, *Annual Reports for 1963, 1964*.

A small number of GPs had access to hospital beds in general practitioner units, chiefly in the small cottage hospitals (which did not usually undertake major medical or surgical procedures) and in GP maternity units. Table 4 indicates that in 1964, 2,174 GPs had access to such units—about one of every ten practitioners—but the proportion appeared to be declining. Furthermore, although the number of beds allocated to GP units was steadily increasing, this still represented a minute proportion of all NHS hospital beds. In 1964 only 4 per cent of all beds in NHS hospitals (excluding those in mental hospitals) were the direct responsibility of general practitioners (Table 5). The Ministry of Health had already set out a policy of consultant responsibility for hospital beds, a policy that still holds. This was a logical decision in the increasingly specialized hospital environment. General practitioners were not trained to utilize the complex facilities of inpatent care. Almost all their experience was in GP surgeries and in patients' homes, and it was in these areas that the GP acknowledged special expertise. If he were to become the consultant's equivalent, a much greater training period in hospitals would be necessary. Meanwhile the GP could not claim a major interest in hospital medicine either through work as a clinical assistant or through admission of his own patients to hospitals.

A third—and in some ways the most immediately useful—link between GPs and hospitals was the encouragement of direct access by GPs to hospital

---

official income received by GPs—was deducted from the "pool," leaving less to be redistributed at the end of the year. Thus the more hospital work GPs undertook, the more did the GP suffer whose income came from capitation fees only. See p. 132.

TABLE 5. *Hospital Beds Allocated to General Practitioners*

Year	Maternity	Other Medical and Dental	Total	Nonmental Bed Complement %
1949			7,684 *	
1950			6,499 *	
1951			6,941 *	
1952			6,735 *	
1953	2,036	6,525	8,561	3.2
1954	2,480	6,667	9,147	3.4
1955	2,664	6,750	9,414	3.5
1956	2,911	6,866	9,777	3.6
1957	3,129	6,828	9,957	3.7
1958	3,373	6,980	10,353	3.9
1959	3,463	7,073	10,536	3.9
1960	3,685	7,108	10,793	4.0
1961	3,811	7,216	11,027	4.1
1962	3,944	7,080	11,024	4.2
1963	4,012	7,114	11,126	4.2
1964	4,090	7,071	11,161	4.2

* Totals are not strictly comparable with those for subsequent years.

Source: Annual Reports, Ministry of Health.

diagnostic departments. Hospital pathological and radiological facilities had never been open to most general practitioners. Partnerships among GPs before the NHS had been small in scale, usually with only two or three partners, no professional supporting staff, and the minimum of diagnostic equipment. The GP who wanted an X ray or a laboratory test for a patient had to refer him to the hospital's own medical staff, who might decide that such tests were unnecessary. Access to these service departments had been one of the points pressed for by the profession's negotiating committee in the 1940s; and after the Act came into effect the Ministry of Health, and later the College of General Practitioners, actively encouraged hospitals to throw open their departments to local general practitioners. As a result, the proportion of hospital pathological and radiological work done at direct general practitioner request rose steadily (Table 6), despite parallel increases in work done for other hospital departments. By 1964 10 per cent of the total workload of X-ray departments and 8 per cent of that of pathology departments were devoted to general practitioners' requests.

Each of these measures—appointment as a clinical assistant, access to

TABLE 6. *Proportion of Work Done for General Practitioners by Hospital Radiological and Pathological Departments; England and Wales, 1953–1964*

	Pathology		Diagnostic Radiology	
	Total work Load,* Millions	Initiated by GPs %	Total Work Load,† Millions	Initiated by GPs %
1953	37.8	4.0	18.2	8.3
1954	42.8	4.3	20.2	8.7
1955	46.9	4.2	21.2	8.6
1956	52.1	4.5	21.6	8.9
1957	56.6	5.0	21.1	9.1
1958	16.0	5.6	20.5	8.9
1959	17.3	5.8	21.1	9.0
1960	19.0	6.2	21.8	9.0
1961	20.6	6.5	22.5	9.1
1962	22.6	6.8	23.5	9.1
1963	24.9	7.2	25.1	9.6
1964	27.6	8.1	26.5	10.0

* From 1953 to 1957 the work load was measured by defined units of work; from 1958 to 1964 by the number of patient requests.

† Number of units of work.

Source: Ministry of Health, *Annual Report for 1955*, p. 27; *for 1956*, p. 148; *for 1958*, p. 270; *for 1964*, p. 141; and Gillie Report, p. 64.

beds, and use of hospital diagnostic facilities—increased the general practitioner's functional relationship with the hospital, but only to a limited degree. The GP seemed fated to continue as a nonhospital doctor with few direct links in his actual practice with the consultant staff of his local hospitals.

Access to diagnostic services reduced the justification for creating well-equipped diagnostic health centers specifically for general practice. At the same time, financial incentives were introduced to stimulate group practice among GPs. This was, however, little more than the extension of financial partnership on the old lines, rather than a new policy. One stimulus was provided by the changes made in the capitation fee structure in 1953 after the Danckwerts award. A "loading" or weighting factor had been introduced which gave additional payments in respect to the 501st to the 1500th person on the GP's list. Partnerships were allowed whatever distribution of patients attracted the greatest loading. For example, if a single-handed principal with a list of 3,000 took a partner, with no addition of patients at all the practice would receive extra pay for an additional 1,000 loadings—in 1959 a sum of £600.[14] This was an inducement for a principal to make his assistant (for whom no loadings were payable) a full partner. Further stimulation was given through the group practice loans plan introduced in 1954 and administered by the Ministry of Health—a group being defined as three to six GP principals working in close association (who were usually but not necessarily also in financial partnership), pooling fees and expenses from common premises, and employing among them at least one nonmedical assistant as a secretary, nurse, receptionist, or social worker. The combination of these measures encouraged a trend away from single-man practice that had already been apparent before the NHS; the marked trend under the NHS is shown in Table 7. But despite a fairly rapid increase in the number of

TABLE 7. *Single and Partnership Practitioners Providing Unrestricted General Medical Services*

Year	No. in Partnership	No. Practicing Single-handed	GP Principals in Single-handed Practice %
1952	9,745	7,459	43
1953	10,863	7,147	40
1954	11,583	6,899	37
1955	12,068	6,715	36
1956	12,514	6,568	34
1957	12,962	6,381	33
1958	13,253	6,346	32
1959	13,535	6,119	31
1960	13,936	5,897	30
1961	14,509	5,598	28
1962	14,879	5,422	27
1963	15,114	5,208	26
1964	15,221	5,000	25

Source: Annual Reports, Ministry of Health.

groups, one of four GPs was still in single practice in 1964, and the most popular size comprised only two partners. Only 600 of more than 20,000 principals providing unrestricted (comprehensive) GP services in 1964 worked in partnerships of six or more. All aspects of general practice taken

14. Ministry of Health, *Annual Report for 1958*, p. 95.

164

together, a considerable body of GPs were still isolated both from hospitals and their fellow practitioners. The financial incentives could thus claim only limited success.

Problems of Communication, Coordination, and Balance

While general practitioners worked in small partnerships outside hospitals, consultants were spending an increasing amount of time working inside. This raised obvious problems of communication. For the one out of ten patients whom GPs referred to the hospital for consultant advice, communication between the GP and consultant was largely by letter. One study of practice in London [15] indicated little personal relationship between GP and hospital staff. Eighty per cent of seventy-three general practitioners interviewed said they never discussed their patients' problems with a consultant, five doctors claiming that it would be unreasonable to take up the time of the hospital staff in this way. Only one third nominated the consultant they wished the patient to see; others merely referred patients to the appropriate department. Moreover, the study indicated a greater degree of personal contact between general practitioners and nonteaching hospital staff than with consultants in the teaching hospitals. Another study of letters from specialists to general practitioners [16] found that in only 6 per cent of these reports was there any indication of what was said to the patient about his illness; in less than four of ten applicable cases was the GP told that an operation was proposed (and in only one of fifty-one cases operated on was he told beforehand); 8 per cent of the outpatient reports arrived *after* the patient had been back to see the general practitioner, and in only 11 per cent of the emergency admissions was a report received by the general practitioner within forty-eight hours. In contrast, when pathological reports or tests were requested from hospitals offering those facilities to general practitioners, 100 per cent of the replies arrived on time. The timing of the arrival of the report, concluded the authors, was a major factor in the success or failure of the specialist–general practitioner relationship. On the other hand, a survey conducted by two GPs and an architect [17] of thirty-three selected general practices within fifty miles of London found morale high and hospital–doctor relations excellent, although there were some complaints of professional isolation. There seemed to be some difference of opinion as to what "good" relations signified.

The relationships between the two branches had implications other than those of personal communication—although this was one important facet that was to be encouraged in the 1960s. One vitally important but as yet barely considered aspect of general practice was the question of numerical balance. The home population of England and Wales rose by 10 per cent between 1949 and 1964; the number of GPs increased by 21 per cent in the

15. R. M. Acheson et al., *Brit. Med. J. ii* (1962), 1315–17.
16. R. de Alarcon et al., *Brit. Med. J. ii* (1960), 1663–64
17. John Fry et al., *Brit. Med. J. ii* (1962), 1311–15.

same period, and the number of hospital staff doctors (reflecting the increased load of hospital work) by as much as 55 per cent. Although both branches of practice were increasing, the numerical gap between them was becoming smaller. The picture is shown in Tables 8 and 9. In terms of the

TABLE 8. *National Health Service Medical Staff,*
England and Wales; 1949–1964

	Home Population (thousands)	General Practitioners	HOSPITAL DOCTORS		
			All	Consultants & SHMOs	Other
1949	42,970	18,165 (est.)	11,940	4,711	7,229
	(100) *	(100)	(100)	(100)	(100)
1954	44,274	21,165	14,644	6,353	8,291
	(103)	(117)	(123)	(135)	(115)
1959	45,386	22,105	16,144	6,841	9,303
	(106)	(122)	(135)	(145)	(129)
1964	47,401	21,903	18,449	7,453	10,966
	(110)	(121)	(155)	(158)	(152)

* Figures in parentheses are proportions as compared with 1949.

Source: Population figures from Ministry of Health *Annual Report for 1950*, p. 163, and *Registrar General's Statistical Reviews of England and Wales*, and *Quarterly Return*, December 1964. Figures for GPs and hospital doctors from Ministry of Health reports and statistics division. GP figures include GP principals, assistants, and trainees. Hospital figures show whole-time equivalents; they exclude honorary and temporary staff, and GPs with part-time hospital posts. Doctors serving in H.M. Forces are not part of the National Health Service and are therefore excluded.

number of doctors per unit of population, GPs still substantially outnumbered hospital staff (there were about forty-six GPs per 100,000 population to only thirty-nine hospital doctors), but the GP ratio had begun to decline. Eventually, decisions would have to be made by the profession and the Ministry of Health about the relative functions, efficiency, and importance of each branch of practice.

General and consultant practice continued to be considered as two parallel disciplines rather than as a cohesive profession. Rarely was the division questioned, although the structural problems of general practice had origins as old as the separate existence of the two branches. The GP claimed, through the capitation system, that he retained his professional independence as a self-employed person; although curiously it was not argued that

TABLE 9. *National Health Service Medical Staff; Number of Hospital and General Practitioners Per 100,000 Population, 1949–1964*

	General Practitioners	HOSPITAL DOCTORS		
		All	Consultants & SHMOs	Other
1949	42.3	27.8	11.0	16.8
1954	47.8	33.1	14.3	18.7
1959	48.7	35.6	15.1	20.5
1964	46.2	38.9	15.7	23.2

Source: See Table 8.

the consultant had lost his independence by becoming employed. GPs accepted a contract of service with the local executive council and, although an average allowance for expenses was made to them through the capitation system, they bore their own practice expenses. Many if not most GPs practiced from their own homes, retaining two or three rooms as their "surgery" premises (the name is a relict of the time of the surgeon-apothecary), but growing numbers were building centers designed for three, four, or more practitioners, with a central waiting area, several consulting rooms, and a secretary or dispenser. Such centers were almost invariably without X ray or any but the most simple laboratory equipment. In some areas the medical officer of health (of the local authority) arranged for a health visitor—a state-registered nurse with additional training in social work—to be attached to a group practice instead of to a district; in this case, the expense was borne by the local authority. The cost of building and staffing was usually borne by the GPs themselves, assisted by the group practice loans program, and the GPs often pooled their incomes and expenditures. Members of the partnership normally received most of their income from the NHS, but any GP might undertake private practice if he chose to do so.

Hospital consultants had a battery of staff at their disposal. If all hospital nurses, technicians, and other professional personnel were averaged out among all consultants irrespective of specialty, each full-time consultant (or equivalent number of part-timers) in 1964 would have had the services of two full-time hospital medical practitioners, thirty-five full-time members of the nursing and midwifery staff, and more than four other full-time trained professional or technical personnel besides secretarial and other supporting staff. The consultant bore none of the cost of this personnel. In contrast, for 21,000 GP principals, there were only 1,020 GP assistants and trainees.[18]

18. Ministry of Health, *Annual Report for 1964*, pp. 71, 144, 152, 154.

Figures for other staff are not available, but it is reasonable to assume that the average GP had the services of well below one ancillary staff member. While the College of General Practitioners was trying to raise the status of that branch, the practical differences between consultants and general practitioners were becoming more clearly marked.

As the consultant had specialized, the GP had been left as the only generalist. General practice was avowedly the foundation on which the NHS had been built, and was becoming increasingly necessary, but it was ill-organized and often inefficient. The hospital and the consultant were the effective organizational hub of the curative services. Instead of the specialties being related to general practice, general practice had to be related to the specialties and therefore (since they were equivalent) to the hospitals.

By forming their own College, general practitioners declared themselves professionally equal to the consultants and specialists. Structurally, financially, and educationally, however, the two branches were still unequal. The primary focus of the NHS between 1949 and 1961 had, not unnaturally, been on the development of hospitals from an uncoordinated jumble to a regional service. As general practitioners became more confident, better informed on organizational problems, and better organized, they became in the 1960s more vocal and more articulate about their position, their expectations, and their relative status. A crisis within general practice and a clash between the two branches was almost inevitable.

12

The National Health Service as an Educational Structure

A joint postgraduate educational structure might have alleviated some of the obvious disadvantages of the divided administration of GP and consultant services and raised the status of general practice. Each hospital region had been deliberately centered on a university medical school. The medical teaching center was thus given implicit regional responsibilities besides its existing functions as an undergraduate school and a local reference hospital. For the first time, virtually all consultants in a geographical area of two or three million population were on equal terms, working in one hospital service.

The university's influence might be expected to extend throughout the postgraduate field, through formal educational programs and informal interchange of staff in the national hospital service, and through responsibility for programs of continuing education for the thousand or more general practitioners working in the regional hospital area. But the universities did not realize the potential as regional educational centers that had been predicted for them by the 1944 Goodenough Committee. One distinguished American visitor is reported to have remarked in 1955 "that no country has produced so many wise reports on the improvements of medical education as Great Britain, and no country has done so little about it." [1]

The separate administration of the teaching and the nonteaching hospitals under the NHS act may have discouraged some universities from embarking on regional training programs. Undergraduate teaching hospitals were recognized as those hospitals, and *only* those hospitals, that were linked through their board of governors to a university medical school. They received their title because they taught undergraduate medical students working toward their university basic degrees or, in parallel, for a Conjoint Board diploma. Each of the twenty-two boards of governors of these teaching hospital groups, of which twelve were the famous London undergraduate schools, had direct access to the Ministry of Health. Nonteaching hospitals

1. Quoted by John R. Ellis in *Lancet i* (1956), 813. Most of the material on undergraduate medical education in this section is drawn from Ellis's papers, delivered as the Goulstonian Lectures for 1956 before the Royal College of Physicians.

were grouped under hospital management committees within a regional hospital area, and matters of policy were channeled to the Ministry of Health through the regional hospital board.

The difference between teaching and nonteaching hospitals reflected their history; it was administrative rather than functional. In Scotland, which had a different educational tradition, all hospitals were teaching hospitals and all were grouped together under the regional hospital boards. In England all hospitals not under boards of governors were called "nonteaching," even though university students were sent for experience to some regional hospitals; even though many provided advanced postgraduate teaching for future consultants; even though most general hospital groups accepted first-year house officers on probation; and even though all hospitals employed staff in the hospital grades originally designated as training grades in the Spens Committee report.

The dual administration was born of compromise and was awkward in practice. Contact between the board of governors and the regional hospital board (which were situated in the same city) was made at various levels through a number of joint committees as well as through informal contact. Nevertheless, the teaching center was not at the organizational hub of the new hospital service. Each board appointed its own consultants and other senior staff. Although arrangements were made for joint appointments between the two boards, these were usually for administrative rather than for educational purposes and had limited application. The board of governors might have only six or seven (teaching) hospitals under its administration, concentrated in a small geographical area. The regional hospital board would be responsible for nonteaching general, mental, and special hospitals in the whole regional area; these ranged from under 100 hospitals in some regions to over 250 in others,[2] spread over diverse areas and sometimes scattered population groups.

It was questionable whether the undergraduate medical school was the most appropriate center for regional postgraduate training—a question that became more relevant under the impact of greater specialization. Revised requirements for undergraduate training had been laid down in 1947 by the General Medical Council, the official watchdog over basic standards in medical education. The Council had recommended that a greater proportion of the student's time be spent on certain special subjects, notably social medicine, pediatrics, and psychiatry; and, as was the custom, it specified the minimum length of time to be devoted to each specialty by the medical schools.[3] As a result of this, and of the questions raised by curriculum content in general, much of the time of medical school faculties in the 1950s was devoted to realigning and reconsidering the details of undergraduate education. Such reforms may have appeared a more urgent need (and were easier

2. Acton Society Trust, *Hospitals and the State. Groups, Regions and Committees. Part II Regional Hospital Boards* (London, 1957), p. 60.

3. See *Lancet i* (1957), 1178.

to approach) than the development of new educational philosophies or a regional postgraduate educational network. Whatever the reason, a curious lethargy paralyzed medical educational programs between 1948 and 1961. The brave words of the Goodenough Committee, which had envisaged the regional hospital concept as part of a great educational design, were scarcely heeded; and many passages in that report calling for reforms were still as relevant in the early 1960s as they had been in 1944.

The Impact of Specialization on Education and Training

Specialization had engendered a crisis in both undergraduate and postgraduate medical education. The whole spectrum, from the undergraduate to the postgraduate level, needed realignment. Undergraduate training could no longer pretend to produce a competent doctor, but once this fact was recognized, many other difficulties arose, extending right along the training ladder; for if the undergraduate course was only an introduction to medicine, or an educational background, the acquisition of skills had to be transferred to the postgraduate level.

British medical education had remained as an undergraduate course, usually of five years. The student entered medical school at the age of 18 years, having already spent two years in the study of chemistry, physics, and biology; this premedical education was narrowly focused, and was largely a factual learning process. There was no such thing as a liberal arts background, or an opportunity for leisurely study of scientific thought. The cultured physician, hallmark of the Royal College, had been replaced by the student of facts, with his brain crammed for the purposes of examination. More than one critic lamented: "The deplorable fact is that medical students now have a less balanced general education than ever before." [4] The first (preclinical) years of university life did little to correct this. In 1963 most medical schools, including all the London schools, retained a basic educational structure little different from that of one or even two generations earlier. The basic sciences were divided from the clinical sciences, and the student was required to spend almost two years in the classroom and laboratory before reaching the patient's bedside. The average preclinical curriculum consisted of five university terms of about 1,200 hours; as much as 60 per cent of the time was devoted to anatomy and histology, another 20 per cent of physiology, and most of the remainder to biochemistry. This left the broader social aspects of medicine—psychology, medical sociology, and statistics—a total of only twenty hours.[5] Yet these were subjects recognized as increasingly important, especially to general practice which even in the 1960s the majority of students would ultimately enter and for which there was no compulsory postgraduate training.

In the three-year clinical course which followed, the student was shunted

4. J. R. Ellis, *Lancet i* (1956), 816.
5. Quoted from British Medical Students' Association data by Prof. C. Wilson in *Psychiatric Education*, Institute of Psychiatry, pp. 34–35.

from one specialty to the next, according to a standard curriculum. Increasing specialization had multiplied staff and departments. A rapid buildup of specialist departments in NHS teaching hospitals, which provided certain specialist services on a regional basis, gave the student a distorted view of medicine as a whole; the teaching hospital was a pole away from the general practitioner's surgery or the run-of-the-mill general hospital. The student was borne along a mass-production line, and it was generally felt that not enough time was available for practical teaching on the wards or in the outpatient departments.[6] Undergraduate education during the 1950s thus appeared to be deteriorating.

The record was by no means all negative. Looking back in 1957 over the previous decade, the *Lancet* recorded "substantial progress" in undergraduate programs. The majority of medical schools had accepted the recommendation of the General Medical Council to include a three-month transitional course between the preclinical and clinical phases. Smaller schools had been enlarged. Full-time university units (professorial units) in the clinical subjects had proliferated. The growth of medical teamwork in hospitals was said to have improved the standard of clinical care displayed before students (there was now group discussion of cases instead of the "oracular pronouncements of the consultant to his houseman"), and interdepartmental teaching had been encouraged.[7] Nevertheless, it was evident that the undergraduate curriculum, supposedly designed (as recommended by the Goodenough Committee) to produce the general practitioner, was no longer fulfilling this purpose. The span of medicine was too broad to fit elements of each relevant specialty into the time available. Second, it was now recognized that general practice was itself a separate species of practice from hospital medicine (if not a specialty), and should be founded on its own general basic principles and appropriate postgraduate study. The emphasis on vocational training was shifting to the graduate stage in general practice, as it had already done in training for the specialties. Undergraduate education was thus increasingly regarded as a mere baseline, not complete in itself.

This factor had been partly recognized by the introduction of the "preregistration" or intern year, directly following the undergraduate clinical period, by the Medical Act of 1950. This compulsory year provided six months of medicine and six months of surgery, and rounded off the official education and training program. Some of the responsibilities for vocational training were thus transferred to the graduate level. The preregistration house officer, although only provisionally registered by the General Medical Council, had passed his university degrees (M.B., B.S.), or a legally equivalent diploma such as that of the Conjoint Board of the English Royal Colleges (MRCS, LRCP), which qualified him for admission to the Medical Register as a licensed practitioner. There was no further examination, but

6. *Lancet ii* (1956), 815.
7. *Lancet i* (1957), 1178.

the graduate had to produce proof of satisfactory completion of the year before full registration became effective, and the year was nominally a university responsibility. When the year was completed, the doctor became a fully "qualified" practitioner, ready to move up to the next hospital grade of senior house officer. The preregistration year could be taken in either a teaching or nonteaching hospital, provided it was approved by the university for this purpose.[8]

During his preregistration year the erstwhile member of the student group became a responsible individual, attached to a medical or surgical "firm" as house physician or house surgeon for a continuous six-month period. He would probably be the only house officer of the firm, and he might work, together with a registrar (and in some cases with a senior registrar), for two or three consultants. As a house officer he would take case histories, order routine diagnostic tests, and treat patients, under supervision, in his consultants' beds. He might also be responsible for minor surgery, and he would bear the brunt of being on call at all hours of day or night to deal initially with any emergency. But even this experience was a mere beginning. It was not pretended, at this level, that the doctor was competent to be a principal in general practice.

Yet at this stage formal training requirements ceased. Future GPs as well as specialists usually took a further hospital post as a house officer or senior house officer. Individual hospitals might set up informal postgraduate teaching programs, demonstrations, and grand rounds, but there was no uniform pattern. No general accreditation or inspection systems existed. The Royal College of Surgeons and the Royal College of Obstetricians and Gynaecologists approved hospitals for training purposes for the FRCS and MRCOG examinations, but this approval was for a limited field and was at best spasmodic.

The university medical schools had appointed regional postgraduate deans and committees at the beginning of the NHS, but some of the committees met infrequently, perhaps once a year, and the role of the postgraduate dean was subject to wide variation. One or two universities appointed retired clinicians who were able to devote a large part of their time to postgraduate

8. Responsibility for recognizing preregistration posts is vested in the universities by the General Medical Council, which issues lists of approved posts. The universities have direct supervision over preregistration posts. The dean of the medical school sits on the regional postgraduate committee that meets once or twice a year to review its preregistration posts according to criteria drawn up by the Conference of Postgraduate Medical Deans (it is emphasized that they are not rigid prescriptions). The criteria suggest that the house officer be responsible for not more than 50 beds, including male and female wards; that there be no posts limited to chronic diseases; and that there be adequate supporting facilities, a library, and adequate supervision. This last is interpreted as at least three sessions a week with a consultant and an experienced resident. On actual teaching, the criteria have nothing to say. *A Review of the Medical Services in Great Britain*. Report of a Committee sponsored by the Royal College of Physicians of London et al. (London 1962) (Porritt report), Appendix 9.

training, but the postgraduate deanship might equally well be an honorary or part-time appointment held by a busy clinical professor in the medical school or by a busy practicing clinician. In the four metropolitan regions (and Wessex) postgraduate advisers were attached to the British Postgraduate Medical Federation of the University of London; in the other regions they were attached to the university medical school. The degree of activity in postgraduate education outside the teaching hospital (the chief function of the postgraduate deans) fluctuated between one university center and another.

The dean's activities included arranging special courses, demonstrations, and ward rounds in the teaching hospital and the main regional (nonteaching) centers. There was little or no attempt to influence the experience or training being given to individual registrars or house officers in the course of their hospital work, nor to advise individuals on subsequent posts in accordance with the edicts on special training abounding in numerous expert reports. The individual registrar was left to fend for himself. If he were working for his FRCS, in a post approved for this purpose by the Royal College of Surgeons, he would have the small satisfaction of knowing that the hospital facilities had been examined by the College at some point within a ten-year period. If he were not a surgeon he did not even have this consolation, since the Royal College of Physicians did not require evidence of experience at an approved hospital. Both house officers and registrars might or might not be fortunate in the teaching ability or interest of the consultant(s) to whom they were attached. There was no one else on the spot to whom they could turn for encouragement, nor anyone who would ensure that they had enough time and facilities to spend on preparation for examinations.

Postgraduate training was complicated because there were other parties involved besides the regional university: the Royal Colleges and other examining bodies, the national specialist institutes in London, and the hospital service, organized through the regional hospital boards and the separate boards of governors. The postgraduate student who decided to specialize worked for the appropriate examination of the Royal College, which he usually took two or three years after full registration. He was employed as a hospital registrar in the National Health Service; and for training he was nominally the responsibility of the regional postgraduate committee whose agent was the postgraduate dean or director appointed by the medical school. At some point in his career he might, for further specialist training, take up an appointment in London under the aegis of the appropriate institute. Finally, having worked his way through the registrar and senior registrar grades, he might be appointed consultant by a National Health Service committee which was guided by criteria formulated by the Royal Colleges.

There was no overall responsibility for education and training. Undergraduate training was wholly the university's responsibility; the intern or preregistration year was partly so. The senior house officer and registrar stages were primarily guided by the Royal Colleges. Once the appropriate membership diploma was gained, the Colleges had no direct control, and this period included the subsequent and vitally important three- to five-year specialist training phase of senior registrar, which was the responsibility of the hospitals. If the universities had made a concerted effort to weave these various strands into one coordinated program, each part might have fitted neatly into the whole, and responsibility might have been more clearly defined. But the introduction of the National Health Service coincided with the need for a completely new look at medical education as a whole. The problems that were already apparent in the 1930s had become intensified, and no ready solutions were available.

By the late 1950s it was clear that the university focus of hospital regions would not of itself provide sufficient general postgraduate stimulus outside the teaching hospital. The movement was all one way. It consisted of an earnest desire on the part of middle-grade hospital staff in nonteaching hospitals in the region to gain an appointment in the teaching hospital and thus to enhance their chances of eventual consultant status. With the buildup of the already prestigious teaching hospitals as specialist centers under the NHS, this kind of focus was almost inevitable. Teaching hospitals were better provided with medical and other professional staff than were nonteaching hospitals of comparable size and on the whole had better facilities. Since the emphasis on training was initially placed on the universities, the regional hospital boards, which were fully occupied with other pressing planning problems, made few efforts to stimulate independent teaching programs in their own (and theoretically nonteaching) hospitals. Furthermore, since general practitioner services were organized apart from hospitals, there was little immediate incentive for nonteaching hospitals to establish schemes which would include GPs as well as hospital staff. Some programs for GPs had been set up, but these sprang from individual consultant initiative rather than from regional encouragement. A number of questions required solving. These ranged from the broad relationship of undergraduate education to postgraduate training, and the immediate need to assign responsibility (to university, college, or hospital), to improved postgraduate training in the nonteaching hospital.

Indications of Organizational Change

If the undergraduate curriculum was to be regarded as broadly educational rather than strictly vocational, elaborate curriculum regulations, designed to ensure that the student was exposed to a wide range of techniques, were no longer applicable. In 1957, the General Medical Council revised its recommendations toward this goal. Instead of describing each stage of training, the Council merely indicated to the medical schools the minimum length of the whole period of professional study, declining to specify the period of study alloted to particular subjects or the sequence in which they should be taught. The new recommendations were an attempt to move away from factual learning toward the development of critical thought; the Council urged schools as far as possible "to instruct less and to educate more." [9]

Under the relative freedom of these new regulations, each medical school was forced to reconsider not only the structure of its own curriculum but the more fundamental problems of medical teaching. Education was central to medical practice, and consideration of curricula had to include analyses of the desired content of medical practice. This included the relative importance of subjects such as psychology and genetics as basic medical sciences, and the arguments for and against including general practice and other aspects of extrahospital medicine not traditionally included in the clinical curriculum. There were also urgent questions of organization and methodology in medical teaching. A period of curriculum revision began in the medical schools, and several began to reorganize their teaching programs. But crucial questions remained. How far should the undergraduate stage be one common to other scientists and professional workers? Of what did medicine consist in the mid-twentieth century? What were the chief distinguishing marks of the good physician? And what was the relationship between the arts and sciences of medical practice and between the generalist and specialist?

Questions on the undergraduate curriculum were paralleled by increasing doubt over the adequacy of experience afforded in the preregistration year. Many consultants endeavored to teach their house officers in their grand rounds and routine rounds of patients on the wards. But the consultant was given no extra time in the NHS contract for teaching purposes, and the house officer might have to scramble along as best he could, learning by imitation. In addition, many house officer posts did not include outpatient work and almost all had no tie-in with medicine outside the hospital. Work loads varied greatly, from the house surgeon who did no minor operations in his six months to his counterpart in another hospital who did several hundred, and there was a marked lack of supervision of patients. Moreover some of the posts—especially those in the teaching hospitals—were highly specialized; one house officer reported in 1962 that he carried responsibility for only twelve beds, and half of these were reserved for patients with tetanus.[10] Some claimed that house officers often reveled in their work: "They love being up to their elbows in blood, sweat and tears, their own and other people's." [11] But the year could be hard labor, and the actual teaching of the graduate ill-organized. Teaching on the job was often left to the registrar, whose mind might well be more on passing his examination in the appropriate Royal College.

The postgraduate examination system had done nothing to clarify relative responsibility for education and training. There were still no diplomas or degrees that testified to specialist status, no training program that automatically conferred on the individual the mantle of the specialist or general prac-

9. *Lancet i* (1957), 1178, 1190–91.
10. P. W. Hutton et al., *Lancet i* (1964), 38–40.
11. D. Stafford-Clark, in *Psychiatric Education,* p. 61.

titioner, and there was still a multitude of postgraduate diplomas of various kinds at various levels of performance, and organized by a variety of examining bodies. Those in the medical specialties normally took the MRCP with perhaps a university M.D.; some might also take a specialist diploma such as one in child health from the Conjoint Board, or one in bacteriology from a university. Surgeons took the general FRCS or its equivalent in ophthalmology or otolaryngology, and frequently also sat for a higher university degree in surgery. Psychiatrists concentrated on the Diploma in Psychological Medicine given by a number of universities and by the Conjoint Boards; similarly, radiologists took one of the diplomas in radiology, while some aspired to a fellowship in the professional Faculty of Radiologists.[12] Thus it went on. Over ninety diplomas or degrees in Great Britain and Ireland were set out for postgraduate students in a BMA handbook of 1962; many similar diplomas were of varying standards.

Concern over specialist and general practitioner training programs became urgent as the brunt of instilling basic vocational knowledge and experience was placed on the hospital middle-grade posts of senior house officer and registrar and on traineeships and assistantships in general practice. As was shown in Chapter 10, at the very time the training period was growing more important, the Ministry of Health, endeavoring to solve hospital staffing problems, was declaring senior house officer and registrar posts to be primarily concerned with the service needs of the hospital rather than the training of the individual, and there was no effective regional system of formal postgraduate training to fill the gap.

Many registrars, appalled at the hurdle represented by professional examinations such as the MRCP or FRCS, took special pre-examination courses at their own expense. In 1961–62 some 3,500 postgraduate students were enrolled at the various institutes of the British Postgraduate Medical Federation of London University, and this by no means included all such students enrolled in courses even in London. Of the 3,500, approximately 2,000 were full-time students and 1,000 held appointments in an institute or postgraduate teaching hospital. Almost 2,000 of them were studying for a specialist diploma of one of the Royal Colleges, and about 400 were studying for university postgraduate degrees or diplomas. Thus the institutes— national university postgraduate schools—were providing a large number of candidates for Royal College examinations and a considerable part of the training of specialists.[13] In the provincial teaching centers, postgraduate specialty courses largely followed the requirements of the diplomas given by the particular university—for example, the Diplomas in Radiology and Radio-therapy (DMRD and DMRT) at Manchester, or in Public Health (DPH) or Psychological Medicine (DPM) at Newcastle.

General practice had no institute. The British Postgraduate Medical Fed-

12. See Additional Notes, pp. 370–72.
13. British Postgraduate Medical Federation, *Handbook for the Session 1962–63*, p. 65. See additional notes, pp. 372–75.

eration took upon itself the responsibility for organizing courses for general practitioners at a number of teaching and nonteaching hospitals, but these tended to be specialist courses for general practitioners rather than courses in general practice itself. An experimental scheme to train general practitioners was begun in the Wessex hospital region in 1959, deliberately aimed at providing a training for the young doctor in the two years after full registration, at the end of which he would be "competent to look after his own list of patients." The trainee spent a year in a rotating post in a local hospital, followed by a second year as a trainee in a practice using the same hospital.[14] But this program was very small; only ten trainees were appointed to it between 1959 and 1962. The lacuna in systematic postgraduate training for general practice was even more pronounced than the deficiencies in formal hospital teaching.

The professional bodies might have organized systematic local educational programs. But the BMA divisions and branches, although they organized local scientific meetings, did not attempt to criticize routine education and training of postgraduates, which was based on the long-held tradition of apprenticeship to consultants. Many of their members were general practitioners whose intrusion into hospital matters might well have been resented by the hospital staffs. Nor did the Royal Colleges provide the answers; they had at that time no regional organization and little direct interest in local hospital standards. More formal links than these were necessary; it was evident that they would have to be based on direct communication between the university centers and the nonteaching hospital groups. Postgraduate education had to be reorganized as a National Health Service function, as well as one pertaining to the universities and the professional bodies.

The responsibility of the National Health Service for training was recommended for senior registrars in the Platt report of 1961, described in Chapter 10: senior registrar training was to be linked with the increased demand for consultants envisaged in this report. Review of the performance of senior registrars was to be streamlined and rotation between teaching and nonteaching hospitals encouraged through a new joint advisory committee set up in each region. It was thought that such committees, jointly staffed by teaching and regional board representatives, might also act as a personnel center for senior registrars, able to give individual guidance on future prospects, especially to those unlikely to obtain consultant posts. The Platt report was emphatic in placing this responsibility on the National Health Service rather than on the professional colleges or the universities. The advisory committees on senior registrars took over all questions concerning senior registrars in teaching and nonteaching hospitals throughout the regional hospital area.

The Platt report thus established an important precept. While the content of training in the specialties was a professional question, "primarily for the

14. George Swift, *Brit. Med. J. ii* (1963), 595–97.

Royal Colleges, the Royal Scottish Corporations and the universities," the responsibility for organization and supervision of training arrangements was recognized as a general management function.[15] The senior registrar was given direct regional supervision. The chief remaining deficiencies in postgraduate training in 1961 lay in the training of hospital junior and middle-grade staff and in general practice, a matter not just of a few hundred but of many thousands of practitioners at various stages of competence. The regional universities alone had not solved the problems inherent in these grades; and at the same time the problems, under the impact of specialization and of increased competition for posts under the National Health Service, had become more acute. Active interest was needed in the nonteaching hospitals. A structure for postgraduate education and training programs needed to be developed, which, it now appeared, ought to be the administrative responsibility of the National Health Service. But also, the content and purpose of medical education and training at all levels needed to be reviewed. This was primarily a matter for the universities and the profession.

15. Platt report on hospital medical staffing, pp. 25–26.

IV

The Impact of
the National Health Service
on Medical Practice: The 1960s

13

Employment in
the National Health Service

Writing on the professions in 1933, Carr-Saunders and Wilson observed that the Minister of Health was already in a position to take the chief means of livelihood from most practicing doctors:

> If the existing system of health insurance is to be preserved without fundamental change, the Minister must continue to control policy; but equally if the medical profession is to continue to order its affairs, the right of the doctor to earn a living must not be revocable at the command of the Minister. Can the system be amended so as to assure to both parties the rights which are desirable? [1]

Since then, the remuneration and working environment of doctors have been increasingly controlled by the Minister. In the early 1930s about half the registered practitioners in practice were on the medical list as "panel" doctors; but in the 1960s the proportion in the National Health Service is little short of 100 per cent, and more than half are employed by the Minister or his agents on a direct salaried basis to work in the nationalized hospital service.

Thus the questions of control, influence, or a balance of authority between the medical profession and the state have become proportionally more important. The prospective specialist in the 1960s has little chance of alternative employment through private practice should he fail to be appointed to a consultant post within the National Health Service. The consultant who is dismissed from his post, for whatever reason, must face the end of his career. The general practitioner may be restrained from NHS practice in the district of his choice through administrative regulation. All these are curbs on individual freedom to practice, but all may be accepted by the medical profession as a necessary part of a national medical service, provided that the exercise of the machinery involved is recognized as reasonable and fair. No responsible consultant, for example, would claim that untrained specialists should be allowed to practice in consultant posts; dismissal of consultants proved to have been grossly negligent would be strongly endorsed; and

1. Carr-Saunders and Wilson, *The Professions,* p. 482.

general practitioners have accepted that in a comprehensive national service there should be some degree of redeployment through administrative means. The question is one of degree. There is a large gray area between what is un-questionably right and what is a questionable use of administrative power or, conversely, of professional influence. In a national health service, the ex-istence of procedures—and the way in which such procedures are applied—thus becomes of paramount importance. The rights of the employer and the employee must be codified in such a way that the exercise of individual pro-fessional judgment is not impaired and that professional advice on questions of policy is not ignored.

The Consultant as a Salaried Employee

Under the National Health Service the consultant, descendant of the honorary unpaid physician or surgeon in the voluntary hospital, became an employee. He signed a contract of service, received a specified salary, and became eligible for the usual fringe benefits that accompany employment in a large organization: a stipulated vacation period, a pension program, and sickness and study leave. This new relationship was to have a substantial impact on consultants; it brought them together under common conditions and it involved them with the administration and development of hospitals at all levels. General practitioners merely agreed with the government to pro-vide certain services. It could be said that they retained their independence whereas consultants had capitulated to bureaucracy. But, in fact, consultants had exercised influence and retained flexibility in their actual working con-ditions; indeed, they have consistently expressed more satisfaction in NHS work than have general practitioners, whose complaints have steadily risen in volume. This is not wholly the result of the National Health Service—the bases for GP unrest were there before—but it was roundly emphasized by the administrative machinery which each branch accepted at the beginning of the service. It is worth examining in some detail the consultant's work conditions, the rules surrounding his appointment, and his involvement with the administrative structure, to discover both his degree of freedom and how his present position has been achieved.

Consultants had entered the National Health Service in July 1948 on temporary contracts while they awaited the decisions of the consultant re-view committees (Chapter 6). Although few details had been agreed upon in advance, most principles of employment had been settled in the 1948 Spens *Report on the Remuneration of Consultants and Specialists*. Consult-ants were to be employed on a standard salary under arrangements similar to those pre-existing in the municipal hospitals. The basic salary scale was identical for all specialties in all hospitals, and the amount of the basic salary was determined by the number of "notional half-day sessions" per week which the individual consultant agreed to work in one or more hospitals. A notional half-day was later spelled out as a period of 3.5 hours, including agreed traveling time; it was "notional" in that it was not necessarily tied to the working day of other hospital personnel. Whole-time employment was equivalent to eleven sessions or a 5.5-day week, and whole-time consultants were not allowed to undertake private practice.

In accordance with Mr. Bevan's promise to the medical profession, the Amendment Act of 1949 confirmed the right of senior staff to part-time instead of whole-time appointment if they so desired.[2] It was decided that the maximum part-time contract consistent with the operation of a private practice comprised nine sessions or the equivalent of 4.5 days per week. Both whole-time and part-time consultants had, however, continuous responsibility for the patients in their beds and might be called in for emergency work at any time.[3] Senior hospital medical officers, the second tenured specialist grade with a lower salary range, were employed on a similar basis. Besides the routine emergency hospital work covered under these arrangements, a domiciliary specialist service was introduced. Consultants were made available, under the NHS and at the GP's request, to visit patients in their homes. This was something quite new: part of the fulfillment of the government's pledge to introduce a twenty-four-hour specialist service. Thus the part-time consultant might have income from his NHS sessions, fees for domiciliary visits, possibly also an NHS distinction award, and a separate private practice; most of his facilities would, however, be provded for him at NHS hospitals. The whole-timer might have all of these except private practice which, by accepting a whole-time contract, he had deliberately eschewed.

These were the broad principles of payment. But there remained in 1948 a multitude of details to be worked out before the final contracts could be made. The National Health Service was specifically excluded from Civil Service arrangements; although the hospitals were nationalized, hospital employees retained a different identity and a completely different grading and payment structure. They become employees of the National Health Service, of regional hospital boards or boards of governors—or for junior staff of hospital management committees—each of which had a corporate identity. The arrangements were in some respects similar to those made in other nationalized industries (for example, the electrical workers, who were also organized through a national and regional administrative framework). This separateness absolved doctors and other professional workers from bearing the label of civil servant, but it also meant that the negotiating bodies had no basic terms and conditions of service on which to operate. These had to be worked out ab initio between the profession and their new employers.

2. National Health Service (Amendment) Act, 1949, Section 12. The Act also prohibited a full-time salaried GP and dental service (Sections 10–11).

3. Under the initial NHS regulations, part-time consultants received a weighted sessional income to include this factor; i.e. somewhat more than the proportional income applicable in relation to the salary of a whole-time consultant. The distinction was abolished for new contracts in 1960, on the advice of the *Report* from the Royal Commission (p. 71).

They included the establishment of a satisfactory pension plan, stipulated vacation periods, and expenses allowable for such items as traveling, lectures, sickness and study leave. One stipulation guaranteed the right of the part-time specialist to undertake private practice in the small number of private beds remaining in NHS hospitals. There was also discussion as to whether any radiologist or anesthesiologist who chose to work whole time under the National Health Service, and was thus not allowed to receive fees from private practice, should be required to treat patients in these private beds. On such matters consultants had considerable room to maneuver in the decisive negotiating period following the passage of the Act, while the review committees were assessing the individual qualities of hospital staffs in 1948 and 1949 and the regional and teaching hospital boards were examining their facilities and formulating development priorities.

Negotiations on these and related subjects would no doubt have proceeded for some time had not the Ministry finally issued a polite threat in July 1949, one whole year after the National Health Service came into effect. It was suggested that if consultants delayed any longer, the Ministry would reconsider its assurance that the financial outcome of the negotiations would be applied retroactively. This had an immediate effect. The Joint Consultants Committee promptly settled its differences with the Ministry and agreed to recommend hospital medical staff to accept permanent employment contracts with the employing boards, and consultants duly signed their contracts with regional hospital boards or boards of governors.[4] They became entitled to six weeks' paid annual vacation and to other leave periods; they contributed to the NHS pension plan. Their conditions of service were carefully specified in a booklet issued to all hospital medical staff and automatically accepted by signing the employment contract. The only major question for decision by the employing boards was the number of sessions that were required at individual hospitals for an adequate service in a particular specialty.

Consultant status was defined by the review committees set up for that purpose at the beginning of the NHS; there was thus no need of further clarification in the terms of service. Because of the staffing structure of British voluntary hospitals, recognition of the consultant through staff appointment was an accepted concept. The replacement of the community as voluntary contributor and customer by the community as taxpayer and consumer, made little difference to this basic philosophy. The consultant still had to compete for an appointment by a hospital board, and the boards, although now agents of the Minister of Health, were still composed of eminent members of the local community. To the individual consultant, however, there were two outstanding differences in his new status. First, he was paid a nationally agreed salary, which was subject to no local variation. Second, unless he was attached to a teaching hospital (when he was em-

4. See *Royal Commission; Minutes of Evidence*, p. 221; RHB (49), no. 102.

ployed by the board of governors) he was appointed by a regional hospital board, serving a geographical area containing some three million people, which would assign him to duties at particular hospitals within the area. The consultant's geographical horizons were therefore automatically widened. He looked to a regional headquarters as his employer, and he was dependent on national arbitrators for the actual amount of money he received and for the determination of fringe benefits. Almost overnight consultants began to become a cohesive national group, irrevocably joined together in common terms of service. This cohesion was to be of major importance in the subsequent pay disputes between consultants and general practitioners.

Salaried service was the only type of employment seriously considered for specialist staff. It was difficult to think of an alternative. General practitioners had come out strongly for a continuation of capitation fees. This was feasible in general practice, where a large number of people registered on doctors' lists. Consultants could not have similar quantitative practices, except in some instances for a relatively small number of private patients. The specialist saw only patients selected for him by general practitioners—when they were sick and when they needed *his* advice rather than the advice of other specialist colleagues—and therefore could not be paid by capitation fees. The only viable alternative to salary would have been remuneration based on a measure of work done, such as a fee-for-service system. However, this had immediate disadvantages. First, it had never been used in a public hospital system, whereas salaries had been used successfully by local authorities. Second, university teaching appointments and all other hospital appointments, from house officer up, were salaried; since consultants were usually to be appointed from the salaried hospital grade of senior registrar, they merely moved upward under the NHS from one salary grade to the next. Third, and finally, salaried employment was infinitely less complicated to administer and, at least to the penurious young consultant, it carried a number of welcome guarantees.

There were, however, certain dangers in salaried employment, not intrinsic to this particular method of payment but to the National Health Service as virtually a monopoly employer. Not only the actual benefits but also the mechanisms of employment for specialists had to be developed. Since the great majority of hospitals—including all the teaching hospitals—were NHS institutions, there was no effective alternative employment. Although the system of part-time employment might provide a generous base for building up private practice, except for the very few there would no longer be a living in private practice alone.

One of the first mechanisms set up was for appointments. Since consultants continued to be thus designated, the system of appointing them was of primary importance. It had to be fair, and it had to be nationally applicable. For his professional status a consultant, unlike a lawyer or an architect but like a university professor or a Member of Parliament, was a consultant only because he occupied a consultant *post*. He could not be self-selected;

consultant status was a rank, not a trade. The first appointments regulations had appeared in June 1948.[5] These regulations were welcomed by the medical profession as a means of widening the choice among appointees. The apprenticeship method of training, as Flexner had pointed out in 1910, had encouraged inbreeding among hospital staffs. Under the NHS, national regulations were to apply. Since consultant appointment would no longer be dependent on locally established private practice and local GP contacts, applicants might be expected in future from all over the country. The new procedure was a "triumph for those reformers who have long been working to make hospital appointments depend more on merit and less on local influence or acquaintance." [6]

Revised regulations along the same lines were laid down by statutory instrument in 1950. All regional hospital boards and boards of governors had to conform to them for each appointment at the consultant or SHMO level, whether whole time or part time. The posts were to be advertised in the medical journals, and canvassing was strictly prohibited. Applications for advertised posts were to be considered by a special advisory appointments committee to each employing board, constituted somewhat differently for appointments by regional hospital boards and by boards of governors of teaching hospitals. The seven-man committee of a regional hospital board was to consist of five consultants and two laymen who were voluntary members of the regional board or hospital management committee; no salaried hospital administrator was to sit on the committee. Teaching hospital boards have a committee of six consultants and two laymen, nominated equally by the board of governors and the university. Similar arrangements were made for appointing a consultant to work jointly in teaching and nonteaching hospitals.

The advisory appointments committees nominate all applicants for new and vacant consultant posts, whether or not applicants are already holding a consultant job in another hospital region. The only exception was made in 1959 for consultants made redundant through changes in hospital organization, who can now be offered alternative employment by the hospital board without going through the hazards of the competitive process against younger and perhaps better qualified senior registrars.[7] The advisory appointments committees are similar in structure and function to the review committees that surveyed existing consultant staffs in 1949. In both, the philosophy was accepted that the consultant be identified by his professional colleagues rather than by his employers, although the final decision legally rests with the regional board or board of governors. Occasionally the employing boards reject the advisory committee's recommendation. But

5. The National Health Service (Appointment of Specialist) Regulations 1948, Statutory Instrument, 1948, no. 1416.

6. *Lancet ii* (1948), 101.

7. The National Health Service (Appointment of Specialist) Regulations 1950, S. I. 1950, no. 1259; and Amendment Regulations 1959, S. I. 1959, no. 909.

usually there is strong professional advice on individual appointments. The power of the profession to perpetuate itself through its hospital appointments is greater than it was under the voluntary hospital system in the nineteenth century, when the common method of appointment was by canvassing the large and influential hospital board, composed primarily of laymen.

The Relationship Between the Consultant and the Hospitals

After his appointment by the regional hospital board or board of governors of a teaching hospital, the consultant signs a contract of service for the stipulated number of sessions per week and for certain duties; and he may decide whether or not he wishes to undertake domiciliary visits. The individual specialist offered a whole-time appointment has also to decide whether he wishes to engage in private practice; if so, he normally chooses the maximum part-time contract of nine sessions per week.

The new consultant has almost invariably spent all his professional life—from student through the house officer and registrar levels to senior registrar—in NHS hospitals. He is usually, but not always, appointed from the grade of senior registrar, designed as a four-year consultant traineeship entered from the grade of registrar, but often of longer duration.[8] The doctor might pass his qualifying examinations at age 24 and become registered to practice at age 25. He might then spend three or four years as a senior house officer and registrar, become a senior registrar at the age of 28 or 29, and begin applying for consultant posts at about age 33. The senior registrar has to apply for posts as they become available and are advertised. Consultant posts are limited in number by the Ministry of Health, thus the new consultant cannot always choose the area in which he would ideally decide to live. In this respect he has far less choice than the general practitioner, whose own mobility is limited by the "negative direction" of the Medical Practices Committee. The prospective consultant may have to apply for an appointment to a group of hospitals which happens, for example, to be situated in a city where there is little or no available private practice in his specialty.

Given a system of identifying consultant status with appointment to a regulated and limited "establishment" of posts, this is inevitable. A senior registrar in, say, neurology at a particular hospital has no guarantee that he will stay on at that hospital as a consultant. There may already be two consultant neurologists in the hospital group, both working on maximum part-time contracts (4.5 days a week); and this may be considered a sufficient

---

8. According to data provided by the Ministry of Health, 528 new consultant appointments were made in England and Wales from 1 Oct. 1961 to 30 Sept. 1962; 100 of these represented extension of sessions or change of location by existing consultants; 214 appointments were from senior registrars; and 70 from senior hospital medical officers. Most others had been full-time clinical teachers or research workers, or had held a post abroad.

number for the work load. Even if the regional hospital board decides that an extra consultant should be appointed, the request has first to be approved by the Ministry of Health; and second, the new appointment is filled after considering all senior registrars who apply for the post. This system, although it may sometimes fall unfairly on particular individuals and although it poses an immense strain on the senior registrar seeking appointment, is generally accepted. Again it stems from the transposition of the old voluntary hospital tradition, of a limited, prestigious consultant staff, into the National Health Service.

Having been appointed, the new consultant has to develop his schedule of NHS work. The regional hospital board assigns him to particular hospitals in accordance with the terms outlined in the advertisements for the post, but it has been a common practice not to specify the exact work the consultant is to perform. Detailed duties still tend to be arranged by the individual in discussion with other consultants attached to the relevant hospitals. One radiologist, whose experience was presented in court in an income tax case in 1961, was appointed by the Birmingham Regional Hospital Board for nine sessions at two NHS hospitals.[9] He became solely responsible for radiology in one hospital, which he attended on four mornings and three afternoons a week, and he went to the second hospital, where there were three radiologists, on one morning and one afternoon a week; private patients were also fitted into this schedule. No permission was sought from or given by any of the administrative staff of the hospital for this arrangement. "The Respondent was entirely responsible for deciding what radiological work he should do and how he should do it." A second consultant in the same case was an ophthalmologist under the board. On his appointment he had an informal meeting with the other two consultant ophthalmologists at the Wolverhampton Eye Hospital, to which he had been assigned. They arranged between them when he should see his outpatients and when he should operate: "No programme of work was ever prescribed for the Respondent by anyone, nor did anyone ever interfere with his work. He was completely free to decide what he should or should not do in his work." Similar statements were made for a consultant pathologist and a psychiatrist. The pathologist was appointed for 31.5 hours a week (nine sessions) but, it was stated, "it was not possible to predict exactly how much time he would spend on National Health Service work and how much on his private practice." The amount of private practice a consultant might do was unspecified.

A consultant obstetrician interviewed for this book explained in more detail how the system worked in his group of hospitals scattered over a small industrial area but with a wide rural coverage; his case is probably fairly typical of the system in general. He was appointed as an additional obstetrician to the group, not as a replacement. The new appointee had

9. *Mitchell v. Ross*, House of Lords, July 6, 1961, Consolidated Appeals and Cross Appeals, Appendix, Part I.

been doubly unfortunate in his career. Like many other young men at the beginning of the NHS, he had expected a greater expansion of consultant services than was actually achieved. He had also chosen a specialty—obstetrics—which was one of the most popular and thus most competitive. As a result he was a senior registrar for nine years before being successful in a consultant appointment; and he was not appointed until the age of 41. The regional board appointed him to the hospital group, giving him the choice of a whole-time or maximum part-time contract. He chose to give full time "because I should be financially better off but as far as the work goes the choice was purely academic." There were already two consultant obstetricians, one of them attached to each of the group's two main hospitals which were several miles apart; the regional hospital board had assigned the newcomer to both hospitals. On the appropriate day he started his work by consulting with his two colleagues on how the work load should be shared among them. There was no difficulty about this. All were on basic salaries and there was thus no financial competition for NHS patients; moreover, the new man had chosen not to do private practice, so there was no threat of competition to the established obstetricians. The three decided among themselves how the available obstetric and gynecological beds would be allocated and arranged the new consultant's outpatient times; GPs in the area had already been informed by letter from their executive council of his arrival and thus knew of his availability. Initially he took all outpatients who were referred to the department with an "open" letter from a GP—that is, addressed merely to the Obstetric or Gynecological Department and not to an individual consultant—and also patients on the waiting lists of the other two consultants, who wished to be seen earlier by the new consultant. As he became known to the local GPs they began to refer patients directly to him.

It is clear that the consultant, although a salaried employee, has considerable freedom to organize his professional life. Once appointed by the hospital board, at an average age of 35, the consultant has a tenured appointment which is only exceptionally terminated before compulsory retirement on pension at age 65. There is little or no routine quality control over his practice. No programs of medical audit and no tissue committees, which exist in the United States, were set up under NHS administration. Indeed, it is often claimed that the rigorous selection procedure for consultants and their high initial standards make any such inspections superfluous. Although consultants have become employees of the state, there is little evidence of that fact in their working conditions. A staff of three or four administrative medical officers exists at the regional board offices, but they are concerned with aspects of medical staffing and planning at a regional level; they do not attempt to impose routine executive authority over individual consultant work.

There is a further factor—commented on as early as the Bradbeer report of 1954—that contributes to local consultant flexibility. By detaching consultants from local employment and attaching them to the regional hospital .

boards, the NHS inevitably weakened the relations between the consultants and the governing body of their own hospital and made it more difficult for them to maintain a "conscious sense of collective responsibility towards any one governing body." [10] Indeed, the local medical hierarchy under the new hospital service was less evident than before, as the old medical superintendents, who had held sway over the municipal hospitals, were reduced in number or were reclassified as consultants.[11] The Bradbeer report recommended the use of strong hospital or group medical committees or the appointment of one consultant as a part-time medical administrator or chief, with oversight of hospital clinical functions. But although most hospitals or groups set up their own medical committees, this last suggestion did not bear fruit. In the great majority of hospitals there is no one consultant with accepted responsibility for clinical standards. For practical purposes consultants continue to behave as if they were still independent professional men, voluntarily donating their services.

This lack of an individual responsible for general oversight of standards and practice within the hospital was to have at least one tragic consequence. In 1960 a consultant anesthesiologist was convicted in the courts for manslaughter which had resulted from his inhaling anesthetic gases during an operation. The implications of this case (the possibility that his colleagues knew of his addiction and thus might have prevented the disaster) were discussed by a national committee on drugs and addiction, headed by Lord Brain. The committee advised that responsibility for detecting such cases and preventing future harm lay in the first instance with a doctor's professional colleagues. It was emphasized that arrangements ought to be made for immediate action by the surgeon if the anesthesiologist appears incapable of carrying out his duties, and that medical staff committees should consider arrangements for dealing with this or any comparable emergency. The Joint Consultants Committee fully agreed that a collective moral responsibility for the safety of patients rested upon the staff as a whole. The Minister thereupon advised medical staff committees of each hospital group to appoint a small standing subcommittee of three or four senior staff to receive and take appropriate action on any report of incapacity or failure of responsibility, including addiction.[12] This subcommittee was to make confidential inquiries to establish the facts in any case and, unless the members were satisfied that they could deal with the situation by the exercise of their own influence,

10. Ministry of Health, Central Health Services Council, *Report of the Committee on the Internal Administration of Hospitals,* (HMSO, 1954), p. 12.

11. In 1948 there were 360 whole-time medical superintendents and 209 deputies, together with 264 part-time incumbents. By 1957, as nonmedical administrators took over much of the work, the time devoted by medical and deputy medical superintendents to administrative duties was equivalent to only 19 whole-time staff. After this date, administrative and clinical duties were not separately considered. Ministry of Health, *Annual Report for 1949,* pp. 356–57; and Ministry of Health Statistics Division (personal communication).

12. Ministry of Health Circular to hospital boards and committees HM (60), no. 45.

they were to bring it to the employing board. The latter would then decide what action should be taken. Thus a collective responsibility for one aspect of clinical standards in British hospital practice was publicly asserted; the subcommittee denoted a new attitude (though one with limited application) in the accepted professional code of nonintervention between consultants.

The absence of local executive responsibility for consultant standards and the traditional independence of the consultant branch also emphasized the more general need for standard disciplinary and dismissal arrangements in case of breach of NHS contract for reasons other than incapacity. Clearly, some arrangements had to be made whereby consultants might be dismissed by boards for offenses or inadequacies or might be disciplined for failing to fulfill the terms of their contracts. At the same time consultants, as other professional staff, had to be protected from unreasonable loss of livelihood.

One of the most serious threats to medical freedom seen by general practitioners during discussions of the National Health Service Act had been the absence of effective machinery to safeguard against unjust dismissal. To answer these objections, the Act had set up the National Health Service Tribunal for GPs and other professions which provide services for the local executive councils. The tribunal, composed of one lawyer, one professional member, and one other member, acts as an appeals body from decisions of executive councils on matters involving the professional conduct of local general practitioners, although final decisions lie with the Minister of Health. Under this system, general practitioners are given rights of appeal similar to those of pharmacologists and the other professionals who provide their skills to the National Health Service through a service contract instead of an employment relationship. The policing by the Ministry of contracted services would be expected to be greater than the policing of standards in hospitals, which are directly under Ministry control. But the result has been that GPs, who sought through their choice of a payment scheme to be independent practitioners, have become more restricted than salaried consultants, who have little or no supervision.[13] Again, consultants and GPs were divided by the type of relationship each entered into with the Ministry of Health.

Consultants and specialists had voiced no demand for an equivalent body and no parallel tribunal was set up to serve them. Disciplinary measures concerning negligent practice, or "infamous conduct," requiring removal or suspension from the Medical Register, remained for consultants and GPs alike the responsibility of the General Medical Council, which was, and is,

13. In 1964, decisions were issued by the Minister or the tribunal on 1,236 cases. Of these, 637—the largest single section—concerned GPs. In 539 of the 637 cases no breach of contract was found or action taken; in 45 cases money was withheld from the GP's capitation and other fees (i.e. he was fined an amount that in two cases exceeded 250 guineas); and in 53 cases a warning letter or other action was taken. In addition, the Ministry of Health's regional medical officers paid over 800 visits to GPs during 1964 to investigate high average prescription costs or one particularly high prescription. Ministry of Health, *Annual Report for 1964*, pp. 104–110.

outside the National Health Service structure. The GMC's functions are in no way usurped by the National Health Service, although hospital authorities are asked to notify the General Medical Council of all cases of dismissal or resignation connected with convictions in the courts. They are also free to report relevant facts of other dismissals. In some cases—for example, gross neglect of patients—the offending doctor is now subject to the disciplinary committees of both the General Medical Council and the hospital boards and also to that of his Royal College, although the Colleges tend to follow General Medical Council rulings rather than make separate inquiries.

The first (1949) and all subsequent editions of *Terms and Conditions of Service of Hospital Medical and Dental Staff*—the handbook of NHS employment—shied away from questions of discipline, except where there was a question of unfair termination of employment. Under section 16 of the handbook, any consultant or SHMO dismissed by his employing board was given a right of appeal to the Minister of Health. The Minister may obtain the written views of the employing board; he then places the case before a special professional advisory committee which consists of representatives of the Ministry and the medical profession. On its advice, the Minister may agree with the employing board or he may reinstate the consultant or come to some mutually agreeable arrangement such as re-employment in a different post. Until this decision is made, the consultant's notice of termination by the board cannot be carried into effect. Thus the consultant who has been dismissed by a primarily lay board (the regional hospital board or board of governors, of whom about one fourth are doctors) may be reinstated by the Minister on the advice of a predominantly professional body.

It might be thought, since the regional and teaching hospital boards are the Minister's agents, that decisions by the Minister would prima facie be decisions by an interested party, and that a tribunal would be a fairer alternative. But the appeals figures have shown no apparent bias in favor of the employing board. Of fifteen appeals against dismissal between 1950 and 1962, in only two cases was the dismissal confirmed. In one of these, termination arose from redundancy and in the other on a question of discipline. In the remaining thirteen cases the Minister accepted the recommendations of the professional committee that the doctor should continue in employment either in his existing appointment, with or without a reduction in the number of half days worked, or in a similar capacity elsewhere.[14] The evidence has shown, first, that it is exceedingly profitable for the dismissed consultant to appeal to the Minister; and second, that the employing authority can rarely succeed in dismissing a consultant. Some of the obvious dangers of monopoly employment have thus been reduced.

Apart from dismissal, no conditions for applying disciplinary action or

14. Of the total of 15 appeals, 3 resulted from disciplinary considerations, 1 from alleged incapacity through illness, and the rest from some modification of the consultant's contract owing to reorganization or redundancy. (Personal communication, Ministry of Health.)

appeals from such action were initially codified in the terms and conditions of service, although the Ministry, through a number of circulars sent out to the employing boards, from time to time suggested various courses of action. There was, for example, no standard procedure with which to approach the consultant who, while leaving his patients adequately covered by junior staff, spent most of his contracted time outside the hospital. During the course of a review of disciplinary and appeals procedures by the Ministry of Health in the early 1960s, one of the questions considered was whether a tribunal —similar to the existing National Health Service Tribunal for general practitioners—should be set up for hospital staff. A decision was made in favor of a less formal type of inquiry. After a great deal of confusion about the powers and duties of boards in particular disciplinary situations, the Ministry issued a circular which attempted to clarify the position in 1961.[15] In cases involving personal conduct, the hospital doctor was given the right to be heard and a right to appeal to the employing authority. He may also approach the Minister as a last resort, but he has no *right* for his case to be reconsidered unless he is dismissed. In questions of professional conduct or professional competence, machinery was recommended in 1961 for preliminary investigation and also for an inquiry, where there is dispute over the facts.

As a result of these measures, tenure of consultants is reasonably secure. Unlike general practitioners, consultants cannot be fined for excessive prescribing or for relatively minor breaches of contract. Hospital employing authorities have the power to suspend doctors from duty, not as a punishment but as a measure dictated by the interest of the service, pending a decision on further action. No formal disciplinary action exists for the consultant who wastes hospital money or who is constantly rude to patients. Patients may of course complain, but there is an impression that they are less ready to complain of specialists than of GPs, whom they see more often and who are more accessible. The regional hospital board medical staff may speak to an offender. Medical staff at the hospital may also raise questions of quality or efficiency among themselves or at their medical committee meetings. But once appointed, a consultant's reputation cannot affect his basic salary. In extreme situations GPs might not send patients to an offending consultant, and it could eventually happen that because of his reduced work the number of a consultant's sessions would be cut by the regional hospital board. But such cases are rare. Generally the consultant works as he thinks best, according to the standards which he himself accepts, and he is entitled to remain impervious to criticism.

Consultant medical practice under the National Health Service continues to be organized in the same basic patterns that were evident at the beginning of the twentieth century. The English hospital system relies on a compact, competitively selected group of specialists who spend their working life in

15. Ministry of Health Circular HM (61), no. 112.

the hospital, who know each other intimately, and whose patients are fed to them (as it were, predigested) by the area's GPs. Each consultant usually comes into the hospital on every day from Monday to Friday, and the consultants usually lunch together in their private dining room. Each clinician has a certain number of beds assigned to him in perhaps one or two large wards, and the sister (charge nurse) in those wards knows the consultant's methods and habits. The clinical consultant may share one or two junior medical staff with another consultant in the same specialty, or he may have a full-time registrar (resident) or house officer attached to him. In addition, a GP may come in once a week to help him in the outpatient department. The consultant, his junior medical staff, his ward nurse, his block of beds and his clinics form a semiautonomous unit within the hospital. This system cuts across other hierarchies, such as the nursing administration. Except that the consultant spends more time in the hospital, the system has changed little from that existing in the teaching hospitals at the beginning of the century.

One effect of this system is a curious relationship between consultant staff and the local administration of nonteaching hospitals. These hospitals were grouped under hospital management committees which are, for administrative purposes, constituents of the regional hospital board. Consultants, on the other hand, are employed directly by the regional board. They are therefore not directly responsible to the local boards (hospital management committees) of the hospitals in which they work. The individual consultant looks for advice to the senior administrative medical officer at regional level —a man of higher status than the administrator of the hospital group, who himself is responsible in an employment relationship to regional administration. The local relationship between consultant and hospital group management is thus one of equality rather than subordination. These patterns tend to reinforce the old feeling of the consultant as an *attending* member of the hospital staff, although a National Health Service employee. The system is strangely reminiscent of the time when physicians, who were gentlemen, gave freely of their time to the hospitalized poor in hospitals run by voluntary boards, whose members were also gentlemen. This is hardly surprising since, although the payment mechanism was that of local authorities, much of the atmosphere of the voluntary hospital system was incorporated into the National Health Service.

The operational flexibility thereby gained has had a considerable impact on the attitude of the consultant to NHS employment. It undoubtedly facilitated his adjustment to employment in a monopoly public service, as did certain other factors: the continued existence of private practice, the curious system of distinction awards, and the major involvement in the machinery of administration and advice.

14

The Consultant, the National Health Service, and the Place of Private Practice

Even before the National Health Service, specialized medicine with its growing array of machinery, facilities, and staff was encouraging consultants to conduct most of their practice from within the hospital. The introduction of a salaried service formalized this trend by making it possible for consultants in all specialties to be paid for the time they spent in hospital. Regional hospital boards, in their advertisements for consultant posts, encouraged specialists to accept a relatively large number of NHS sessions. As early as 1949 almost a fourth of consultants employed in the NHS were on whole-time contracts, and the average number of half-day sessions of whole-time and part-time consultants combined was well over seven per week.[1]

Since then the proportion of whole-time consultants has scarcely changed; just over one fourth (28 per cent) of NHS consultants worked whole time in 1963 (Table 10). Specialties that attract whole timers appear to fall into two groups: those that were traditionally whole-time appointments as they developed under municipal authorities (chest diseases, infectious diseases, geriatrics, mental illness); and those tied to the hospital because of their need for staff or facilities (radiotherapy, pathology). In both of these categories there is little private practice. Indeed, the continuance of private practice is an important factor influencing the choice of part-time contracts, for although the relative number of whole-time consultants fluctuates widely, the average number of sessions or proportion of time contracted to NHS hospitals is remarkably consistent among the specialties. About 90 per cent of general surgeons are on part time, but the average part-timer in that specialty has a contract for over eight sessions (four days) a week. With one or two exceptions it is clear that a substantial proportion of part-time consultants is on "maximum part-time" contracts of nine sessions a week, and

1. There were 1,310 whole-time consultant appointments in 1949, out of a total of 5,189 consultants, including honorary NHS staff and those appointed by the Board of Control (since abolished) and the Public Health Laboratory Service. The sum of sessions undertaken by consultants represented a work load equivalent to 3,549 whole-time staff (the total number of sessions divided by 11). Ministry of Health, *Annual Report for 1955*, p. 168, *Annual Report for 1960*, p. 187, and Ministry of Health Statistics Division.

TABLE 10. *Percentage of Paid and Honorary Whole-Time Consultants by Specialty, 1963*

Specialty	Total Number	Whole Time Number	Percentage of Whole Time	Percentage of Working Week Committed to NHS hospitals *
All Specialties	7,802	2,146	27.5	79.8
General medicine	786	123	15.6	75.2
Pediatrics	227	51	22.5	78.9
Infectious diseases	30	23	76.7	83.3
Chest diseases	272	170	62.5	89.7
Dermatology	142	8	5.6	73.2
Neurology	95	8	8.4	74.7
Cardiology	37	4	10.8	73.0
Physical medicine	95	22	23.2	77.9
Venereal disease	75	33	44.0	82.7
Geriatrics	104	77	74.0	94.2
General surgery	845	93	11.0	78.9
Ear-nose-throat	310	7	2.3	75.5
Traumatic & orthopedic surgery	385	27	7.0	79.5
Ophthalmology	302	2	0.7	70.9
Urology	40	1	2.5	72.5
Plastic surgery	53	6	11.3	81.1
Thoracic surgery	91	14	15.4	81.3
Dentistry & orthodontics	290	69	23.8	61.7
Neurosurgery	66	10	15.2	81.8
Gynecology & obstetrics	467	36	7.7	77.9
Anesthesiology	886	164	18.5	80.9
Radiology	508	186	36.6	85.6
Radiotherapy	135	73	54.1	89.6
Pathology	758	438	57.8	82.7
Blood transfusion	13	13	100.0	100.0
Mental illness	593	382	64.4	87.2
Mental subnormality	75	69	92.0	97.3
Mental illness (children)	108	37	34.3	75.0
Social medicine	9			22.2
Other	5			20.0

* Total number of NHS sessions for each specialty, divided by number of sessions possible if all consultants were whole time. Whole time work is assessed at 11 sessions (half days) per week.

Figures in this table include honorary staff, for example full-time university teachers or research workers with hospital privileges, and exclude temporary staff on paid appointments.

Source: Ministry of Health, Statistics Division.

such contracts are frequently considered equivalent to whole-time employment.

Recent employment figures are shown in Table 11. If anything, there appears to be a slight trend toward whole-time appointments and a tendency for part-timers to increase their sessions. In 1959 the average part-time paid consultant had a contract for 7.9 sessions; the comparable figure

TABLE 11. *Employment of Paid Consultants in the National Health Service; England and Wales, 1959–1964*

	PAID CONSULTANTS				AVERAGE NO. OF SESSIONS OF PAID CONSULTANTS	
	Total No. of Consul- tants (1)	No. of Paid Consul- tants (2)	No. in Full- time NHS Employ- ment	Per Cent Full Time	All	Part Time Only
1959	7,052	6,572	1,772	27.0	8.8	7.9
1960	7,200	6,701	1,824	27.2	8.8	8.0
1961	7,456	6,900	1,918	27.8	8.9	8.1
1962	7,645	7,059	2,009	28.5	9.0	8.2
1963	7,944	7,221	2,146	29.7	9.0	8.2
1964	8,161	7,355	2,249	30.6	9.1	8.3

Column 1 includes honorary staff, and also temporary locum staff who are not included in Table 10. In 1962, for example, there were 42 incumbents of consultant posts in a locum tenens capacity, 544 honorary staff, and 7,059 paid consultants on regular contracts (column 2), a total of 7,645 including locum appointments. As far as possible, inconsistencies in base data have been removed from the tables given, but this has not always been practical because of the different forms in which official data are presented. Figures before 1959 are not available.

Source: Annual Reports of the Ministry of Health.

five years later was 8.3. Taking all consultants together, the average number of sessions in 1964 was 9.1, or over 4.5 days a week. The neurologist contracted for the same number of sessions as the average consultant in pediatrics, gynecology, or radiotherapy; and the average 40-year-old consultant had a contract similar to that of the man of 60. Whole time or part time, the consultant spends most of his time in the NHS hospital.

It is because of this concentration on the hospital that there are still relatively few consultants compared with the number of doctors as a whole, despite the great increase in hospital work and the growing sophistication of hospital techniques. The underlying reasons for this British pattern are historical. Its implications may, however, be general to other societies in which professional patterns have developed differently.[2]

To the English GP the hospital is on the periphery of medical care. An average of less than one of ten patients seen by the GP is referred to the hospital outpatient department, primarily for treatment or advice, although there are wide variations in referral rates among practitioners.[3] Precise figures are unavailable, but the average number of consultations between patients and GPs appears to be about four per listed person per year. This would indicate, in the crude terms of doctor–patient contacts, less than one visit by a patient to a consultative outpatient department to every six visits to a GP, and one visit to an emergency or casualty department to every fourteen or fifteen GP consultations.[4] Even without allowing for the selectivity of those patients who have hospital contact, and who may therefore weight the number of attendances at outpatient and emergency clinics, the strong GP element of practice is evident. Hospital care—and thus consultant care—is merely the top of a widely based iceberg.

Some of the effects of a system in which general practitioners outnumber consultants by almost three to one and consultants spend most of their time on hospital work, can best be described by illustration. There is a city in the south of England, which (let us say) is called Southhaven. The city itself has a population of a quarter of a million people, but the city's hospitals—grouped under one hospital management committee (HMC)—cover a suburban and rural population of a much larger size. There are two large general hospitals, each of over 500 beds (one an ex-municipal hospital, the other an ex-voluntary hospital), three smaller hospitals in the city, and several rural cottage hospitals and maternity homes, all of which were in existence before the National Health Service. The group laboratory and the hospital X-ray departments are open to all local general practitioners.

In Southhaven itself there are just under a hundred GPs, typically practicing in small partnerships from specially built centers, lockup surgeries, or from their homes, with the minimum of on-the-spot professional and technical assistance. Outside the city but within the hospital service area are probably another fifty GPs who make some use of Southhaven's hospitals.

---

2. Roemer has illustrated a trend toward employment of full-time chiefs of service in general hospitals in the United States, not only in radiology and pathology but increasingly in the clinical specialties. It seems probable that this trend will continue as the hospital increases its technological expertise. In the long term the proportion of physicians with control of inpatient hospital facilities in the United States may contract, and British experience may be peculiarly relevant. Milton Roemer, *Am. J. Pub. Health,* Sept. 1962, p. 1453.

3. See D. L. Crombie and K. W. Cross, *Lancet ii* (1964), 354.

4. In 1963 there were 47,325,431 names on GP lists. If, on average, each listed person paid four visits to a GP in that year, 189,301,724 visits were paid. There were 30,002,000 attendances at consultative outpatient departments and 12,894,000 to hospital accident and emergency departments. Ministry of Health, *Annual Report for 1963,* pp. 66, 130.

General practitioners admit their patients to beds in the cottage and small maternity hospitals, but not to the major hospital in the city. About forty of the GPs also work part time in the hospitals, usually as clinical assistants at a consultant outpatient session once or twice a week. No health centers have been built by the city authorities and none is planned; like other local authorities their attitude to health centers is cautious. A number of GPs do, however, conduct antenatal sessions for the city, and those on the GP obstetric list work closely with the local domiciliary midwives. All draw on other municipal services such as home nursing, home help, or health visiting for the treatment of their patients in the community. GPs undertake the great majority of all medical episodes, treat common illnesses, and offer advice on a much wider range of subjects, including marriage guidance and housing problems, than is available at the local hospitals.

In contrast there are only forty-eight consultants over all specialties in Southhaven, all employed by the regional hospital board, which is in a different city. They have beds or facilities assigned to them in the group's hospitals and they accept their NHS patients primarily through GP referral. There are another seventeen specialists in the SHMO grade, plus sixty-five hospital doctors from the senior registrar down to house officer level. The small group of consultants is privileged; their work is selected and their standing is high. Southhaven has only one consultant pediatrician for the whole area of perhaps 400,000 people. He works with a registrar and a part-time GP clinical assistant and shares a house physician with a consultant in another specialty, spends most of his time in the group hospitals, regularly attending four hospitals, and visits the outlying hospitals when called in. He is responsible for sixty-eight NHS hospital beds, holds four consultative outpatient clinics a week, makes an average of three to four visits a week to patients' homes, and says he is "mildly" overworked. In addition he has a small private practice.

Similarly, there is only one dermatologist, one thoracic surgeon, and one consultant in orthodontics serving the hospital group; the forty-eight consultants span eighteen different specialties. All concentrate on cases GPs do not feel competent to handle. Each has an assigned number of hospital beds, assigned junior medical staff and GP assistants. Other specialties are provided elsewhere in the region at strategic regional centers. These include the psychiatric specialties, plastic surgery, and neurosurgery. In turn the Southhaven group has its own radiotherapy unit with two consultants, which draws patients from other groups without this facility. All the consultants are employed on identical terms of service; some have more NHS sessions than others, some hold NHS distinction awards, some undertake private practice.

A consultant in general medicine described his weekly schedule as three mornings or afternoons a week on ward rounds and another three on scheduled outpatient sessions. The remainder of his time might be spent on the wards, dictating notes or letters to GPs, conferring with the social worker, visiting the general practitioner hospitals attached to the hospital group, making domiciliary visits (an average of three a week), attending meetings, or "general odds and ends." The consultant had thirty beds in general medicine at one hospital and had the services of a half-time registrar—a full-time man whom he shared with a second consultant physician—and a full-time house physician. Another consultant in the same specialty but in a different hospital group had a similar schedule. He shared responsibility with a consultant colleague for forty general medical beds and a hundred geriatric beds together with a geriatric day hospital; the two men had the services of one full-time registrar and two house physicians. In addition, this being primarily a rural group stretching over a wide area, the consultant visited a number of GP and maternity hospitals and paid occasional visits to a neighboring hospital for the mentally subnormal. The first had a maximum part-time NHS contract, the second worked whole time.

The keys to the system—besides the existence of the general practitioners —are the organization of hospital staffing and the consultative role of the outpatient department. Hospital staffing patterns ensure the personal attachment of junior to senior staff, and thus the potential for regular delegation by the consultant of certain medical duties to other members of his team. The consultant's responsibilities go much farther than the work he himself performs. He may, for example, see all new patients referred to his outpatient clinic, but delegate most of the return consultations to his registrar, house officer, or clinical assistant. The function of the hospital outpatient department is to provide a specialist consultation service for all sectors of society at the request of GPs; walk-in patients are seen only in the emergency room.

The Consultant's Work

So much is the professional independence of consultants taken for granted that, although they are employed by the hospital boards for the great majority of their working week, there are virtually no data on how they spend their time or how work is assigned among the consultant's team. Undoubtedly, practice varies considerably. The Platt report gave as an illustration the work load associated with eighty occupied beds in 1957 in two groups of similarly matched hospitals. At Hospital A, in the specialty of general medicine, 83 new outpatients and 267 old outpatients were seen on the average each week; at Hospital B the comparable figures were 23 and 90. At Hospital C 125 operations were performed a week in general surgery; at Hospital D the figure was only 38.[5] There is thus great variability even within a specialty, the reasons for which may be partly functional and partly historical.

Revans has suggested that each hospital has a character of its own, linked with various factors including staff attitudes and length of patients' stay.[6]

5. Platt report on hospital medical staffing, p. 18.
6. R. W. Revans, *Standards for Morale, Cause and Effect in Hospitals* (London, 1964).

Feldstein has shown that in areas where there are fewer hospital beds, fewer people are admitted to hospital, rather than a larger number admitted for shorter periods.[7] There are also marked variations in the rates of GP referrals to consultative outpatient sessions and in the proportion of outpatients to inpatients.[8] The ratio of senior to junior medical staff and of medical staff to nurses obviously also influences the amount and character of consultant work. Operational research in medical care in Britain is, however, still in its infancy. For example, there has been no definitive study of the effect on the GP's work of a relatively greater or smaller number of consultants in particular specialties—or vice versa. Existing indicators of consultant work are de jure, rather than de facto; they measure the responsibility of the consultant rather than what he actually does.

The national number of beds, discharges, and outpatient clinics averaged in relation to each broad specialty group is shown in Table 12. The data are

TABLE 12. *Consultant Work Loads by Specialty Group; England and Wales, 1963*

Specialty Group	No. of Full-time and Part-time Consultants	Average No. of Beds	Average Annual No. of Discharges and Deaths	Average No. of Clinics per Year	Average No. of Attendances per Clinic
		PER CONSULTANT IN EACH SPECIALTY GROUP			
Medicine *	2,174	58	509	207	19.7
Surgery †	2,215	32	824	237	28.6
Obstetrics & gynecology	467	61	2,060	323	29.7
Psychiatry	776	266	223	241	7.6
Other specialties ‡	2,170	2	17		

* General medicine, pediatrics, infectious diseases, chest diseases, dermatology, neurology, physical medicine, venereal diseases, geriatrics, chronic diseases.

† General surgery, urology, ear-nose-throat, orthopedics, ophthalmology, plastic and thoracic surgery, dentistry, neurosurgery, radiotherapy.

‡ Anesthesiology, radiology, pathology and subspecialties, blood transfusion, and other specialties.

The average number of beds refers only to those in specialist units. It excludes beds in general practitioner medical, dental, and maternity units; pre-convalescent and convalescent beds; and staff and private beds.

Source: Ministry of Health, *Annual Report for 1963*, pp. 128, 130, 136.

7. Martin S. Feldstein, *Brit. Med. J. ii* (1964), 562.
8. See R. F. Logan in *Problems and Progress in Medical Care,* ed. Gordon McLachlan (London, 1964).

crude and hide considerable variations among the specialties. Thus the medical group includes such specialties as venereology, which has a relatively small number of inpatient beds and a large outpatient service, and specialties like geriatrics which have one consultant responsible for several hundred beds. Nevertheless, the broad pattern of consultant care under the NHS is shown: a substantial block of beds (whose number per physician or surgeon is not too dissimilar to that existing in the larger voluntary hospitals at the beginning of this century), a large consultative outpatient practice, and a fairly busy schedule of domiciliary consultations at the request of GPs.

A domiciliary consultation is defined in *Terms and Conditions of Service* as a "visit to the patient's home, to advise on the diagnosis or treatment of a patient who on medical grounds cannot attend hospital." Over 130,000 such consultations were made in 1949, and by 1963 the annual rate was over 320,000.[9] Any GP can call any consultant (or SHMO) who has agreed with the employing board to undertake domiciliary visits, and the consultant merely fills in a claim form to collect his payment for them. Eighty per cent of consultants were available for domiciliary consultation in 1962, and in that year they made, on average over all specialties, one such visit per consultant per week. The great majority of domiciliary consultants were in the field of general (internal) medicine, general surgery, and general (adult) psychiatry—a factor that may indicate a major use of such visits for diagnostic purposes. In 1962 these three specialties accounted for over half the domiciliary visits made by consultants. The figures are given in Table 13. Other specialties that had a large proportion of domiciliary visits relative to their size were pediatrics, chest diseases, geriatrics, orthopedic surgery, and gynecology–obstetrics—all fields which are to some extent GP specialties, routinely handled by general practitioners.

Interviews with consultants indicated a wide range of practice and attitude to the domiciliary service. One pediatrician, who made about 170 domiciliary visits a year, spoke of the difficulties of communicating with the GP: "The GP phones up and says I've got a child for you to see—and I make the visit to keep the child out of hospital, although many of them could be seen as outpatients. I go in my own time and the GP isn't usually there."

Some consultants appear to regard such visits not as true consultations but as an extension of, or an alternative to, hospital practice, when the GP is not present; some may not wish to call the GP out on an extra visit; and in some cases the GP himself may not desire to attend. Others disagree. One consultant obstetrician, for example, said he was called in for home visits "because the GP wants to discuss his patients with you—a *real* consultation." A general surgeon discerned three main reasons in GP requests for him to visit: advice on the management in the home of inoperable cases in the elderly, decision on whether the patient's abdominal pain is grounds for hospital admission, and cases in which the patient is a friend of the GP and

9. Ministry of Health, *Annual Report for 1963*, p. 124.

TABLE 13. *Domiciliary Consultations by Consultants in Contract with Regional Hospital Boards in the Year Ended 30 September 1962 by Specialty*

	No. of Consultations	Percentage
General medicine	69,546	23.8
Pediatrics	13,214	4.5
Infectious diseases	855	0.3
Chest diseases	13,080	4.5
Dermatology	7,111	2.4
Neurology	2,519	0.9
Cardiology	1,432	0.5
Physical medicine	3,254	1.1
Venereal disease	72	*
Geriatrics	13,435	4.6
General surgery	50,308	17.2
Ear-nose-throat	7,677	2.6
Traumatic & orthopedic surgery	17,818	6.1
Ophthalmology	7,552	2.6
Radiotherapy	1,569	0.5
Urology	644	0.2
Plastic surgery	116	*
Thoracic surgery	391	0.1
Dentistry	148	*
Neurosurgery	879	0.3
Anesthesiology	847	0.3
Gynecology & obstetrics	21,898	7.5
Pathology	12,861	4.4
Radiology	11,130	3.8
Subnormality & severe subnormality	452	0.2
Mental illness	33,091	11.4
Mental illness (children)	244	*
Orthodontics	7	*
Total	292,150	100

* Less than one tenth of 1%.

Senior hospital medical officers, although able to undertake such visits, are not included in this table; SHMOs made 23,823 visits during this period.

Source: Gillie Report, p. 60.

the domiciliary visit saves him from spending time in the outpatient department or seeing the consultant as a private patient. Such comments can be multiplied. They may not be representative of consultants' views in general, but they indicate some of the uses to which home visits are put. How far the free domiciliary service does keep patients out of hospital, provides a better service, is a forum for direct communication between consultant and GP, or saves certain patients the embarrassment or inconvenience of a hospital appointment cannot yet be quantitatively assessed. The potential exists for all such claims, and the growing number of consultations indicates their attractiveness to general practitioners. The domiciliary service, like other aspects of consultant work, is not rigidly policed by hospital administration. The only barrier is the amount of money for basic domiciliary fees which the National Health Service will pay; there is a ceiling of £960 (200 paid visits) per specialist per year.

The Extent of Private Medical Practice

Apart from this inpatient, outpatient, and domiciliary work, all part-time consultants and SHMOs in the NHS are free to undertake private practice. Conversely, all patients may receive either NHS or private medical care at their own volition, or both in a variety of combinations, simultaneously or at different times. A patient may be referred by his GP under the NHS to a consultant whom, for reasons of convenience, he decides to see privately; or the same situation might exist in reverse. For both specialists and general practitioners, NHS work forms the major part of their practice, but for both, private practice exists as another kind of practice. Because it provides an alternative—and for many doctors an additional source of income—private practice has an importance disproportionate to its size. Its presence or absence may indicate a degree of dissatisfaction or acceptance of NHS practice on the part of the doctor or the patient. It may have some value as a gauge of NHS standards. It may be relished by some practitioners as a more relaxed or a more invigorating type of work. Possibly, as is sometimes claimed, it gives the doctor a feeling of greater freedom or flexibility; or some may have inherited a vague belief from the past that those who served part time (in a voluntary hospital) were thought of more highly than those who served whole time (in the municipal hospitals). The tantalizing fact of all these possibilities is that they must, for the present, remain only speculative.

Little is known of the extent or the nature of private medical practice as it now exists in England. Figures given by the Royal Comission on Doctors' and Dentists' Remuneration were inconclusive. GPs reported average incomes of £2,129 in 1955–56, when the target net income from the NHS capitation system was £2,222. Consultants reported an average income of £3,391 where the basic NHS scale ranged from £2,100 to £3,100 for a whole-time employee; [10] but the Commission did not disclose how much of

10. *Royal Commission; Report,* pp. 62, 113.

this represented additional NHS payments such as distinction awards or fees for special services (such as domiciliary fees), and it is therefore impossible to estimate by elimination how much the consultant earned outside NHS practice. Even in fiscal terms, therefore, the relative importance of private practice is unknown.

The amount of private practice by GPs is particularly difficult to assess. A survey of 14,580 GPs in 1955–56 indicated that about 10 per cent regarded private practice as the main part of their work, and another 26 per cent regarded it as subsidiary.[11] Recent events in the pay structure disputes in general practice (described in Chapter 21) have emphasized the development of private practice as an alternative to the NHS, but have revealed no new data on either present or potential levels.

Private practice by specialists can be measured in one respect; the only well-documented gauge, and this may be misleading, is the utilization of pay beds in National Health Service hospitals. These include both private and "amenity" hospital beds, identified by the section of the NHS Act that applies to them. Private or "section 5" beds are fully private in that the patient is responsible for payment of both hospital bills and medical fees; the patients are usually accommodated in specifically designated single rooms. With certain exceptions, consultants are not permitted to admit private patients to beds other than those so designated. Besides occupying a single room, the private patient normally receives a different diet but does not necessarily receive better or more frequent nursing care. The chief medical advantages appear to be flexibility in admission date (including possible avoidance of a long waiting period for hospital admission) and, particularly in obstetrical and surgical cases, a greater degree of certainty that the consultant himself and not one of the juniors will supervise or undertake major procedures. The private patient pays hospital charges on an average charge scale. This is in no way related to the cost of services received but is merely an average cost of patient care per week over the whole hospital. Medical fees are normally subject to ceilings for various procedures laid down by the Ministry of Health. Amenity or "section 4" beds are also beds outside the main wards, but all services provided, including medical services, are supposedly identical with those on the general wards. The patient pays a small fee each week for the amenity of privacy obtained; no medical fees are payable.

Table 14 indicates that the number of private beds in NHS hospitals has remained relatively static since 1948. In 1963 private beds represented only 1 per cent of all staffed NHS hospital beds. Not only were they few, but private beds were on average only half filled with private patients on any one day; there was little change in this low rate of occupancy between 1953 and 1963, and none in the proportion of all hospital beds occupied by private patients (shown in column 7 of Table 14.) It cannot be argued that

11. Figures refer to Great Britain. *Royal Commission; Supplement to Report, Further Statistical Appendix,* Cmnd. 1064 (HMSO, 1960), p. 102.

TABLE 14. *Private and Amenity Beds in National Health Service Hospitals, England and Wales, 1949–1963*

	Total Occupied NHS Beds Thousands	AMENITY BEDS			PRIVATE BEDS		
		No. of Designated Amenity Beds	Average Daily Occupancy by Paying Patients %	Beds Occupied by Paying Patients as Per Cent of all NHS Occupied Beds %	Staffed Beds Allocated	Average Daily Occupancy by Paying Patients %	Beds Occupied by Paying Patients as Per Cent of all Occupied Beds %
	(1)	(2)	(3)	(4)	(5)	(6)	(7)
1949	397.6	5,901			6,647		
1950	402.6	5,388			6,402		
1951	406.8	6,030			5,960		
1952	416.1	6,086			5,726		
1953	424.1	6,257	46.2	0.7	5,793	49.7	0.7
1954	427.6	5,900	48.9	0.7	5,787	48.5	0.7
1955	426.0	5,997	45.9	0.6	5,656	49.4	0.7
1956	423.8	5,942	44.1	0.6	5,634	50.8	0.7
1957	420.2	5,400	48.0	0.6	5,609	50.8	0.7
1958	417.6	5,449	42.4	0.6	5,645	49.9	0.7
1959	412.6	5,425	42.2	0.6	5,713	47.9	0.7
1960	410.3	5,345	39.1	0.5	5,595	49.8	0.7
1961	404.4	5,143	37.4	0.5	5,593	50.1	0.7
1962	403.0	5,012	34.6	0.4	5,622	50.3	0.7
1963	404.0	4,996	31.9	0.4	5,623	51.2	0.7

To give as realistic a picture as possible, the figure for private beds is the number of "staffed beds allocated." This is slightly lower than the number of beds officially designated as Section 5 accommodation. In 1962, for example, there were 5,663 designated private beds; from this figure the average daily occupancy by paying patients was 49.9.

Source: Ministry of Health, *Digest of Health Service Statistics*. This table includes all NHS beds in general, mental, special, and cottage hospitals, and in NHS convalescent homes.

private practice in NHS hospitals is increasing.[12] If anything, it appears to be slowly decreasing in relation to utilization of NHS beds as a whole, for the turnover in nonprivate beds has increased faster. The use of amenity beds by paying patients fell between 1953 and 1963. On average, of every 1,000 patients in all NHS general, special, and mental hospitals on any one day in 1963, 7 chose to be private patients, 4 to occupy amenity beds (paying only a nominal charge), and 989 were liable to no hospital charges or medical fees.

Although private practice forms a minute and apparently stationary part of work in NHS hospitals, there may be some increase in other forms of private practice. Seventy per cent of NHS consultants were on part-time contracts in 1963, and it is possible that the majority conducted at least a token private practice besides this work. Some specialists practice completely independently of the NHS, but it is not known to what extent. One estimate in 1961 was that 700 doctors (GPs and specialists) were employed wholly in private practice in England, Wales, and Scotland,[13] the equivalent of under 2 per cent of all doctors engaged in clinical or hospital work in the National Health Service. But this figure is admittedly the product of guesswork; it could be more but it may well be less.

There are many private nursing homes, some of which are equipped as full-scale hospitals. Nursing homes are not controlled by the National Health Service. The Nuffield Nursing Home Trust, a private nonprofit organization, opened eight nursing homes of between twenty-five and forty beds between 1958 and 1962 and had plans for seven more.[14] These are very small numbers, but they reveal some demand for private care outside NHS hospitals. There may also be a flourishing consulting practice from private offices, which certain aspects of the NHS may actively encourage. The professional ethics and administrative rules that obtain between private and NHS services are not clear. Although private patients must pay for their drugs, some GPs send private patients to hospital for free diagnostic X-ray and pathological services under the NHS or refer them for NHS outpatient advice. The existence of a free GP and hospital service has undoubtedly also influenced the kind of private practice now demanded. Patients in private nursing homes may sometimes benefit from the free diagnostic services of a neighboring hospital; or a patient may live in a nursing home and be transported to a NHS hospital for free radiotherapy or other forms of treatment. Some people may prefer to carry insurance for private convalescent care after hospitalization under the NHS. The relatively low fee schedules for private procedures undertaken in private accommodation in NHS hospitals may keep down the medical fees charged by consultants for other private

12. For a different view see D. S. Lees and M. H. Cooper, *Brit. Med. J.* i (1963), 1531–33.

13. John and Sylvia Jewkes, *The Genesis of the British National Health Service* (Oxford, 1961), p. 56.

14. *Brit. Med. J.* i (1963), 1531.

patients, and thus encourage nursing home care. Equally, however, they may discourage consultants from all kinds of private practice.

Nor is health insurance an accurate guide. The British United Provident Association, the largest single voluntary contributing insurance agency, estimated in 1963 that its own membership covered about 1.8 per cent of the total population and that about 3 per cent of the population was covered by some source. Even though the number insured continues to rise, the actual proportion is thus still insignificant. Moreover, the total includes insurance for different kinds of health service (for example, hospital or convalescent care alone); the proportion of total health service covered is inevitably less.[15] On the other hand, the extent of private practice may not be related to the number insured. An unknown degree of "intermittent" or "convenience" private visits are made by patients who accept most services under the NHS (and do not carry health insurance) but in particular situations seek private advice. Whether this type of consultation becomes more frequent as the population becomes more affluent, is unknown. Even if such practice is increasing, however, it seems clear that although a few GPs and consultants can undoubtedly make a living on private fees, it is equally certain that the great majority will not be able to do so unless public attitudes to medical care radically change. If private consultant practice were developing substantially, there would probably not be a movement toward more NHS sessions and to full-time rather than part-time NHS work. The question remains of how far individual practitioners can or cannot actively stimulate their private practice if they wish to do so.

The medical profession's Porritt report (1962) spoke of private practice as an incentive and a stimulus to good work, and suggested measures through which private practice should be encouraged. But at the same time, the members of the Porritt Committee concluded that "basically, the concept of a comprehensive national health service is sound." [16] Similarly, the results of a Gallup poll conducted in conjunction with the Porritt report, indicated that 82 per cent of a population sample said they received "good service" from the National Health Service; 41 per cent of the sample thought their GPs also had private patients; and 32 per cent considered that the doctor made the same arrangements for private patients that he did for those treated under the NHS.[17]

There is no lack of criticism of the NHS. General practitioners are particularly vehement about their income and their working conditions. Many consultants are bitterly incensed at the poor physical structure and lack of money for maintenance of many hospital buildings and facilities. Nevertheless, the NHS is not generally regarded as a second-class service vis à vis private practice—either by doctors or by patients. Such evidence as there is suggests the continuation of the National Health Service and private prac-

15. British United Provident Association (personal communication).
16. *A Review of the Medical Services in Great Britain* (Porritt report), p. 14.
17. Ibid., pp. 216–17, 223.

tice side by side, with private work providing a relatively minor part of the practitioner's total load. For consultants there may be a continuing trend toward full-time NHS contracts in all specialties. All the advantages of consultant status—access to hospital beds, and professional recognition through the distinction awards system—lie within the National Health Service. Private consultation is a real alternative for the prospective patients; to the doctor it means only that for some part of his time he sees patients to whom he sends medical bills.

The continuation of a system in which there are relatively few consultants and relatively many general practitioners—with a system of referral operating between them—enhances the consultant's operational flexibility within the National Health Service. The hospital is confirmed as the base of a relatively small number of experts who concentrate the great majority of their time on referred specialist work. Even in a large city there may be just one pediatrician or one dermatologist who focuses only on the rare or more sophisticated branches of his subject. Naturally this degree of rarity adds eminence, and eminence of itself presupposes certain operational freedom. From the consultant's point of view the system has much to commend it. Its disadvantages refer not to the relationship between the consultant and the hospital authorities or to some vague menace of bureaucracy, but to the relationship between the consultant in the hospital and the GP in the home.

15

The Distinction Awards System

In theory, and to some extent in practice, a free medical market has built-in financial incentives. Doctors operate on a fee-for-service basis in a system more or less conforming to the dynamics of supply and demand. The two gauges of the specialist's market value, and hence the fees he can command, are his popularity with patients and the respect of referring colleagues. Medical incomes are therefore unequal, and material and professional success tend to develop hand in hand. A salaried service is based on different criteria, on peer or employer judgment rather than on consumer demand; payment for time replaces payment for work done. Under a nationalized system the two methods had to be reconciled.

The National Health Service took over a large group of specialists, badly distributed and with a wide range of income. There were large variations among specialist groups and among individuals in the same specialty. Of a sample of specialists practicing in London in 1938–39, 13 per cent of those aged between 40 and 49 had net incomes of less than £1,000, and 87 per cent earned less than £5,000; yet 2 per cent earned net incomes of more than £10,000.[1] The range of incomes represented about a tenfold difference between the highest and the lowest.

The wartime hospital surveys had shown that the competitive system, whatever its merits as a professional morale booster, had not succeeded in providing an efficient specialist service throughout the country; specialists were concentrated in the major cities, particularly in London. The Ministry of Health and the profession were faced with the dilemma of remunerating NHS specialists in such a way that a more even distribution of specialists could be achieved without, at the same time, destroying a financial incentive for good work or upsetting those consultants—some of whom were leaders of the medical profession—who were earning considerably more than average. The Spens Committee of 1948, which established the present payment mechanism, was limited in scope by being specifically enjoined to take notice of what specialists were earning before the war; it could thus not be particularly original. Not surprisingly, the committee skirted the psychological problem of whether financial inducements do in fact improve professional work and concentrated on the practical problem of integrating several

1. Spens Report on Consultants and Specialists, p. 24.

thousand specialists, already earning unequal incomes, into some kind of income pattern acceptable both to the profession and to the state. The result was a curious and unique system of professional patronage in a public service.

The uniform salary scale satisfied the need for standardizing salaries among specialties and among hospitals. Through the basic salary, every full-time consultant was assured a comfortable income but not a lavish one. Approximately one third of all specialists were, however, to receive more than the basic scale through the award of additional money on the basis of merit. The solution was an ingenious answer to reconciling unequal incomes with egalitarian principles. Distinction awards, it was claimed, would provide "sufficient incentives to stimulate effort and encourage initiative." The present whole-time salary scale (from April 1963) for consultants at age 34 or on appointment is £2,910, rising by nine increments to £4,445; the maximum of the scale can be reached by age 44. With a top distinction award a whole-time consultant may receive £9,000. A considerable range was thus built into the NHS system.

The crux of the distinction awards system was the definition of individual distinction or merit. With a reduction in private practice, the general public and referring GPs were largely removed from deciding relative merit in financial terms. Salary levels are usually decided by employers, but government, in its role of employer, was not to assign the awards even though the money involved was public money and part of the operating budget of the National Health Service. This was left by the Spens Committee to the medical profession. For the first time, since the new awards would be payable as extra salary tailored to the number of NHS sessions undertaken by the consultant, the profession was to have direct administrative control over the income of its most eminent members and was to adjudicate their relative worth.

The distinction awards system was created as, and has remained, an intra-professional matter at a very high level. The overall number of awards is centrally controlled, but decisions on the allocation of awards are made by an advisory committee appointed by the Minister of Health. This committee is in effect a symposium of the English and Scottish consultant bodies, including among others the presidents of the three English Royal Colleges and senior representatives of the Scottish Colleges. The committee dispenses considerable patronage; in 1964 it made 12 new A-plus awards (an annual sum of £4,550 each), 29 A awards (£3,425), 58 B awards (£2,000), and 106 C awards (£850). A consultant keeps his award until he retires, when he receives additional pension in lieu of it. Altogether there are 100 A-plus awards available, together with 300 A awards, 850 B awards and 1,700 C awards.[2] Table 15 shows the actual distribution of awards in 1964; the

2. B awards were increased from 800 to 850 and C awards from 1,600 to 1,700 as an interim measure; *Review Body on Doctors' and Dentists' Remuneration,* Fourth Report, Jan. 1965, Cmnd. 2585 (HMSO, 1965).

Distinction Awards Committee (even allowing for reduced awards to part-time consultants) is ultimately responsible for the distribution of several million pounds a year through additional salary awards.

TABLE 15. *Distinction Awards by Type, 1964*

	Number of Consultants *	%
All consultants	8,082	100
On basic scale (£2,910–£4,445) †	5,609	69.4
With: C award (+ £850)	1,413	17.5
B award (+ £2,000)	707	8.7
A award (+ £3,425)	265	3.3
A-plus award (+ £4,550)	88	1.1

* Includes honorary consultants.

† Figures in brackets relate to the amount of distinction award applicable to a consultant on a whole-time salary. Part-time consultants receive a scaled-down award according to their contracted number of sessions under the National Health Service.

Source: Minister of Health, *Annual Report for 1964,* p. 163.

The structure and extent of the distinction awards system has meant that in effect the awards are less prizes for distinction than salary raises graded according to proficiency. The age structure of award holders bears this out, as is shown in Table 16. Most C awards are given to consultants in the age range 40 to 50, most B awards in the 45–55 group, most A awards to those between 50 and 65, and A-plus awards after age 55. For many consultants —about one third at any one time—the distinction awards system carries on an incremental pay structure where the basic scale leaves off. Yet it is the profession, not the employer, that makes the choice, and the award is based on personal ability rather than on job responsibility.

The System in Operation

That the distinction awards system was able to function was due almost entirely to the indefatigable efforts of Lord Moran, Dean of St. Mary's Hospital Medical School (1920–45), President of the Royal College of Physicians (1941–50), physician and friend of Sir Winston Churchill, member of the General Medical Council, consultant adviser to the Ministry of Health, member of the Spens Committee, and the first chairman of the Advisory Committee on Distinction Awards. Without him the scheme might never have come into existence. Lord Moran controlled the distribution of distinction awards until 1962 when he was succeeded as chairman by Lord

Brain, who was president of the Royal College of Physicians from 1950 until 1957. The power of Royal College rather than BMA leadership was thus again asserted.

TABLE 16. *Age of Medical and Dental Consultants (Including Honorary Staff) Receiving Various Categories of Award for the First Time, 1961–1964*

Age	A-plus Awards	A Awards	B Awards	C Awards
Under 40			1	45
40–44			35	114
45–49		9	57	116
50–54	3	26	53	68
55–59	17	26	38	28
60–64	10	29	8	11
65–69				
	—	—	—	—
Total	30	90	192	382

Consultants aged 70 or more are not eligible for awards. Source: Ministry of Health, *Annual Reports for 1961, 1962, 1963,* and *1964,* pp. 243, 206, 152, 162 respectively.

Lord Moran came to the conclusion that the distinction awards system should be organized on a personal basis rather than through a network of local, regional, and national nominating committees or through a system of election.[3] Candidates for the awards were to be selected by their seniors, not by their peers. The full committee, after the first year of operation, met only twice a year, when its report was drawn up for presentation to the Ministry. In the meantime, Lord Moran and his vice-chairman, Sir Horace Hamilton, would tour the country to identify outstanding medical talent. They sought advice from a number of small and informal local committees and from individuals in the hospitals; and also from the Royal Colleges. For specialties not covered by the Colleges, two or three assessors were consulted:

> For example, in mental health we get one of the heads of the Maudsley, or somebody like that, and somebody who will be on the teaching hospital as their mental hospital teacher, a man who is familiar with the practice and familiar with the medical superintendents of these mental hospitals.[4]

3. See *Royal Commission; Minutes of Evidence* (Lord Moran), Question 917, and passim.
4. Ibid., Question 1009.

There were no hard-and-fast rules; different kinds of selection were applied to different areas and to different specialties. All were based on personal judgment as well as objective criteria. The senior surgeon and senior physician of a hospital were usually marked as likely candidates and so was the senior eye or ear specialist who perhaps had three other staff specialists working with him. Laboratory, radiology, and pathology chiefs were always carefully considered, but were not automatically given awards. Of pathologists, Lord Moran said,

> The difficulty in this branch is that since they have not got out-patients, or things like that, they are rather expected to write something to lift them out of the ordinary rut and not just carry out routine pathological duties, so it makes it a little more difficult to assess.

Anesthesiology was also reportedly a difficult specialty in which to assess special merit.

Good work by itself was not necessarily sufficient consideration for a distinction award. Lord Moran quoted the example of a thoracic surgeon who was a borderline case for some years. He was not initially given an award because, although he was competent, another man in his region immediately had gone to the local medical school to master the technique of cardiac surgery when it came in, but he had not. Initiative was thus a contributing factor. There are undoubtedly many other factors that influence the committee's judgment in particular cases, since the choice is inevitably made on the basis of general professional and personal opinion. This has opened the committee to charges that the most popular or best-known consultants are more likely than others to receive awards—those, for example, who join regional committees or are active in their specialty associations. The secrecy surrounding the names of awardees makes any analysis impossible, but such predilection might be expected in almost any payment system.

The committee has neither to justify its individual choices to the government nor to publish its recommendations. In the first year of the committee's operation, there was a large majority in favor of secrecy. The reasoning behind this was obscure. Although it had been quite obvious before the National Health Service—and was still to some extent—which consultants were the top men of Harley Street, it was now thought unwise that patients be able to judge the quality of their medical treatment by the rate of remuneration of the consultant. "It gets into the Medical Journal," said Lord Moran before the 1957–60 Royal Commission, "and then these lay people search every week and I have suffered bitterly from this." [5] Doctors seemed not to object if the profession knew, but had the greatest objection to letting the public know which consultants were most highly esteemed by the profession.

5. Lord Moran raised the difficulty of a patient who might think a consultant was a better doctor because he had an award, when in fact his award was given for research. Such comments again pose the question of the purpose of the award system. Ibid., Question 1063.

Certain medical groups have been uneasy about the secrecy, because the public is unaware of how its money is being spent or because they felt the distribution of awards is unfair. The Socialist Medical Association has recommended instead some type of responsibility allowance related to a particular post rather than to individuals; [6] and some younger consultants have re-echoed this view in personal interviews. An anesthesiologist claimed: "Distinction awards are a dreadful system—they are *not* given on merit. And no one is worth an A-plus award. . . . A salary of £9,000 means too great a differential." He had no award himself. In contrast, a consultant with a top award, practicing in the same city, spoke out in favor of the system: "When you take half a dozen people, and you say, 'Do you think X should have an award?', they all agree." Such comments illustrate an ambivalent attitude toward the distinction awards system within the profession; in some ways *as a system,* it is untenable. It puts immense patronage into the hands of the profession; its possibilities for abuse are enormous; there is no relief for the man who feels he has been wronged; and there is a rigid insistence on secrecy which demands that elaborate precautions be taken in the offices of the employing boards that disburse salaries. There has, however, been no criticism of the integrity (if there has been some of the judgment) of the members of the committee. Personal admiration of members of the committee has stilled the most vehement of critics. One illustration may suffice. The British Medical Association passed a resolution at its representative meeting in 1956 in favor of abolishing distinction awards. Later, Lord Moran was asked to address the consultant committee of the BMA; in his own words, "at the end when I had left they passed unanimously in favor of it." Subsequently the BMA Council ratified this decision, and in 1957 the Representative Body also changed its mind.[7]

Lord Brain, the new chairman of the Distinction Awards Committee, is continuing the system bequeathed to him by Lord Moran. But in addition, small regional committees have been set up, nominated by regional consultants and specialists committees to sift the candidates for the lowest awards in their particular areas. These committees send their recommendations for C awards directly to the Awards Committee, and their recommendations remain unpublished. By this action the system has been opened to local participation. Since the awards are generally given in stages (first a C, then a B, and so on), in future many distinction award holders will pass through these local committees. This is by no means the only method of recommendation, but it is assumed that it will be of increasing importance in the future.[8] The Central Consultants and Specialists Committee of the BMA received Lord Brain's suggestions with enthusiasm. It "felt well satisfied that the system Lord Brain proposed was as good as any that could be devised, and

6. Ibid., Question 56. Similarly it was later claimed: "The real charge against the committee is not that justice is not (on the whole) done but that it is not *seen* to be done." *Lancet i* (1962), 897.

7. *Royal Commission; Minutes of Evidence,* Question 923.

8. See *Brit. Med. J.* Suppl. *i* (1963), 74.

any disquiet the Committee may have had was put to rest." [9] Despite its peculiarities, the awards system has survived the scrutiny of a Royal Commission and continuous criticism from certain members of the profession.

The system has certain major advantages. It gives consultants an opportunity to create its own prima donnas; and it relieves the Ministry of Health from haggling with the profession over which posts should be graded higher than others. It is probably true that without the distinction awards system, the basic consultant scale would have to be raised very considerably; without distinction awards, there might well have been much more outcry from consultants over their salary levels than there has in fact been. Consultants with awards have the best of both worlds, and they are spared the competitive market for patients.

Because of distinction awards, incomes of specialists under the nationalized system are still unequal. If the awards are made solely on the basis of renown, then in a situation where the more brilliant men consistently enter particular specialties or where some specialties are more professionally fashionable, it is to be expected that the distribution of the awards will favor those specialties. Generally, the people in the "lesser" specialties, said one physician, "are those who gave up the competitive race to the top. Therefore," he continued, "they do not deserve distinction awards." One of the lesser specialties he had in mind was psychiatry. Clearly, membership on the Distinction Awards Committee must influence decisions between one specialty and another—a factor that was to be taken up, among others, by pathologists and psychiatrists in their pressure for increased status and their own colleges. The distribution of distinction awards among the specialties is shown in Table 17. In 1964 about six of ten thoracic surgeons, cardiologists, neurologists, neurosurgeons, and general physicians had awards. At the bottom of the scale were geriatrics, anesthesiology, and psychiatry. These three specialties accounted for over 22 per cent of all consultants, but they received fewer than 10 per cent of all awards. The average chance of all specialists of receiving an award at any one time was a little under one in three.[10] For nearly half of all consultants, however, because of their fields, the chances of receiving an award were nearer to one in six. General medicine, general surgery, and obstetrics and gynecology were still among the

9. The disquiet arose from the need to reconcile a potentially dangerous system of patronage with the ingenuity of the actual scheme. The *Brit. Med. J.*, e.g., while expressing distrust, concluded: "However, it works; and is accepted even by the Treasury." *Brit. Med. J. i* (1963), 630.

10. But a much higher proportion over the average consultant career, since the awards are weighted towards the older age groups. For example (assumed that the average age of gaining an A-plus award is 59, the average length in the consultant grade is 30 years, and retirement is at 65), although there are only 90 A-plus awards, during one individual's consultant career five times this number will be granted. The A-plus award is the extreme example, but the principle is true of all awards. The average chance of getting an award at some time is nearer two to three than one to three. See *Royal Commission; Minutes of Evidence,* Question 541.

TABLE 17. *Distribution of Distinction Awards by Specialties, 1964*

	PERCENTAGE DISTRIBUTION		
	Of Consultants by Specialty	Of Awards by Specialty	Percentage of Consultants in Each Specialty Holding Awards
Anesthesiology	11.3	4.8	13.1
Cardiology	0.5	0.9	57.5
Dentistry	3.6	2.1	17.8
Dermatology	1.8	1.8	30.7
Diseases of chest	3.5	3.5	31.0
General medicine	10.4	19.0	56.9
General surgery	11.0	17.9	50.7
Geriatrics	1.4	0.6	12.7
Infectious diseases	0.4	0.7	48.6
Psychiatry	10.0	4.2	12.9
Neurological physiology	0.2	0.1	15.4
Neurology	1.0	2.0	60.5
Neurosurgery	0.8	1.6	59.7
Obstetrics & gynecology	6.0	7.6	39.3
Ophthalmology	3.8	3.0	25.0
Orthopedic surgery	4.9	5.3	34.1
Ear-nose-throat	3.8	3.5	29.2
Pediatrics	2.9	3.9	41.7
Pathology	10.6	7.3	21.5
Physical medicine	1.2	0.6	15.3
Plastic surgery	0.7	1.3	54.1
Radiology	6.5	3.9	18.5
Radiotherapy	1.6	1.4	26.3
Thoracic surgery	1.2	2.5	63.0
Venereology	1.0	0.7	21.7
All specialties	100.0	100.0	

Source: Ministry of Health, *Annual Report for 1964*, pp. 164–65.

most popular specialties; they accounted for only 27 per cent of consultants, but they appropriated 45 per cent of all the distinction awards.

These same trends are shown in the distribution of awards by size of award. Although one in five of the eighty-three venereologists in England and Wales held a distinction award of some kind in 1964, all but one was in the C category. In contrast, of a total of ninety-one A-plus awards given to consultants in all specialties (which doubled their annual NHS salary), twenty-three went to physicians practicing in the field of general medicine, fourteen to those in general surgery, and eleven to obstetricians—more than half of all top awards to three out of a field of twenty-five listed specialties.[11] *The Economist* and others have questioned whether this position really represents the distribution of merit among the different specialties:

> Or does it, at least in part, reflect the composition of the selection committee, with its membership almost exclusively drawn from fellows, including the presidents, of the three royal colleges of physicians, surgeons, and obstetricians and gynaecologists? [12]

The question is impossible to answer for the same reasons that "distinction" is undefinable as a single attribute equally applicable to all specialties. How, for example, ought distinction to be measured in relation to a single radiologist in a large rural area, a thoracic surgeon in a major teaching unit, and a part-time gynecologist with a flourishing private practice in a large urban center?

Part-time consultants (those with private practice) are more likely to have awards than those who are whole-time. In 1958, over 36 per cent of part-time and under 20 per cent of full-time consultants held awards; the proportion of those with top awards was eight times as great for those who were

TABLE 18. *Distribution of Distinction Awards by Hospital Affiliation (Teaching and Nonteaching), 1964*

	Total No. of Consultants	AWARDS				
		A-plus £4,550	A £3,425	B £2,000	C £850	Total
With teaching hospital appointments only, or joint appointments*	2,309	80 (3.5)[†]	207 (9.0)	443 (19.2)	533 (23.1)	1,263 (54.7)[‡]
With nonteaching hospital appointments only	5,773	8 (0.1)	58 (1.0)	264 (4.6)	880 (15.2)	1,210 (21.0)[‡]

* There were 1,371 consultants with teaching hospital appointments only; 938 had appointments at both teaching and nonteaching hospitals; 49% of the former and 63% of the latter held distinction awards.

† Percentage of consultants with awards is noted in parentheses.

‡ Difference of 0.1% is due to rounding.

Source: Ministry of Health, *Annual Report for 1964*, p. 163.

11. Ministry of Health, *Annual Report for 1964*, pp. 164–65.
12. April 28, 1962, p. 333.

part time as for those who were full time.[13] There is no evidence to suggest that these proportions have radically changed. Similarly, teaching hospital consultants are more likely to hold awards than are those in nonteaching hospitals (Table 18). Consultants holding nonteaching hospital appointments only (that is, employed wholly by a regional hospital board on a full-time or part-time contract) had one chance in five of holding an award in 1964; those with teaching hospital affiliation had a more than even chance. The difference was especially marked in the high awards. Less than 2 per cent of consultants who worked only in nonteaching hospitals had A or A-plus awards, compared with 13 per cent of those with teaching hospital appointments. These proportions apply to the situation at one point in time. Over his whole career period, the chance that the individual will gain an award is much higher than this, and the gap between the two kinds of hospital must be widened considerably. Finally, although efforts were made to allocate the distinction awards evenly among the fifteen hospital regions, some areas held a greater proportion of awards than others. This is illustrated in Table 19. Thirty-seven per cent of consultants in London and the four metropolitan hospital regions stretching out from London held awards

TABLE 19. *Distribution of Awards by Hospital Regions, 1964*

Region	Percentage of Total Number of Consultants in Region Who Have Awards				
	A-plus £4,550	A £3,425	B £2,000	C £850	Total
Newcastle	0.4	2.9	9.2	15.6	28.1
Leeds	0.7	2.8	8.1	14.6	26.2
Sheffield	0.4	3.1	7.4	15.3	26.2
East Anglia	1.2	2.4	7.7	15.3	26.6
Oxford	3.3	3.9	8.2	18.0	33.3 *
South Western	0.7	3.0	7.8	19.6	31.0 *
Wales	1.0	3.0	7.3	15.8	27.1
Birmingham	0.6	3.3	7.8	12.9	24.6
Manchester	0.5	2.9	7.3	15.3	26.0
Liverpool	1.0	3.0	7.9	12.9	24.8
Wessex		1.1	8.7	18.1	27.8 *
Metropolitan regions	1.6	3.9	10.4	20.7	36.7 *

* The difference of 0.1% is due to rounding.

Honorary consultants are included. Consultants with appointments in more than one region are included in each.

Source: Ministry of Health, *Annual Report for 1964*, p. 163.

13. *Royal Commission; Report*, p. 79, Table 28.

of some kind in 1964. But in the Liverpool and Birmingham regions, in contrast, the proportion was only 25 per cent.

The characteristics of award holders can be enumerated: the holder is more likely to belong to a small exclusive specialty such as neurosurgery, or to one of the "big three"—general medicine, general surgery, obstetrics. The consultant with an award is more likely to engage in private practice than not; and he is much more likely to have a teaching hospital appointment, than a nonteaching hospital appointment alone. If it is assumed that distinction awards accurately represent the distribution of high-quality practice—and there is no reason to doubt this—the highest level of medical skill is still found in the teaching hospital, in the south of England rather than the north, and in the traditionally popular career choices. Consultants attached to teaching hospitals in London clearly have the best possible chance of gaining a distinction award. The figures are carefully guarded, but it is probably not too inaccurate to assume that the chance that such a consultant will be given an award at some time during his career is of the order of 70 or 80 per cent.

These points have been emphasized to show both the function of the distinction awards system and the influence of the consultant hierarchy. Monetary awards could have been used to reward consultants in outlying areas for heroic work under adverse conditions, or to attract consultants to those specialties where there was the most need. They could have been used to encourage whole-time work in hospitals or to raise the academic status of the nonteaching hospital. To some extent, the system does attempt to do these things. But it is not being used to barter for policies of this kind. The professional committee has interpreted its function as rewarding personal distinction. The effect has been to perpetuate differences in financial status among specialties and among hospitals.

Coincidentally, and this is one of the most interesting aspects of the awards system, the power of the Royal Colleges was once more asserted. Indeed, it was remarkable how quickly College representatives had moved from the wholly professional into the administrative and executive spheres of practice. They sat on appointments boards and the Joint Consultants Committee (and thus as specialist representatives on the Whitley Committee concerning pay awards) as well as on the Distinction Awards Committee; they were enmeshed in the effective operation of the nationalized hospital system. Through the National Health Service the government had enlisted professional self-government as its delegated authority.

16

The Machinery of Planning and the Distribution of Doctors

One major reason for establishing a national health service was to increase the availability of medical services to the whole population. This meant not only the removal of cost barriers that might prevent the individual from seeking or accepting medical treatment but also the careful deployment of medical staff and facilities to provide readily accessible services of reasonable quality. Once the principle of free medical care to patients was accepted and a new system of financing and administration evolved, socioeconomic questions were replaced by straightforward business issues—primarily, the amount of money made available for the health service by the government and the efficiency with which this money was used. Geographical redistribution of services was more complex and more sensitive. It inevitably included some form of assignment (or at least persuasion) of health service personnel to understaffed areas. Machinery for redistributing the supply of doctors could mean increased controls over the individual's choice of practice area. It thus played an essential part in professional acceptance of public employment.

The geographical redistribution of general practitioners and the development of a regionalized hospital service in the early years of the National Health Service implied the gradual upgrading of substandard facilities. In both cases this was accomplished through a minimum exercise of directive authority, because of the steady expansion in the number of doctors. The extended capitation system for general practitioners encouraged new entrants to set up practice in areas where there were few doctors in relation to the population served. Indeed, the effect of this alone on the distribution of GPs was noted as early as 1948.[1] Meanwhile, the regional hospital boards were advertising specialist posts in understaffed districts at the same salary as those in the major teaching centers. There was thus a certain economic attraction of doctors towards substandard districts.

When the Medical Practices Committee circularized the new local executive councils in 1948, almost all indicated that their GP services were adequate. The committee, set up by the National Health Service Act to regulate

1. Medical Practices Committee, *First Report,* June 1949.

the distribution of GPs (and officered by civil servants), was therefore not called on to take drastic redeployment action. Instead, it began to develop criteria against which adequacy might be measured, and it concentrated on the two staffing extremes. In 1952 11 per cent more doctors than in 1948 were practicing in areas classified by executive councils as underdoctored; and there were nearly 10 per cent fewer doctors in relatively overdoctored areas. In prosperous Bournemouth, for example, there were ninety-seven GP principals in 1948 and only seventy-two in 1952.[2] This was effected merely by discouraging new entrants from practice in such areas and was welcomed by other GPs—the fewer doctors there were, the larger their practices and the higher their incomes.

After the award by Mr. Justice Danckwerts in 1952 (one element of which was to discourage large list sizes) the Medical Practices Committee was asked to revise its classifications. The committee classified districts within executive council areas as "restricted" (where the average list size was 1,500 or less), "intermediate" (between 1,500 and 2,500) and "designated" (over 2,500). A fourth grade was added in 1962, when part of the intermediate category was split off to describe so-called "open" areas. Any doctor, after very little experience, might set up practice in a designated area. He was encouraged to do so by a financial incentive known as the initial practices allowance: a four-year grant to enable him to establish his facilities. In the open areas, admission to medical lists was automatic, but initial practices allowances were not paid; in intermediate areas, applications for admission might be refused. A restricted area was one considered adequately staffed by the committee, and a doctor was admitted only in exceptional circumstances, even as a replacement for an outgoing practitioner.

In 1963, some 3,300 National Health Service GPs were in designated (underdoctored) areas, 12,900 in open areas, and 2,400 in intermediate areas. Only 1,800, or fewer than 9 per cent, were in areas that were termed restricted or overdoctored. The great majority of GPs practiced in areas in which no limitations applied. They might take on a partner or an assistant without restriction. Thus the "negative direction" was not so great as the machinery might suggest.

Negative direction worked reasonably well while the number of incoming doctors was increasing. The figures are given in Table 20. In 1952 over half of all people registered with GPs were in areas classified as designated or undoctored. By 1957 the proportion had fallen to under 20 per cent. At the same time, the average number of patients per GP in underdoctored areas steadily decreased. Thus the individual GP work load, inflated in many of these areas because of the lack of doctors, began to fall. The average GP in a designated area in 1957 had a list of about 2,660 people, or 200 fewer patients than the average GP of 1952—but this still represented more work than that of the GP in intermediate or restricted areas.

2. In July 1948, 6,648 principals were said to be practicing in underdoctored areas and 1,176 in overdoctored areas; the figures for the same areas in 1952 were 7,397 and 1,062. Ibid., *Fourth Report,* January 1953.

TABLE 20. *Distribution of National Health Service Patients by Medical Practices Committee Classification; England and Wales, 1952–1964*

| | PERCENTAGE OF PATIENTS IN AREAS | | | AVERAGE NO. OF PATIENTS PER PRINCIPAL IN AREAS | | |
	Designated	Open and Intermediate	Restricted	Designated	Open and Intermediate	Restricted
1952	51.5	44.1	4.4	2,851	2,184	1,581
1953	38.9	56.4	4.5	2,726	2,183	1,594
1954	27.3	67.5	5.2	2,741	2,228	1,546
1955	23.4	72.0	4.6	2,736	2,229	1,554
1956	21.7	73.4	4.9	2,711	2,234	1,548
1957	19.4	75.6	5.1	2,659	2,264	1,517
1958	18.6	76.4	5.0	2,672	2,247	1,594
1959	19.9	74.9	5.2	2,745	2,251	1,575
1960	20.1	74.5	5.4	2,737	2,257	1,603
1961	17.1	78.3	4.6	2,742	2,272	1,563
1962	17.6	76.4	6.0	2,744	2,297	1,608
1963	19.2	74.6	6.2	2,748	2,313	1,652
1964	20.9	70.6	8.5	2,768	2,359	1,747

Changes in the medical practices classifications and regrouping of districts make these figures not exactly comparable from year to year, which may account for some differences in the figures.

Source: Annual Reports, Ministry of Health. Figures for 1952–59 also appear in Jewkes, *The Genesis of the British National Health Service,* 1961, p. 61.

In the late 1950s, however, the situation changed. The number of GPs was not increasing as fast as the general population, and thus the average number of patients per GP began to rise. Areas that suffered first were those that were least attractive to incoming practitioners; the average GP in an underdoctored area in 1963 had more patients on his list than he had in 1954. Part of the change among the different kinds of areas might be a result of changes in the classifications used by the Medical Practices Committee. But the general trend was clear. From the patient's point of view the distribution of GPs did not materially improve in the late 1950s and early 1960s; and the general shortages of GPs, as would be expected, was felt most keenly in the areas most in need: sparsely populated rural areas and the northern industrial cities.

It became clear that the Medical Practices Committee would have to exert a more positive pressure on new entrants to general practice if the overall staffing pattern were not to deteriorate. The committee had made changes in its classification in 1962. In June 1964 it informed the medical profession that it proposed to tighten its basic criteria further in the light of an increasing shortage of general practitioners; a greater number of districts would be classified as restricted or intermediate.[3] Admission of applicants to many of the restricted and intermediate areas, even as replacements for outgoing practitioners, would in future be the exception, and only areas in which the average list size was over 2,100 would be open to all new applicants. This policy would strengthen the directive power of the committee by diverting new applicants from a greater proportion of "desirable" areas.

Generally, the activities of the Medical Practices Committee have been accepted as inevitable and useful. They have also been relatively cautious, and there has been little sense of compulsion among GPs. In a situation of manpower shortage, the committee may, however, be compelled to tighten its control further; if so, this may raise questions of practice choice. Up to 1961 about 7 per cent of all GPs practiced in restricted areas (Table 21). Changes in classification in 1962 and 1964 increased this proportion to well

TABLE 21. *Distribution of General Practitioner Principals by Areas Classified by the Medical Practices Committee, 1952–1964*

| | NUMBER | PER CENT OF PRINCIPALS IN EACH YEAR | | |
		Designated	Open and Intermediate	Restricted
1952	17,272	44.0	49.2	6.8
1953	18,044	33.2	60.2	6.7
1954	18,513	22.8	69.5	7.7
1955	18,817	19.5	73.7	6.8
1956	19,180	18.2	74.7	7.2
1957	19,437	16.6	75.9	7.6
1958	19,685	15.8	77.1	7.1
1959	19,745	16.6	75.9	7.5
1960	19,928	16.8	75.5	7.7
1961	20,188	14.3	79.0	6.7
1962	20,325	14.7	76.6	8.6
1963	20,349	16.2	75.0	8.7
1964	20,246	17.9	70.7	11.4

Figures not exactly comparable from year to year, as in Table 20.

Source: Annual Reports, Ministry of Health.

3. The criterion of a restricted area was to be an average list size of 1,800 people or less (instead of 1,600, as it had been since 1962); in intermediate areas the cut-off figure was to be 2,100 instead of 1,900. *Brit. Med. J.* Suppl., *i* (1964), 262.

over 11 per cent. The proportions are small, but they may be indicative of a change in policy. If relatively large numbers of areas which were the most congenial places to live were closed to new entrants, the question of a more positive direction of GPs might arise.

Such terms as negative and positive direction, however, being relative, depend on historical perspective and professional expectations. The term "negative direction" has not been applied to consultants (or for that matter to prospective Members of Parliament or university professors), yet they have for long been tightly restricted in their choice of practice area, since they may apply only for posts that are available or advertised. If no consultant post is available to the senior registrar in the areas of his choice, he has to decide whether to apply for posts elsewhere, or wait and hope; and even if a post is advertised he has to compete for it. His location is likely to be determined by the appointments that appear at the time he is ready to apply. General practices on the other hand are still run as small independent business concerns. Although the buying and selling of practices was abolished with the NHS, the monetary partnership remains. While it would be unthinkable to suggest that a consultant have the right to nominate his successor, GPs claim precisely this for outgoing partners, and regard the system as a vestige of former independence. This curious mixture—the traditions of private practice and the demands of a public service—sometimes leads to conflicts and is only gradually being modified. But the Medical Practices Committee itself is a curious mixture: part Ministry agent, part professional body, and part—perhaps a growing part—a kind of supernumerary appointments board.[4]

The Medical Practices Committee consists of seven doctors, including the chairman, nominated by the profession; a lawyer recommended by the Lord Chancellor; and one other member representing executive councils. All are appointed by the Minister of Health, and the committee operates as the Minister's agent: another example of the enlistment of medical committees as administrative bodies. A doctor who wishes to set up in general practice applies to the local executive council. In the case of a new practice falling into the appropriate classification, the executive council draws up a short list of applicants, who are interviewed by the Medical Practices Committee. With other vacancies the executive council usually nominates the candidate, and the central committee accepts this nomination. Since the executive council is invariably guided by its local medical committee, the whole process has a strong professional flavor. The appointment to GP vacancies is little different from the appointment of specialists to consultant posts. It may

4. One executive function of the Medical Practices Committee is the granting of certificates of sale. Before a GP may sell his premises to the incoming candidate he must have a certificate, based on a district valuer's report of the worth of the premises. This system was set up to prevent outgoing GPs from including any elements of practice goodwill (the sale of which was abolished under the NHS) as part of the purchase price.

become necessary in a situation of continuing manpower shortage for GPs, like consultants, to have a relatively small choice of practice area in the future and be subject to a standardized local appointment procedure. The Medical Practices Committee was built around the capitation system. Much will depend on the payment system on which GPs ultimately decide.

Consultant Establishments and the System of Rationing

There is no equivalent of the Medical Practices Committee for consultants and specialists. Consultants are limited by the number of posts made available, rather than by choice of practice area. It was originally intended that consultant vacancies be filled solely by the regional hospital boards and boards of governors of teaching hospitals. Not until the manpower crisis of 1950, when national staff planning became essential for budgetary reasons, were specific measures taken to provide any form of national control. But the Advisory Committee on Consultant Establishments, which was set up in 1953, was not primarily intended to redistribute senior hospital medical staff. Its chief function was to ration the available supply of consultants in the face of increasing demands from the employing boards.

The Advisory Committee on Consultant Establishments consists of three components: the Minister's consultant advisers in general medicine and surgery, representatives of the Joint Consultants Committee, and members of the medical staff of the Ministry of Health. It meets every two months under the chairmanship of a deputy chief medical officer of the department. Like the Medical Practices Committee, it is a medical committee acting as agent for the Ministry of Health. The committee considers all applications for extra senior medical staff from the regional and teaching hospital boards. Taking into account the number of doctors in the various specialty fields, and balancing one area or one field against another, it then decides whether or not to approve them. The Advisory Committee therefore does not suggest new posts; it waits for applications to be made and judges each on its merits. The medical staff in one group of hospitals might, for instance, agree that there was an acute need for an extra consultant in pediatrics. This request would go to the senior administrative medical officer of the regional hospital board, and would be considered by the board's committees. If the request were thought reasonable it would be passed on to the Advisory Committee at the Ministry of Health; and if it were subsequently approved by that committee, the regional hospital board would be allowed to increase its establishment by one pediatrician, and an appropriate advertisement for candidates for the new post would be inserted in the medical press.

Almost all applications are approved by the Advisory Committee. Between the middle of July 1953 and the end of 1961, 1,351 new consultant posts were approved—the equivalent of 1,060 whole-time appointments. Eighteen per cent of all consultant posts in 1961 had been approved as new posts by the Advisory Committee in the eight years of its existence, and additional posts had been approved in all specialties except the declining field of infectious diseases.[5] Applications may be deferred for several reasons, but the most likely cause of deferment is a shortage of consultant material in a particular specialty, and it is here that the Advisory Committee exerts its authority. The Sheffield Regional Hospital Board, for example, reviewing its progress from 1957 to 1962, spoke of particular difficulties arising from this system, as it affected its own requests for staff in the specialties of anesthesiology, radiology, and adult and child psychiatry, in all of which there were comparative shortages of senior registrars.[6] In the specialties where the supply of consultants has equaled the demand, rationing has not been necessary. Planning of specialist staff has thus rested on two criteria: recognition of local need by the employing boards, and a post facto national rationing process according to the available supply of manpower assessed by a selected medical group.

It will be recalled that the initial lack of national planning at the senior registrar level led in the 1950s to a glut of senior registrars in the major specialties, for whom no consultant posts were available.[7] The resulting discontent impelled the Ministry to supervise the number of these training posts instead of leaving the problem to the regional boards. The Advisory Committee now has as one of its basic guides the annual number of senior registrars in all specialties. There is, for example, a serious shortage of consultant anesthesiologists and a limited number of senior registrars in anesthesiology. Rather than encourage maldistribution or drastically lower standards among new entrants, the Advisory Committee agrees only to the most essential additions of these consultants, while it attempts to increase the number of senior registrars so that the shortage will be temporary. This is done, in the typical nonauthoritarian voice in which the Ministry speaks to the regional hospital boards and boards of governors, by asking the boards to review their programs to provide additional senior registrar training posts in anesthesiology. This means that there is a limitation on the number and distribution of senior registrar posts: they are approved only when adequate and full training can be given, according to the assessment of the Advisory Committee.

The ideal number of consultants for each specialty for each unit of population was not pursued after the overoptimistic 1948 circular on the development of specialist services. Despite the continuous expansion of consultant services after 1948, almost all the specialties in 1962 were well below the levels suggested in that circular. This was true not merely of specialties such as infectious diseases and chest diseases, that had become relatively less important, but also of those that had become relatively more important, such as pediatrics, pathology, physical medicine, and anesthesiology. The Advisory Committee, in considering the cases put to it, uses its collective judgment rather than numerical standards to approve or defer each applica-

5. *Brit. Med. J. ii* (1962), 1393.
6. Sheffield Regional Hospital Board, *Quinquennial Report 1957–1962*, p. 54.
7. See Chap. 10.

tion. In the large specialties the Ministry refers applications to its relevant consultant advisers for their recommendations before sending them to the committee. Since there are no numerical yardsticks, the adviser, drawing on his experience in the field, considers each case according to his own experience, on the basis of existing supply and demand.

Proceedings of the Advisory Committee are not published, and the names of its members are not public property. As a wholly medical committee (consisting of consultants together with Ministry medical staff), it once more reflects—even in its relatively limited capacity—the influence of the profession on official medical matters. It also indicates the peculiarly domestic way in which the National Health Service is run. One member of the Ministry's medical staff said:

> We are at a great geographical advantage compared with, for example, the United States. In London we have contact with all senior members of the profession—the Colleges, the Associations, the Faculties. If one doesn't know something at first-hand, one can learn it second-hand.

The Chief Medical Officer of the Ministry is a Fellow of the Royal College of Physicians and a member of the General Medical Council; he knows, personally, eminent men in all the specialty fields. Consultant advisers, members of the various negotiating and advisory bodies, and leaders of the professional associations form a relatively small professional group. Time and again, looking at one planning or policy committee or another, one finds familiar names. The judgments of its advisers are more highly regarded by the Ministry than figures from its statistical department. Since the advisers may also be influential members of their specialty organizations, the body of opinion built up by the profession is of great importance in decisions eventually taken by the government.

The Advisory Committee on Consultant Establishments, however, like the Medical Practices Committee, is a regulatory rather than a planning agency. It applies judgment in particular situations instead of acting as a consultant manpower center. Like the Medical Practices Committee, it is more certain of success when the manpower situation is expanding than it is in a general manpower shortage. In a time of shortage only those areas likely to attract new staff will request additional consultant posts, whereas the relatively unpopular areas will be unable to fill posts they already have available. Both committees operate more through the power of veto than the power of initiative. The most obvious results of this method have been the lack of national standards for size of staff, the belated and limited acceptance of financial and other incentives offered the individual to work in unpopular areas or unpopular specialties, and above all the lack of investigation to determine the major problems and the best solutions. On the other side, the system has had the advantage of maintaining maximum flexibility in relation to individual choice of area by GPs and to the wishes of the hospital boards.

Specialist Planning within the Region

The employing boards reach their manpower decisions in a number of ways. Each regional hospital board has a medical department, headed by a senior administrative medical officer (SAMO) with, typically, five or more other whole-time doctors and both senior and junior administrative staff. The medical department is undoubtedly the most influential section of the board's staff, which in 1964 averaged 290 whole-time staff per board, and bears the major responsibility for planning both medical staff and facilities. Besides doctors, the regional hospital board includes administrators, architects, engineers, legal advisers, accountants, nurses, and a full supporting staff.[8] Among the medical officers, responsibilities may be shared by function or by geographical area or both; one medical officer might be responsible for all matters relating to hospital maternity services in the region and also oversee all general medical matters of one regional sector.

A senior officer of one regional board described how requests for additional consultants develop into a formal application to the Advisory Committee in London. A report might come through a formal resolution from a hospital management committee, which had itself received a resolution from its group medical advisory committee. Alternatively, an area consultants committee might make a request directly to the regional board or an individual might approach the regional board medical officer assigned that particular area, to ask for help; or the medical department itself might initiate a request on the basis of hospital statistics. The board considers the extra facilities that will be needed if the request is approved: extra outpatient facilities, hospital beds, and surgical time. One of the board's medical officers may discuss the question fully with the local medical staff, work out a program with them, and see whether they are willing to give up some of their hospital beds to a newcomer. Here the traditional system of bed assignment intervenes. "If a reasonable number of beds cannot be found" commented one board official, "the scheme is stillborn." When this phase is cleared, a formal proposal is made to the board. The next step is for the area doctor to get the SAMO's support, and for the board's medical advisory committee to approve it. This last committee might, for example, dismiss a suggestion for an extra part-time consultant in a district where there were already several part-timers who might be able to increase their number of NHS sessions and thereby carry the extra load. If the proposal passes the board's medical committee it goes to the regional hospital board itself, and from there is submitted for approval to the central Advisory Committee on Consultant Establishments.

The most striking aspects of redistribution of specialists in this system are the deployment of staff within the regional hospital area under the direction of each regional hospital board: the development, first, of regional specialty centers to concentrate particular specialist services, and second,

8. Ministry of Health *Annual Report for 1964*, p. 159.

of a network of consultant services available to the whole population, no matter where they live. Regional specialist centers act as reference units in scarce or expensive specialties such as cardiac and plastic surgery, neuro-surgery, and radiotherapy, which would not form a normal part of a local hospital's facilities. One region might have three or four radiotherapy cen-ters, strategically placed, two or three centers for neurosurgery, and so on, functioning as units in nonteaching hospitals and in the regional teaching hospital. Area facilities serving several hospital groups (in a population of, say, 500,000 or more), particularly for laboratory services, have also been developed in some areas, and major accident centers are being developed on the same principle. The second planning aspect, the buildup of "peri-pheral" consultant services, or those away from the major towns in the region, is perhaps the greatest success of the National Health Service. Un-fortunately, neither of these organizational patterns lends itself easily to statistical measurements; nor, indeed, do the appropriate statistics exist, since consultant statistics are published only on a regional basis. One or two illustrations may, however, suffice. It is hoped that they will indicate the potential of regionalized services and the need for detailed studies of their effect.

The Sheffield Regional Hospital Board, which has the lowest staffing ratios of all hospital regions, inherited under the National Health Service 394 specialists who were graded as consultants or senior hospital medical or dental officers by the review committee in 1949. They were to work in non-teaching hospitals serving a population of about four million people.[9] There were certain areas in the region, with populations over 30,000, which had only cottage hospitals staffed by local general practitioners. But at the other end of the scale, the region contained three major centers for thoracic sur-gery and a radiotherapeutic service. In the first years of its existence the board had to weld together these services into a unified whole. There were 174 general and special hospitals with their annexes, 11 mental hospitals, and 15 hospitals for mental subnormality, together with a blood transfusion and clinical pathological service focused on major hospitals, which had been developed during World War II. One of the immediate priorities in all re-gions was the development of consultative outpatient departments. Accord-ing to the board's criteria, there was not one "adequate" outpatient depart-ment in the Sheffield region, most of the existing departments being badly designed and too small. By the end of 1962 the Sheffield Regional Hospital Board employed 576 consultants and senior hospital medical and dental officers, of whom 239 were on whole-time contracts. The region was divided into thirty-three constituent hospital management committee areas and con-sultant staff were available to, or responsible for, all hospital beds. In ad-dition there were regional centers for cardiology, infectious diseases, neu-rology, neurosurgery, plastic surgery, radiotherapy, spinal injuries, and

9. Sheffield Regional Hospital Board, Quinquennial Reports.

thoracic surgery. In sixteen years the health services—particularly the hospital services—were transformed. Perhaps the transformation was not as great as was hoped in the optimistic enthusiasm of the immediate postwar period; but the record was honorable. Almost every hospital had been absorbed as a unit of a hospital group, with a common consultant staff. The same consultant had beds or held clinics in what used to be a voluntary hospital and the old workhouse infirmary; and he visited and sometimes supervised work in the little units in the small outlying towns run by local GPs. He was paid one salary for all this work. Both the population and the medical profession had generally accepted free GP and hospital services.

In particular groups the change has been dramatic—and this is true of the relatively prosperous as well as the relatively deprived areas. In the rural southwest of England, for example, the West Dorset Hospital Management Committee (part of the Wessex region) acquired in 1948 two ex-voluntary general hospitals of about 100 beds each in Dorchester and Weymouth, together with two smaller voluntary hospitals, a small eye hospital, three small infectious disease hospitals, and two hospitals for the chronic sick.[10] The Dorset County Hospital had had the services of full-time specialists in otolaryngology, ophthalmology, and radiology by 1939, but all the general physicians, general surgeons, and anesthesiologists to both the primary hospitals were general practitioners. The two main hospitals had only three residents between them. In 1963 the West Dorset group had a total hospital medical staff of 71, of whom 31 were consultants and SHMOs. They included specialties such as physical medicine, geriatrics, dentistry, and child psychiatry, besides the more usual specialties, and provided hospital services for a population of 140,000. In addition, specialty centers for particular services were available to all patients at other centers in the hospital region, all services to patients being without charge. Consultants appointed to such groups were appointed by the regional hospital boards concerned, which used the same criteria for appointment and offered the same terms of service as those in all the major cities.

It appears from such examples, which can be multiplied many times, that planning within hospital regions has been more effective than the redistribution of specialists between one regional area and another; for under the existing planning system, marked variations may persist between regions and among the regional and teaching hospital authorities. Application for new consultant staff in the past (and apparently also today) is generally initiated by the consultant on the spot, and confirmed or not by the employing board. One board officer put the planning mechanism in a nutshell: "You must staff round your existing staff." At least to some extent, the patterns of employing boards are thus self-perpetuating.

The figures for teaching and nonteaching hospital staffs provide an ex-

10. A.M.H. Gray and A. Topping, *The Hospital Surveys of London and The Surrounding Area,* p. 175; and Wessex Regional Hospital Board (personal communication).

ample of the effect of decentralized planning initiative. Between 1949 and 1955 the medical staff rose much faster in nonteaching hospitals than in teaching hospitals. The figures are given in Table 22. Indeed, in teaching hospitals the number of junior staff actually declined in this period. Senior staff increased by almost 30 per cent in the hospitals taken over by regional

TABLE 22. *Teaching and Nonteaching Hospital Medical Staff in National Health Service Hospitals, 1949–1964; Whole-Time Equivalents; Whole-Time, Part-Time, and Honorary Staff*

A. NUMBER

	1949	1955	1962	1964
Consultants, SHMOs, Senior Registrars				
All hospitals	6,163	7,685	8,568	8,936
Teaching hospitals	1,535	1,686	1,924	2,102
Nonteaching hospitals	4,628	5,999	6,644	6,834
Other Medical Staff				
All hospitals	5,814	7,645	9,700	10,212
Teaching hospitals	1,690	1,601	2,538	2,664
Nonteaching hospitals	4,124	6,044	7,162	7,548

B. PERCENTAGE CHANGE

	Percentage increase or decrease		
	1949:55	1955:62	1962:64
Consultants, SHMOs, Senior Registrars			
All hospitals	+ 24.7	+ 11.5	+ 4.3
Teaching hospitals	+ 11.0	+ 14.1	+ 9.3
Nonteaching hospitals	+ 29.6	+ 10.8	+ 2.9
Other Medical Staff			
All hospitals	+ 31.5	+ 26.9	+ 5.3
Teaching hospitals	− 5.3	+ 58.5	+ 5.0
Nonteaching hospitals	+ 46.4	+ 18.5	+ 5.4

A similar table on the 1949–55 figures appears in the Acton Society Trust booklet, *Creative Leadership in a State Service,* 1959, p. 75; but the 1955 figures there shown do not include honorary staff.

Source: 1949 and 1955 data from *Sixth Report of Select Committee on Estimates 1956–57,* pp. 361–62; 1962 and 1964 figures calculated from data supplied by the Ministry of Health. All figures exclude general practitioner staff working in hospitals; hospital dental staff are included.

hospital boards, and by only 11 per cent in those run by boards of governors of teaching hospitals. After the mid-1950s, when regional boards were experiencing staffing shortages, the situation changed. Between 1955 and 1962, teaching hospital staffing increased more rapidly than that of regional hospitals; the difference was most marked in junior staff, where the increases were respectively 59 per cent and 19 per cent. In terms of totals, the trend continues. It is apparent that in the early years of the National Health Service there was a great expansion of staff in nonteaching hospitals, but that these hospitals in recent years seem to be losing ground. In both senior and junior grades of staff, the teaching hospitals have been widening the staffing gap. These changes do not follow changes in the overall work loads of the teaching hospitals.[11]

The undergraduate and postgraduate teaching hospitals in 1962 accounted for 6 per cent of all National Health Service hospital beds; they employed 22 per cent of the National Health Service senior medical staff and 26 per cent of junior staff; these proportions were not so radically different from those of 1949. They were much better staffed than nonteaching units and, as the distinction awards system indicates, contained a greater proportion of distinguished consultants. The recent trends are disconcerting.[12] As teaching hospitals become district or community hospitals, as is now planned, the only legitimate difference in the staffing ratio between those hospitals and other district hospitals will be in respect of research and teaching. Detailed studies may have to be undertaken to gauge how great a staffing difference this ought to imply.

Similarly, staffing differences have persisted between hospital regions. Regional trends are shown in Table 23. Over the period 1954 to 1964, although all regions showed a marked increase in consultant staff, the same differences between them that were apparent at the beginning of the period still existed at the end. Indeed, the gap between the highest and lowest areas —Sheffield and the combination of the Metropolitan and Wessex regions—

11. The number of inpatients discharged (or died) from teaching hospitals was 441,354 in 1949, and 587,935 in 1962, an increase of 33.2%. Between 1949 and 1955 the increase was 17.0% and between 1955 and 1962 it was 13.9%. Nonteaching hospital discharges rose from 2.5 million in 1949 to 3.8 million in 1962 (52.4%); the increase between 1949 and 1955 was 25.6% and between 1955 and 1962, 21.3%. The outpatient figures for nonteaching hospitals rose much faster. New outpatients at teaching hospitals rose from 1.6 million in 1949 to 2.6 million in 1962 (60%). Comparable figures for nonteaching hospitals rose from 4.5 million to 10.8 million (137%). All outpatient attendances rose in the same period by 22% in teaching hospitals and by 80% in nonteaching hospitals. Source: 1949 figures from Ministry of Health, *Annual Report for 1950*, p. 163; 1955 figures are given in *Sixth Report from the Select Committee on Estimates*, Session 1956–57, *Running Costs of Hospitals* (HMSO, 1957) pp. 357, 359; 1962 figures calculated from data supplied by Ministry of Health Statistics Division.

12. J. A. H. Lee et al. have noted a higher fatality per case for certain conditions in nonteaching than in teaching hospitals, and have pointed up the difference in staffing ratios as a possible contributing factor. *Lancet i* (1960), 170.

TABLE 23. *Whole-Time, Part-Time, and Honorary Consultants by Hospital Region; England and Wales*

	1954	1957	1962	1964	Target 1967
A. Number					
All regions	4,913	5,279	6,010	6,732 *	8,670
Newcastle	363	393	414	457	694
Leeds	267	282	332	350	508
Sheffield	313	349	406	433	609
East Anglia	137	156	181	197	263
Metropolitan & Wessex	2,104	2,212	2,518	2,639	3,355
Oxford	174	196	216	230	318
South Western	287	299	328	358	470
Wales	263	267	313	322	510
Birmingham	443	486	558	605	795
Manchester	332	385	440	461	667
Liverpool	230	254	304	322	481
B. Per 100,000 Population					
All regions	11.1	11.8	12.9	13.4	18.5
Newcastle	12.4	13.3	13.6	14.9	22.8
Leeds	8.7	9.2	10.6	11.1	16.2
Sheffield	7.5	8.2	9.1	9.6	13.7
East Anglia	9.3	10.4	11.6	12.3	16.8
Metropolitan & Wessex	14.2	14.7	16.0	16.5	21.3
Oxford	11.8	12.9	12.9	13.1	19.0
South Western	10.3	10.7	11.3	12.0	16.2
Wales	10.1	10.2	11.8	12.0	19.3
Birmingham	9.9	10.6	11.5	12.3	16.5
Manchester	7.6	8.8	9.8	10.2	14.9
Liverpool	10.9	11.9	13.8	14.5	21.9

* The difference of two whole-time equivalents is due to rounding from official figures, which are expressed to one decimal point.

These populations do not necessarily represent the exact "catchment areas" of the hospitals staffed by the consultants of each region. The Liverpool region, for example, draws patients from all over North Wales. But this factor would not alone explain the differences in the ratios between regions. Figures include staff of both teaching and nonteaching hospitals.

Source: Figures for 1954 and 1957 are from Jewkes, *The Genesis of the British National Health Service,* Table XIX; 1962 and 1964 figures from Ministry of Health. Table B is calculated according to the home population in each region in each year; regional populations are to be found in Registrar General's *Quarterly Return for England and Wales,* December issues. 1967 figures represent estimates made by the regional Platt review committees, given in *Lancet ii* (1964), 352.

actually widened over the ten years. The difference in ratios of consultants to population between these areas was 6.7 per 100,000 in 1954 and 6.9 in 1964. The activities of the Advisory Committee have thus not taken from the rich regions to give to the poor, nor have they even kept the better-staffed areas static while the rest caught up. This point is stressed not to deny the considerable improvement of consultant services since 1949 but merely as a comment on the work of the Advisory Committee. Largely because of its policy of decentralized planning initiative, it has tended to perpetuate pre-existing staffing differences. Target figures for 1967, the result of the review committees set up after the Platt Committee reported in 1961, indicate how widely regional patterns would diverge if each region was enabled to meet its self-styled requirements.

The Distribution of Medical Practitioners

Taking the whole of England and Wales there were in 1963, 47 general practitioners to every 100,000 population. The ratio of GPs to population ranged from 43 in the Birmingham regional hospital area to 53 per 100,000 in the South Western area (Table 24). The northern and midland regions— Newcastle, Leeds, Sheffield, Manchester, Birmingham, and Liverpool—had fewer GPs than the south. The range of hospital medical staff was wider than that of general practitioners. There were only 27 hospital doctors per 100,000 population in Sheffield in 1963; in contrast, there were 45 in the Liverpool region and 53 in the four Metropolitan regions, which include the London teaching hospitals. The figures show no striking relationship between numbers of general practitioners and numbers of whole-time equivalent hospital staff. Logically it is arguable that the more GPs in an area, the fewer the number of hospital staff required, and vice versa. The Newcastle region, for example, was among the four lowest in respect of GP staffing and among the four highest in respect of hospitals; and the reverse was true for Wessex where there were relatively more GPs and fewer hospital doctors. Alternatively, it might be thought that the more GPs in a region, the more specialist work would be referred to hospitals, and thus there would be a demand for a greater number of hospital staff. The Metropolitan regions, which were among the best staffed in both categories, and Sheffield and Birmingham which are among the worst, might illustrate such a factor. Again, this was not an observation that was true for all regions, and it was much more likely that existing variations were due not to absolute needs but to some totally different circumstances.

Regions well staffed with consultants tend also to be well endowed with junior hospital staff. The four Metropolitan regions together in 1964 had a junior staff, from registrar down, equivalent to almost 29 full-time posts per 100,000 population; Sheffield had to manage with under 14. There were also differences between the regions in the internal distribution of specialists, some aspects of which are shown in Table 25. The Newcastle region, for example, had the highest consultant staffing ratio outside the four Metropolitan regions but had relatively fewer general physicians and geriatricians,

TABLE 24. *Hospital and General Practitioners by Regional Hospital Area; England and Wales, 1963*

	1963 Home Population (thousands)	Doctors per 100,000 pop.	
		General Practice	Hospital
All regions	47,023	47.2	39.2
Newcastle	3,054	43.8	37.7
Leeds	3,148	44.9	32.2
Sheffield	4,477	43.7	27.1
East Anglia	1,585	46.6	31.7
Metropolitan	14,036	50.5	52.9
Oxford	1,712	46.6	37.5
South Western	2,932	53.2	33.1
Wales	2,662	50.8	34.9
Birmingham	4,893	43.1	31.0
Manchester	4,493	43.9	33.5
Liverpool	2,212	45.3	44.8
Wessex	1,818	48.4	30.7

These figures must be interpreted with caution; they are not strictly comparable, owing to the lack of generally accessible statistical information. Figures for general practice relate to the numbers of principals, assistants, and trainees (a total of 22,203) on Oct. 1, 1963, assigned to regional hospital areas by statistical staff at the Ministry of Health. Doctors practicing in more than one hospital area have been apportioned according to the percentage of the population of the executive council area living within the boundaries of each regional hospital area. The ratio is calculated according to the population given in the table, which refers to June 30, 1963.

Hospital staffs (18,424) include all doctors except general practitioners. Data refer to Sept. 30, 1963, and are calculated in relation to the population of June 30, 1963. The data refer to the whole-time equivalent of senior staff (not the actual number), and the number of junior staff, who are almost invariably on whole-time appointments; honorary staff are included. Source: Basic data from Ministry of Health Statistics Division.

pathologists, and psychiatrists than many regions which had much lower overall totals. On the other hand there were twice as many anesthesiologists to population in the Newcastle region as in Manchester or Sheffield. Liverpool had twice as many general surgeons as Sheffield, but only 50 per cent more anesthesiologists and 33 per cent more pathologists.

Pathology was interesting in the internal breakdown of its specialties (not shown in the table) as well as in broad regional differences. The Wessex regional area included fewer pathologists per 100,000 population than, for example, Birmingham, but most of the latter were under the category of

TABLE 25. *Distribution of Consultants by Selected Specialty and Region; Whole-Time Equivalents Per 100,000 Population; England and Wales, 1964*

	All	General Medicine, Geriatrics	General Surgery	Anesth.	Path.	Psych.	Other	Staffed Beds per 1,000 pop.* Non-psychiatric	Psychiatric
Newcastle	14.9	1.3	1.6	2.1	1.3	1.4	7.1	5.4	3.8
Leeds	11.1	1.2	1.2	1.2	1.1	1.2	5.2	6.1	4.6
Sheffield	9.6	0.9	1.0	1.0	0.9	1.3	4.5	4.6	3.3
East Anglia	12.3	1.3	1.1	1.3	1.0	1.7	5.9	4.9	4.0
Metropolitan	17.0	1.9	1.6	2.0	1.9	1.8	7.7	6.0	5.1
Oxford	13.1	1.4	1.1	1.6	1.2	1.4	6.5	5.2	3.5
South Western	12.0	1.3	1.4	1.3	1.1	1.3	5.6	5.8	5.6
Wales	12.0	1.4	1.5	1.4	1.1	1.2	5.5	6.1	4.3
Birmingham	12.3	1.4	1.6	1.4	1.3	1.5	5.2	5.0	3.9
Manchester	10.2	1.2	1.0	1.0	1.1	0.8	5.1	5.4	4.1
Liverpool	14.5	1.8	1.5	1.8	1.2	1.7	6.5	7.3	4.0
Wessex	12.3	1.3	1.2	1.6	1.1	1.5	5.5	5.0	4.6
All regions	13.4	1.5	1.4	1.6	1.4	1.5	6.2	5.6	4.4
Total number	6,372	693	662	739	649	692	2,937	264,615	207,487

* At December 31, 1963. Both consultants and beds include the appropriate teaching hospitals.

Totals may not add exactly, owing to rounding of figures at one decimal point.

Source: Basic data supplied by Ministry of Health Statistics Division.

"general pathologists." For its population of 4.9 million, the Birmingham Regional Hospital Area had equivalent whole-time services of less than two designated biochemists and only one bacteriologist; the Wessex region on the other hand had four whole-time biochemists, four hematologists, and four morbid anatomists as well as a bacteriologist and a number of general pathologists, for a population of only 1.9 million. In psychiatry also there were variations in subspecialty distribution. The Sheffield and Manchester regional areas covered approximately the same population, but the equivalent of eight whole-time child psychiatrists were employed in Sheffield while in Manchester there were only four. The list can be extended. Taking the psychiatric specialties together (subnormality and severe subnormality, mental illness, and child psychiatry) there was a marked difference in the regional figures. Liverpool and East Anglia had proportionally twice as many consultant psychiatrists as had Manchester; and this did not follow the proportional distribution of psychiatric beds. Taking hospital beds as a whole, there was only a minimal relationship between the proportion of beds in an area and the proportion of consultants and other senior medical staff.

Such differences can be accounted for in various obvious ways. The area may be vastly different in the kind of medical care demanded, hospital care be more or less intensive in terms of the length of patient stay, or distances may vary; supporting services may be more or less effective; the distribution of hospitals (in large, small, or scattered units) may be more or less wasteful of staffing time; it may not be possible to recruit doctors; or the employing boards and doctors in the area may just be accustomed to particular staffing levels. The four Metropolitan regions, which embrace a total population of over fourteen million, are strongly influenced by the density of population and of medical facilities in the Greater London area. London itself includes twelve undergraduate medical schools, with their hospital complexes, and fourteen postgraduate schools and hospitals, compared with only ten undergraduate schools in the whole of the rest of England and Wales. This concentration of specialist services, research, and teaching naturally inflates the proportion of specialist staff in relation to other areas of the country. But the influence of teaching hospitals is clearly not the only influence on general variations in ratios between one region and another. Wessex Regional Hospital Area, which alone of the regions contains no university medical teaching center, had a higher proportion of senior medical staff in 1962 than five other regions, all of which included university medical schools. But none of these reasons for variations, either alone or in concert, entirely accounts for existing staffing fluctuations. The proportion of general practitioners is not subject to such marked variations; there is no evidence for substantial differences in health demands between regions; and distances do not appear significantly to affect staffing—Sheffield, one of the largest regions geographically has the smallest proportion of senior hospital staff.

While a regional hospital service was being developed, and while GP services were being redistributed to provide maximum patient coverage, there was every advantage in having separate administrative and planning mechanisms, each of which could concentrate on a relatively straightforward issue. The regrouping of facilities and the development of regional specialist centers were undoubtedly facilitated by reliance on regional rather than national responsibility for planning; and a similar argument might be used for the development of consultant services separate from those in general practice. Indeed, the advantages of regional flexibility may still outweigh any disadvantages that may accrue from having no planning norms for national manpower. It is clear that the Newcastle Regional Hospital Board, to take perhaps the most marked example, has concentrated much of its activity on building up specialist services. Other regional hospital boards may have preferred, in the early years of the National Health Service, to develop different aspects of the hospital service, such as physical plant or other categories of hospital staff.

What is now urgently needed is a series of studies on the operational effect of such variations, and experiments with different patterns. It may be that the regions with the lowest staffing ratios are providing as good service as those with the highest. It may be that areas with fewer general practitioners utilize the hospitals more fully than do those with more general practitioners. The information is not available. These questions become more urgent as the total manpower position becomes more strained. Questions of distribution of doctors—by geographical area, by teaching or nonteaching hospital, or by type of practice—take on a new light. In each of these aspects the redistributing tendency apparent in the first decade of the National Health Service appears to have halted and in some cases to have regressed. Given the choice, the average graduate may prefer to work in a particular geographical area, in a teaching instead of a nonteaching hospital, or as a consultant rather than a general practitioner. There is some evidence that he is influenced in his choice of career not only by his teachers at medical school but by the location of the school. This points to the desirability of building new schools in areas where the staffing ratios are lowest, and to including a strong inducement to general practice in the medical curriculum. To some extent these needs are beginning to be met.

In summary, the machinery of planning for medical staff has been, for both GPs and hospital staffs, a system of negative direction according to a national rationing process. This was successful only where the number of doctors expanded steadily in relation to demand. In a situation of manpower shortage some of the previous advantages have been reversed, and it has become clear that more positive planning norms need to be developed. Equally clear is the conclusion that the machinery of manpower distribution provided through delegated authority to the Medical Practices Committee and the Advisory Committee on Consultant Establishments has not provided the central planning leadership that is now required and that is only gradually being assumed by other sections of the Ministry of Health.

17

Medical Manpower:
Responsibility and Definition

By the early 1960s there was not only concern at the distribution of doctors: there was also an acute shortage of doctors in both general and hospital practice, and at junior and senior levels. Only ten years before, there had been alarm that too many doctors were being produced. The Ministry of Health had then accepted responsibility for the geographical distribution of specialists, as well as general practitioners, and for the proportion of senior registrars. It was becoming clear that now it would also have to accept responsibility for the overall number of doctors and for their internal distribution among the different kinds of practice. Gradually the Ministry was assuming a more positive role in the national planning of medical practice.

The Report of the Willink Committee

The number of doctors is governed by complex factors which include the number and size of university medical schools, the cost of medical education, the age distribution of doctors, and the rate of "wastage" through emigration or retirement. To some extent these aspects can be manipulated by increasing the number or size of training centers for students; by initiating scholarships; by raising the retirement age of those in post; by attracting married women back into medicine; or by discouraging emigration. Similarly, it is possible to reduce the number of doctors. The basic question of manpower is not the means to produce it but the responsibility for determining the number of doctors required.

The concept of supply and demand is not always applicable to professional services. Medical fees are relatively inelastic. Often they are governed by professional ethics or agreements, or by fee schedules or other payment mechanisms, which prohibit the doctor from raising his charges to discourage patients or from lowering them to attract custom. At this point professional influence intervenes. The capitation system provides an illustration. The GP cannot, like any other entrepreneur, cut his prices to attract more business. He may offer better services, but his ethics do not allow him to advertise this fact, and the public is unaccustomed to shop for medical services which, to be most effective, rely on an association of trust between the individual GP and the patient. If the GP is to retain or expand his income under the NHS, he has to do it by exerting influence, as a member of a professional group, to raise capitation fees, to give each doctor a guaranteed income, or to limit the number of doctors in relation to the total amount of money available. The community may be willing to spend a certain amount of money for medical services; but the profession, by influencing the output of doctors, may be able to determine the number of doctors among whom the money shall be shared. The *Lancet* put this point of view clearly during debates in 1957 on the number of doctors required in the National Health Service, at a time when doctors in both general and hospital practice were pressing urgently for substantial increases in pay. The question was "simply of the number for whom the nation is willing to offer the kind of livelihood and conditions of work which professional people consider necessary." [1] Medical manpower, although limited by economic factors, is thus inevitably influenced by questions of professional status and professional expectations. It follows that the profession itself has some responsibility, however informally exerted, for the total number of doctors at a given point in time.

Under the National Health Service, the Minister of Health formally assumed responsibility for providing comprehensive medical services. He thus tacitly accepted responsibility for providing an adequate number of doctors, distributed in such a way that comprehensive services would in fact be available to the whole population. But there were no gauges of how many doctors of each kind there ought to be. General practice had three indicators of trends: the maximum size of list allowed per NHS practitioner, the average list size, and the classification of areas by the Medical Practice Committee. But each of these terms had been arrived at arbitrarily, and each could only be compared with a previous or hypothetical situation. They were measurements that bore little resemblance, except in relative terms, to concepts of an actual superfluity or an absolute need. The concept of adequacy was thus largely a matter of opinion; and as opinion changed, so did the demand for manpower. In great part this opinion, not unnaturally, stemmed from within the medical profession.

"Ideal" ratios for the number of consultants and specialists had been set out by the Ministry of Health in its circular on the development of specialist services at the beginning of 1948. When it became clear that the money would not be available to pay this number at the agreed salary scales, the circular was quietly forgotten; the choice seemed to be between a limited number of well-paid doctors and a larger number of doctors with smaller incomes. As late as 1957 the *Lancet* warned: "From the public as well as from the professional standpoint an excess of doctors would be a bad thing." [2]

The Ministry of Health showed no signs of taking the lead in overall

1. *Lancet ii* (1957) 1043.
2. Ibid., and see Lindsey, *Socialized Medicine in England and Wales*, p. 176.

medical staffing policy and chiefly restricted its activities to redistribution of available manpower. The universities controlled the enrollment of medical students. They were in no way subject to the Ministry of Health, although they were linked with the University Grants Committee—an independent public body set up to channel government money into the universities—and with the Ministry of Education. Even if the Ministry of Health had assumed responsibility for the total number of doctors, its responsibility would have been pragmatic. It had no overall standards for guides. After the unhappy reception of its suggestions in 1950 for a rapid reduction in the number of senior registrars, the Ministry of Health retreated. As a result, there was no positive planning of medical numbers as a whole. It seemed to be felt that staffing policy was an internal matter to be dealt with by the medical profession, not by the central administration. One senior administrator of the Ministry of Health revealed this reticence when asked to comment on aspects of the senior registrar problem in 1958. He said it would be a little unfair to the professional witnesses, "if anyone like myself expressed a view of what was right or wrong," adding that it would be "a little presumptuous if a lay civil servant was too dogmatic about how you organize the professional or clinical staffing of a hospital." [3] Yet without such dogmatism, either from the profession or from the Ministry, it was impossible to predict the number of doctors that might be required in the future. Meanwhile, the demand for medical staff, particularly in the hospitals, was increasing rapidly.

By 1955 two points of view were held simultaneously by leaders of the medical profession. The first was that too *many* doctors were being trained, in terms of the positions likely to be available to them within the National Health Service. The second was that too *few* doctors were being trained to give an adequately manned and comprehensive service. Both opinions were valid but both were relative: they depended partly on the financial expectations of the medical profession and partly on the projected financial status of the Health Service. At this point no long-term plans existed, and there was no one in a position to make an authoritative pronouncement one way or the other. But in 1955, when it was clear from the hospital staffing situation alone that more effective plans for manpower were needed, the Minister of Health (Dennis Vosper) and the Secretary of State for Scotland appointed a committee to estimate the number of medical practitioners (and consequently the number of medical students) required in the immediate future. Seven of the eleven-man committee were eminent members of the medical profession and the chairman was an ex-Minister of Health, Sir Henry Willink. This committee took evidence from numerous bodies, including the Royal Colleges, the medical schools, the BMA, the drug industry, and an array of public administrative bodies and government departments including even the Ministry of Supply and the Ministry of Transport, and from organizations as relatively small as the Conference of Missionary Societies of Great Britain; and the full statistical resources of the government were made available. From this study the Willink Committee con-

3. *Royal Commission; Minutes of Evidence,* Questions 3766–67 (Sir John Hawton).

cluded in 1957 that the medical schools in Britain had not been producing too many doctors, but that they soon would be. It called for an immediate 10 per cent reduction in the enrollment of medical students.[4]

There were many reasons to accept the Willink Committee conclusions. The profession was receptive to the idea of limiting their numbers. The Government Actuary had emphasized the high proportion of doctors in the younger age groups. The armed services were undergoing a planned reduction in size and were abolishing the draft, thus making more physicians available for the NHS. The Commonwealth Relations Office had warned the Willink Committee that opportunities for employment in the self-governing countries of the British Commonwealth had been declining and would shrink still further in the future. The missionary societies foresaw no explosive expansion in their medical activities abroad. The Ministry of Health produced tables to show a sharp reduction in the annual increase of consultants and SHMOs in 1953, 1954, and 1955. Finally, the general birth rate appeared to have stabilized after the postwar bulge. Taken together, these findings might well, all other things being equal, indicate an equilibrium in the demand for medical practitioners.

By the following year, however, it had become abundantly clear that the findings of the Willink Committee were unsound. The committee had relied on statistics relating to the period 1953–55. Official statistics of 1958 emphasized the acute shortage of junior hospital staff then being experienced in hospitals as well as a continued imbalance between senior registrars and consultants; and at the same time the rate of emigration of doctors was also receiving attention, although the exact figures were unknown. The number of university students had already declined prior to the Willink report, and the medical schools made no move to decrease it further. It now seemed as if the number would need considerable expansion. Thus the Willink Committee report was consigned to obscurity, owing partly to unfortunate timing, deficiencies in official statistics, and a misguided concentration on the immediate situation rather than on general trends—a fault the committee apparently shared with the Ministry of Health. Perhaps the most important factor in the committee's miscalculation was the rapidly changing social environment, particularly in respect of population growth and the increased demand for hospital junior staff. But the report was also rendered obsolete by rising professional expectations in an inflationary economy. If both income and numbers could rise together, the professional demands for additional staff would grow in concert. Hence the Platt report on hospital medical staffing (1961) revealed a shortage of consultants, when there had been a supposed surplus of senior registrars (the consultant training grade) only a few years before. From an administrative point of view, the vital question was partly economic and partly a question of social values. Was it more important to develop staffing ratios or to provide better physical sur-

4. Ministry of Health, Department of Health for Scotland, *Report of the Committee to Consider the Future Numbers of Medical Practitioners and the Appropriate Intake of Medical Students* (HMSO, 1957).

roundings and equipment, or more secretarial or technical assistance? What was the appropriate level of medical care expected—and financed—by the community in the affluent society of the 1960s?

Responsibility for Manpower in the 1960s

The year 1961 was a turning point in centralized control of the National Health Service. At about this time the Ministry of Health finally decided to take the initiative in long-term planning and policy issues that had previously either been ignored or regarded as professional rather than administrative affairs, or as regional rather than national problems. Neither the BMA nor the Royal Colleges had manpower plans of their own. The Ministry of Health had already assumed responsibility for the geographical distribution of general practitioners and specialists. It had ultimately set up a research and statistics division and collected basic information on medical numbers for the entire country. The Ministry of Health, under the leadership of Enoch Powell, was the obvious body to assume manpower responsibility.

In July 1961 the Minister of Health formally, but cautiously, accepted the need for more doctors by announcing that the prospective demand for medical services would justify a rise in the university acceptance of preclinical students to 10 per cent above the levels set out by the Willink Committee four years before. This statement was accepted by the government; the universities and the University Grants Committee together decided that this increase could be effected without building new teaching centers, and it was agreed to make available extra money for expansion within existing medical schools. This new decision was, however, somewhat unrealistic in that the number of medical students had been steadily declining. Between the academic years 1956–57 and 1961–62 alone, the number of medical students in Britain had fallen by over 5 per cent.[5] The increase in university enrollment might make good the absolute losses in relation to population growth, but it did not necessarily solve the acute shortages which were suddenly being discovered at all levels and in all categories of medical staff. The contrast with ten, or even five, years earlier could not have been greater.

By 1962 the pressure for a substantial increase in medical staff, particularly hospital staff, had become intense. The review committees, set up in each hospital region as a result of the Platt report—to collect information on the adequacy of existing hospital staffs and the extent of future needs—were revealing serious deficiencies in the number of consultants. At the same time growing discontent among general practitioners was being expressed in demands for shorter hours, better working conditions, more pay, and more GPs. The two branches of practice were competing for the same scarce manpower. As the virtual monopoly employer of both branches, the Ministry of Health ultimately had to make crucial decisions that would affect both the

5. University Grants Committee, *University Development 1957–1962*, Cmnd. 2267 (HMSO, 1964), pp. 24, 157.

future of general practice and the relationship of one branch with the other.

The first long-term national hospital plan appeared in 1962; the first local health plan, and the first serious efforts to come to terms with general practitioners' problems came in 1963. All these moves were sponsored by the Ministry of Health, motivated by a new determination to provide leadership of the National Health Service; but none of the reports made any major pronouncement on medical manpower policy. The Hospital Plan detailed the proposals for each National Health Service hospital in the country up to 1975; [6] it made no reference to the number or ratio of doctors required to staff this program, either in hospitals or in general practice, although the implementation of the recommendations would have a marked impact on medical staffing patterns. The plan accepted a norm for the number of hospital beds of various kinds for a given population and applied these generally to the long-accepted concept of a large multipurpose district hospital (600 to 800 beds) serving a population of 100,000 to 150,000. The district hospital would include, besides the usual specialties found in larger general hospitals, a maternity unit, a short-stay psychiatric unit, a geriatric unit, and facilities for the isolation of infectious disease. Some of the existing cottage hospitals or small general hospitals would be retained under the plan. Some would be converted into maternity or geriatric units, and some would be closed. Thus, eventually, the hospital system would be streamlined; in this program the number of hospitals beds would be reduced, the biggest decrease being in beds assigned to mental illness.

But if hospitals were to be reorganized and the number of beds reduced in this way, general practitioners, supported by local health workers, would have to bear an increased load of community-based care. The hospital plan skated over the next logical step—changes in general practice—merely observing that the number and distribution of GP principals had improved in the previous decade. It showed a similar optimism in contemplating trends in the community supporting services—health visitors, home nurses, and mental welfare officers—organized by local health authorities. Thus, while there were agreed bed ratios per population unit, there were no nationally agreed staffing ratios or any detailed consideration of the interdependence of general and hospital medicine in the new hospital environment.[7] With hospitals organized more efficiently in large units, there might be a case for fewer rather than more consultants, and a renewed emphasis on general practice. Yet the emphasis in 1962 and 1963 was on the demands of the hospital service for more consultants, and no detailed studies were being undertaken on the GP manpower situation. Never had the deficiencies of the tripartite administrative structure of the NHS been so clearly illustrated.

6. National Health Service, *A Hospital Plan for England and Wales,* Cmnd. 1604 (HMSO, 1962).

7. For criticism in relation to the mental health services see PEP, *Psychiatric Services in 1975* (London, 1963).

The report of the medical profession's Porritt Committee, published in November 1962, also skirted the question of manpower shortage.[8] Instead, it made recommendations for the reorganization of the structure of the National Health Service through the formation of area health boards. These would apparently have fallen somewhere between the regional hospital board and the hospital management committee, although the Porritt Committee refused to specify the possible size of population served. The area health board was envisaged as a multipurpose health authority which would take over the work of both regional hospital boards and local executive councils; and specialists and general practitioners would thus for the first time be combined under one reasonably local administration. But the actual recommendations were vague and, although the medical bodies which had sponsored the report accepted the conclusions, no serious stand was taken. It was by now recognized that the immediate problems of the National Health Service were of deeper import than its administrative structure—they related to functional balance among the various aspects of the system, particularly to the question of balance between general practitioners and specialists. Although there was an underlying concern that too few doctors were being produced, there was even greater anxiety about the specific future of each branch of practice. At the same time, insufficient information was available on which clear-cut decisions could be made.

The Hospital Plan was followed by a parallel plan for local health and welfare services in the spring of 1963.[9] This, like the Hospital Plan, was in effect the amalgamation of the plans of all constituent planning bodies. In this case it was the amalgam of 146 health authorities rather than a nationally conceived design. Indeed, it was stressed that the purpose of the document was not to set out a standard pattern nor to state principles and objectives dogmatically: "Rather it is, by showing the picture as a whole, to stimulate discussion, study and experiment, and make it possible for local authorities to consider and revise their own intentions in the light of what others are doing and proposing." Because of this, the health and welfare proposals did not relate community health facilities directly to the demands that would fall on these facilities from the restructuring of the hospital service. Thus, though each plan—for hospital and for local authority—described a feasible planning situation and acknowledged the existence of the other, the result was not a carefully interwoven master plan of facilities and manpower. Each section—hospital, GP, and community care—detailed its own needs, with only peripheral reference to the other two branches. Such planning as there was stemmed from a continuous drift along pre-established lines.

The Local Health and Welfare Plan was followed in the autumn of 1963

8. Royal College of Physicians of London et al., *A Review of the Medical Services in Great Britain* (London, 1962).

9. *Health and Welfare—The Development of Community Care,* Cmnd. 1973 (HMSO, 1963).

by recommendations on the future of general practice, produced by a special committee chaired by Dr. Annis Gillie.[10] The Gillie report was neither a plan nor a statement of intent; it was merely an advisory report by a group of doctors working under the auspices of the Central Health Services Council to the Ministry of Health. Why an official Ministry committee on general practice was not set up at the time the medical department was considering the future of hospitals is obscure. Possibly the Ministry did not feel competent to design a comprehensive plan for general practice. The hospitals were nationalized institutions and specialists were public employees; general practice was outside this structure. At least in theory, GPs had remained professional entrepreneurs who happened to draw part of their income from public sources. Whatever the reason for this kind of committee, the Gillie report concentrated on guiding principles. It stressed the long-overdue need for "objective examination" of the work of the family doctor, and its conclusions reflected the deficiency; they were general rather than specific. The report emphasized the central position and the vital importance of general practice, commented on the advantages of group practice for GPs; stressed the need to keep the maximum size of doctors' lists under review; and set down suggestions for better cooperation between GPs and other members of the medical team, both in local authority service and in relation to the hospital. These suggestions included access to such hospital services as pathology, radiology, and autopsy facilities and recommended part-time hospital appointments for GPs. But while providing a useful background for detailed discussion of GP services, the report did not commit itself to quantitative assessment of the need for GPs nor did it discuss the apparent doctor shortage.

A final official report which had implications for medical manpower in 1963 was the Robbins report.[11] But again its value was limited, this time because its aims were somewhat different from those of medical manpower planning. While surveying the whole field of university and other higher educational facilities, the report made little reference to the immediate numerical problems in the medical schools, and even at this level the Robbins report analyzed primarily the availability of students rather than the demands of the National Health Service. This may have been a sensible criterion for the purpose of the report, but it was one that did not clarify the supposed manpower shortage then being experienced by the medical profession. "In 300 pages," said Lord Brain, "there are six lines of text and 6½ lines in two footnotes devoted to a branch of higher education which is vital to the welfare of the country." [12]

10. Central Health Services Council, Standing Medical Advisory Committee, *The Field of Work of the Family Doctor,* Report of the Sub-Committee (HMSO, 1963) (Gillie report).

11. Committee on Higher Education, *Higher Education,* Report of the Committee appointed by the Prime Minister under the Chairmanship of Lord Robbins, 1961–63, Cmnd. 2154 (HMSO, 1963).

12. The Robbins report suggested that the number of medical students would

Thus while the Ministry of Health had accepted responsibility for the number of doctors, it had little formal information on the functional relativities between general and specialist practice; there were no adequate definitions of manpower needs, and there were no accepted staffing ratios. Finally, although there were two detailed official reports on hospital services—the Hospital Plan and the Platt report on hospital staffing—neither had taken general practice into account, and there were no detailed plans for future GP services.

The Need for Definitions

In 1959 the average number of patients registered per GP principal had begun to increase. The numbers are given in Table 26. The Ministry of Health explained at the time that this position might be temporary, and the figures might be misleading because of inflation of lists through patients registered with more than one doctor. But the upward trend continued. The

TABLE 26. *Average Number of Patients Per General Practitioner Principal Providing Unrestricted Services, 1952–1964*

	No. of General Practitioners	Annual Increase	Average No. of Patients per Principal
1952	17,272		2,436
1953	18,044	772	2,324
1954	18,513	469	2,293
1955	18,817	304	2,283
1956	19,180	363	2,272
1957	19,437	257	2,273
1958	19,685	248	2,267
1959	19,745	60	2,282
1960	19,928	183	2,287
1961	20,188	260	2,292
1962	20,325	137	2,304
1963	20,349	24	2,326
1964	20,246	− 103	2,362

Unrestricted practice means that the GP does not restrict his work to staff of a hospital or an institution, provide GP maternity services only, or restrict his work for other reasons; 662 GP principals restricted their lists in some way at October 1, 1964.

Source: Annual Reports, Ministry of Health.

expand from 16,500 in 1961–62 to 21,000 in 1980–81 (ibid., p. 165). Lord Brain's comment, made in the House of Lords, December 11, 1963, was reported in the *Brit. Med. J. ii* (1963), 1598.

average GP in 1963 had a slightly larger list of patients than he had in 1953, and the position appeared to be deteriorating. In addition, the number of entrants to general practice was falling off. The Gillie report pointed out that the number of applicants per advertised practice vacancy had dropped from forty-three in 1956 to seventeen in 1962. Since, in the earlier year, there was still concern that there were too many doctors, the drop in applicants was inconclusive evidence for a real shortage in 1962. But the complaint represented a growing anxiety about the manpower position. Between October 1, 1962, and October 1, 1963, the number of GP principals providing unrestricted general medical services increased by only 24, or 0.1 per cent. This was by far the lowest increase since the beginning of the National Health Service. The following year, 1963–64, there was the first net loss of principals since the National Health Service began.

In addition, the number of assistants and trainees in general practice had been gradually decreasing. The number of doctors in general practice as a whole, including assistants and trainees, and GP principals providing restricted as well as unrestricted services (such as a GP list limited to the staff of an institution or the rare GP who provided maternity services only), reached a peak in 1961 and then began to fall. Table 27 shows the numerical position from 1952. There were fewer doctors in general practice in England and Wales in 1964 than there were in 1957. Again, the GP position seemed

TABLE 27. *Doctors in National Health Service General Practice; England and Wales, 1952–1964*

	All Doctors	Principals *	Assistants	Trainees
1952	20,162	18,164	1,689	309
1953	20,801	18,908	1,596	297
1954	21,165	19,365	1,504	296
1955	21,461	19,642	1,515	304
1956	21,865	19,951	1,546	368
1957	22,005	20,191	1,465	349
1958	22,170	20,444	1,394	332
1959	22,105	20,473	1,357	275
1960	22,234	20,626	1,345	263
1961	22,259	20,889	1,169	201
1962	22,232	21,006	989	237
1963	22,173	21,020	947	206
1964	21,903	20,883	855	165

* Includes principals in unrestricted and restricted practice. For definition see Table 26. Source: Annual Reports, Ministry of Health.

to be deteriorating. If there was a shortage of doctors generally, it followed that the shortage was more acute in general than in hospital practice. Taking into account both the trends in general practice and the possible extra demands to be made on general practice in the future under the combined effect of the Hospital Plan and the optimism expressed by the Gillie report, general practice needed at least the effort that was being put into demands for hospital staff through the Platt review committees.

Meanwhile, although it was being claimed that there were already too few doctors to go around, each of the fifteen regional hospital boards and thirty-six boards of governors of teaching hospitals in England and Wales and the five Scottish boards were busy through their Platt review committees collecting statistics, evaluating opinions, and interviewing department heads, preparatory to submitting to the appropriate health department their claims for more staff at all levels. As the English reports came into the Ministry of Health in London during 1963, it became clear that demands were being made for vast increases in hospital medical staff that could not possibly be met in full and, even if met in part, would impose a further strain on recruitment to general practice.

By the end of 1963 all the regional reviews had been completed. Despite the care taken to brief the assessors who joined the various review committees, there was a wide diversity among the regions as to how many hospital posts each thought it should have. Additional staff in the consultant grade (including those SHMOs who were paid an extra allowance for undertaking recognized consultant work) proposed during the next five years ranged, in terms of the population, from a 9 per cent increase in one regional hospital area (S.E. Metropolitan) to a 49 per cent increase in another (Newcastle). Excluding the London metropolitan areas, the number of half-day sessions per 100,000 population envisaged at the end of the five-year period varied from 151 (the equivalent of thirteen full-time consultants and one part-timer with eight sessions) in the Sheffield region, to 251 proposed by the neighboring Newcastle region. All the employing boards taken together, a 26 per cent increase in the whole-time equivalent of staff of consultant standing was being requested within five years.[13]

Clearly this demand could not be accomplished within the five-year target period: the manpower was not immediately available, and it took at least five years to train a doctor. To be useful the figures had to be pruned; otherwise, they would be discarded as impractical. The Ministry of Health decided that a "realistic" measure would be to take the median figure of the boards' proposals as a national target. All proposals above this level were reduced to the median; all lying below would remain as they were. But even after this scaling down, some 1,100 additional whole-time consultants (or their part-time equivalents) were called for in five years, and natural wastage in this period was thought to account for another 1,400. Thus, in the short

13. The figures are given in *Brit. Med. J. ii* (1964), 438, and *Lancet ii* (1964), 352.

space of five years, the number of extra whole-time consultant posts (or their equivalent in part-time posts) had to be stepped up from the current yearly increase of under 200—the increase was only 181 between 1962 and 1963—to a steady 500 a year.

The final irony of the staffing situation was that the annual output of senior registrars would meet only half this demand. For senior registrars the proposed increase of consultants had come ten years too late. Since then their numbers had steadily been whittled away. There were under 1,200 senior registrars in training in 1963. Assumed that the majority of new consultants would come from the senior registrar grade, some 1,900 senior registrars were needed to provide the extra consultants. The vital secondary consideration was thus an expansion in the number of senior registrars.

While these complexities were being discussed by the Central Consultants and Specialists Committee and the BMA prior to consideration by the Joint Consultants Committee—with no figures or statement officially published by the Ministry of Health—the Scottish Health Department, which had proceeded independently with its own reviews, quietly sent its detailed proposals to press.[14] The Scottish committee had decided to approach the review problem from different criteria. It specifically argued against the methods (used in the English surveys) of permitting laissez-faire estimates from each employing board. Instead it made a real effort to include in the surveys an element of what should be an "agreed work load" for categories of staff, using this as one indicator of future specialist needs.

As the *British Medical Journal* pointed out on the report's publication (February 1964), "It was doing something that had not been done before." [15] For each specialty, certain benchmarks of activity were recorded, which followed on clearly defined principles. These included the acceptance of the "firm" system; the possibility of enlarging the firm to include associated specialties; the desirability of exchange of beds between firms; and the allocation of both beds and outpatient duties to each consultant. It further indicated that consultant contracts should be for whole-time or maximum part-time (nine-elevenths) duties, limited as far as possible to one main hospital but including time (and facilities) for clinical research. Following from these, the number of consultants and supporting staff for each specialty was detailed in relation to numbers of beds, population, or services given, and these were extrapolated with allowances for special circumstances to give the estimated requirements for each hospital region. The resulting document came to the conclusion that some 350 more consultants and 140 more junior staff were needed in Scottish hospitals, although no specific time period was laid down. This increase was the equivalent of 14 per cent more than the existing total of 3,150, but only half the rate of increase proposed for England and Wales.

14. Scottish Home and Health Department, *Medical Staffing Structure in Scottish Hospitals* (HMSO, 1964).
15. *i* (1964), 387.

With the publication of the Platt review data, the extent of the staffing shortage could be more clearly seen. Not only was there a shortage of consultants, and thus of senior registrars, there were also acute shortages in general practice and the junior hospital grades, in both of which the position appeared to be worsening. The registrar and junior and senior house officer grades, which included all full-time doctors between house officer and senior registrar or over one fourth of all hospital medical staff, were heavily bolstered by foreign-born doctors. The proportions were steadily increasing; by 1964, 54 per cent of senior house officers and 45 per cent of the registrars working in NHS hospitals were born outside Britain (Table 28). It was

TABLE 28. *Hospital Medical Staff, Selected Grades, by Place of Birth; England and Wales, 1964*

	Number in Grade *	Percentage Born Outside British Isles †
Senior registrar	1,133	14.8
Registrar	3,794	44.6
JHMO	608	46.9
Senior house officer	3,027	54.1
House officer ‡	2,428	27.8

* The figures given are in whole-time equivalents of paid staff and relate to 30 September. There is no reason to doubt that they also give an accurate picture of the proportion of foreign graduates in terms of persons, since almost all staff in these grades are on whole time.

† United Kingdom and Eire.

‡ Both preregistration and postregistration posts are included.

Source: Ministry of Health, *Annual Report for 1964,* p. 144.

reasonable to suppose that many of these were only temporary residents and would not be available for future senior staffing either as consultants or as general practitioners.

Publication of the first detailed study of emigration of British doctors, by Brian Abel-Smith and Kathleen Gales, in June 1964 did little to allay the anxiety of those who saw emigration as a major staffing problem.[16] The Minister of Health had estimated in 1962 that between 6 and 7 per cent of British doctors who graduated during the 1950s were then resident abroad. The new study indicated that nearly 17 per cent of doctors registered on the home list between 1950 and 1954 were resident outside the United Kingdom in July 1962, together with over 11 per cent of those who were

16. *British Doctors at Home and Abroad* (London, 1964).

registered between 1955 and 1959. Of all those in the sample of doctors who received their medical education in the United Kingdom between 1925 and 1959, 16 per cent were resident elsewhere in 1962. The number of doctors, born and trained in Britain, who were leaving the country appeared to have reached a peak in 1959 and since then to have declined; but the estimated rate of leaving between January 1955 and July 1962 was 392 doctors a year. It was not, however, known from this study how many of those who emigrated ultimately returned, or whether this overall position was radically different from that of fifteen years or even fifty years before, when large numbers of British doctors worked in the Indian Medical Service and in other parts of what is now the British Commonwealth. Nevertheless, the findings added a further source of alarm and a further argument for increasing the supply of home-trained practitioners.

Although enrollment in British schools rose from under 1,800 in 1960–61 to over 2,100 in 1963 it was still, as the chairman of the Joint Consultants Committee observed, "obviously inadequate to meet the overall demands." [17] In July 1964 the Minister of Health announced the establishment of a medical school at Nottingham—the first since the inauguration of the National Health Service. A 1,200-bed teaching hospital was to be built, and the school would annually accept 100 students. At the same time it was announced that existing medical schools would be expanded to produce a further 150 students by October 1966.[18] But, as Kenneth Hill pointed out in an analysis of the medical manpower position in September 1964, these proposals together would increase the number of doctors only by 250 a year; [19] according to the demands in the Platt reviews, additional consultants alone would absorb 500 doctors a year. There were indications that the wastage of doctors in 1964 was greater than the input of new students; and there was concern that the supply of foreign-born doctors might be reduced by restrictions on emigration imposed by their own countries—particularly by India, whose doctors furnished a large proportion of hospital staff in certain areas of the country. Dr. Hill considered that twelve new medical schools were required and that the situation was sufficiently urgent to merit a crash training program.

Despite the cries of manpower shortage, however, the total number of doctors had steadily increased under the National Health Service both in absolute terms and relative to population increases. The demands had to be seen in perspective; but it was not clear what this perspective should be. It was still not known how effectively existing doctors were being utilized. The relative function of general and specialist practice needed urgent attention; for although hospital planning indicated a greater burden to be placed on general practice, the Platt reviews had indicated an equally urgent need for more consultants. The divided structure of the National Health Service did

17. *Brit Med. J. ii* (1964), 816 (T. Holmes Sellors).
18. *Hansard* (H of C), 1964, no. 151, col. 699.
19. *Lancet ii* (1964), 517–19.

not facilitate combined study. Finally, a new look needed to be taken at the whole planning process.

There was clear cause for investigating a manpower situation that apparently moved from a surplus of doctors to an acute shortage in the space of ten years—during which more information was available than ever before on the numbers and characteristics of doctors in the country, routine committees had been set up with the power of veto over applications for new consultant and GP posts, and the overall ratio of doctors to population had steadily improved. Either the demand for manpower had changed far more rapidly than could possibly have been foreseen year by year or the planning machinery had been grossly deficient.

The responsibility for manpower questions now clearly rested with the Ministry of Health. The number of doctors could no longer be left to laissez-faire arrangements or be subjected to the sometimes unreliable gauge of general professional opinion. But there were as yet no definitions and no effective machinery for positive manpower scrutiny. The Ministry's role was just beginning. It had accepted the need for a hospital plan; manpower planning was the next logical step and one which the Ministry was being forced to take through the increasing demands of general practitioners for better and more attractive conditions and the question of balancing the number of doctors between general and consultant practice. There was now an important need in almost all planning fields to discover the value of different staffing patterns, the cost of alternatives, and the actual work done by doctors at different levels and in different kinds of practice.

Of all the outstanding manpower questions, the most important concerned the rift between GP and hospital, which by 1965 had become one of extreme urgency. It concerned the future of general practice—its function, its organization, its planning, and its relative monetary value; this arose primarily from the outcries of GPs. A related question was the corollary to the general doctor shortage. What were the most valuable interrelationships of the two branches of practice in terms of manpower utilization? Was it, in crude terms, more expedient to develop consultant or GP services, and what criteria should be used? Could the efficiency of either branch be improved—and how? Was the generally recognized shortage of doctors a question of overall expansion or could it be relieved by further, and perhaps drastic, redeployment? Finally, were the two branches, with their long history of conflicts, a master-stroke—in terms of providing a ready-made "personal" doctor to interpret and coordinate the team of specialists—or were they an anachronism?

V

The Medical Profession

18

Professional Participation in the National Health Service Structure

There would have been an increasing need for cooperation between public bodies and representatives of the medical profession whether or not a National Health Service had been introduced: on the issues of the number and distribution of general and specialist practitioners, on the cost and availability of medical services, and on the most effective means of ensuring the highest quality of medical care. The medical profession has become more intimately involved in questions of public policy as specialized medicine has developed; and at the same time society has become increasingly interested in the availability of health services, and thus in the intentions of the medical profession. But control of the means of practice by the state, whether through a scheme of insurance, prepayment, nationalization, or by any other means, adds a further dimension: an acute and immediate need to formalize and codify professional advice.

The professional viewpoint may be formally obtained in a number of ways. Doctors may be employed as specialized administrators, for example, in the Ministry of Health or in regional hospital boards, or they may become voluntary members of management or other special committees with delegated administrative authority; in these cases the doctor is an active administrative or executive participant in the operation of various aspects of the health service. Alternatively, or in addition, the administration may set up advisory committees or panels to give a professional opinion on administrative and policy-making matters, and the profession may exert influence through committees set up by its own organizations. Under the National Health Service, each of these methods has been, and continues to be, used.

One early effect of the National Health Service was the replacement by career administrators in England and Wales (but not in Scotland) of physicians who superintended unit hospitals or groups of hospitals. Hospital administration developed its own body of skills, and there was little to be gained by employing clinicians in these posts. The teaching hospitals had long been accustomed to nonmedical clerks, house governors, and treasurers; moreover, the "firm" system of hospital staffing was not conducive to the incorporation of clinical chiefs of service on the American pattern. The administrative duties of medical superintendents in ex-municipal hospitals were rapidly whittled away.[1] Although mental hospitals still tend to include a part-time medical superintendent as well as a career administrator—apparently on the assumption that the hospital as a therapeutic community should itself be under psychiatric guidance—this pattern too is beginning to change. General use of doctors as full-time administrators is confined to the Ministry of Health, regional hospital boards, and local health authorities.

The medical department of the Ministry of Health employs about 175 doctors as civil servants through its own divisions and in the separate Welsh Board of Health, besides its full complement of nonmedical administrators. Regional hospital boards also have a medical section as part of their secretariat.[2] The senior administrative medical officer of a regional board is paid more than the nonmedical administrator or secretary, and the board is run as a joint venture. Their functions range over all aspects of development within the region. Since all major policy decisions on hospitals are taken regionally or nationally, the influence of the profession through their employment in an administrative capacity is substantial, both in the planning and operation of specialist services.

The medical profession is also closely involved in the voluntary committee structure of hospital administration. The physician may sit on the hospital management committee of his own hospital, whereas the pharmacist or the nurse may not. Consultants may also sit on committees of the regional hospital board that employs them. Indeed, of the first 364 appointments to regional boards made in 1947, more than 120 were doctors. A 25 per cent limit was introduced as the result of the Guillebaud Committee's recommendation in 1956, following the discovery of the extent of medical membership on regional boards; in one board 42 per cent of the members in 1954–55 were medical practitioners. By 1959 they represented a little over one fourth of the membership of hospital boards and a slightly smaller percentage of membership of hospital management committees.[3] The structure is not one of laymen on the one side and doctors on the other, but of close involvement by the profession in decision-making; this continues the use of the profession as an executive arm in a public function, that was effective during World War II.

Advisory Bodies to the Ministry of Health

Nevertheless, those doctors involved in such administrative capacities are comparatively few compared with the size of the profession, and they

1. In 1949 the administrative work of medical and deputy medical superintendents represented the equivalent of 261 whole-time staff; by 1955, it represented only 16. Ministry of Health Statistics Division. And see chap. 13, n. 11.

2. 101 whole-time and 3 part-time administrative medical officers were employed at regional hospital board headquarters in 1964. Ministry of Health, *Annual Report for 1964*, p. 159.

3. Guillebaud report, p. 97; Ministry of Health Circular HM (56), no. 111; Lindsey, *Socialized Medicine in England and Wales*, p. 91.

may not be representative of the profession at large. A much more significant aspect of professional participation is the reliance by administrative committees and personnel on the recommendations and in some case delegated authority of medical advisory bodies. This is particularly relevant to the hospital service. The nationalized hospital structure is studded with professional committees from local to national level. There are standing committees with particular expert functions, such as the Advisory Committee on Distinction Awards, the Medical Practices Committee, and the Advisory Committee on Consultant Establishments; [4] committees set up for special purposes of investigation or review; and regular advisory committees at each level of administration. The Ministry of Health also retains a regular panel of "consultant advisers," who are teachers and clinicians in a broad spectrum of specialties, chosen by the Chief Medical Officer of the Ministry to provide guidance as required on topics concerning a particular specialty area. In 1964 the panel consisted of thirty-nine persons representing thirty specialties, from biochemistry to mass radiography, malaria, and rehabilitation of injured miners. There was also a separate special adviser on general practice.[5] In each of these cases medical practitioners are directly available to the NHS administration.

The main channel of formal advice is a standing professional advisory committee at each level of the hospital hierarchy (Figure 2). At the top, the Minister of Health may draw advice from the Central Health Services Council, set up under the National Health Service Act. The full council, a prestigious body drawn from a spectrum of health professions, has forty-one members, including the presidents of the three English Royal Colleges, the president of the General Medical Council, and the chairman of the councils of the BMA and of the Society of Medical Officers of Health. Apart from these six members, who serve ex officio, the membership represents medical and dental practitioners, registered nurses, midwives, pharmacists, and other persons with health service experience.

The Central Health Services Council, which proffers advice over all aspects of the National Health Service, is broken down into nine specialized standing advisory committees, including a Medical Committee and a Maternity and Midwifery Committee. Recommendations are collected from these committees as the need arises, often with additional expert members. The Council, lacking its own statistical and research unit, draws on Ministry staff for the compilation and analysis of relevant data, but in fact, Council reports have tended to be the combined result of the opinions of its members rather than the outcome of specific research projects. Early reports included those on treatment of tuberculosis, hospital administration,

4. See Chap. 15 for a discussion of the distinction awards system and Chap. 16 for the Medical Practices Committee and the Advisory Committee on Consultant Establishments.

5. Ministry of Health, *On the State of the Public Health,* the Annual Report of the Chief Medical Officer of the Ministry of Health for the year 1963 (HMSO, 1964), p. 240.

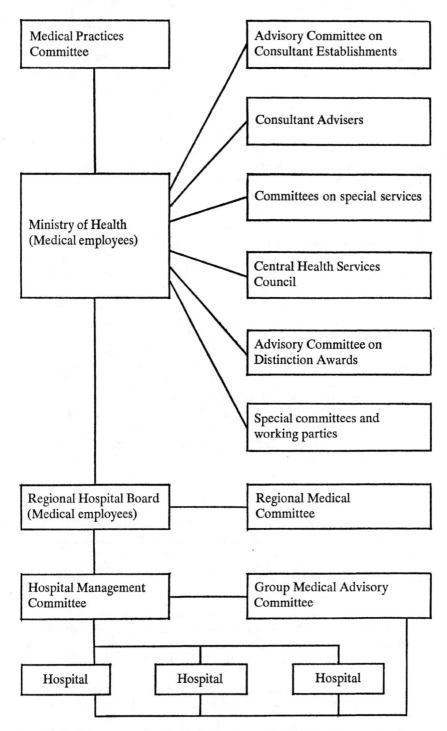

FIGURE 2. *National Health Service: Medical advisory bodies*
262

prescription of drugs, and health centers. Recent published reports have included consideration of the hospital inpatient's day (by a nursing subcommittee, 1961), human relations in obstetrics (by the Standing Maternity and Midwifery Advisory Committee, 1961), the future organization of accident and emergency services (by the Standing Medical Advisory Committee, 1962), problems of communication among doctors, nurses, and patients (by a joint subcommittee of the medical and nursing advisory committees, 1963), and the future field of work of the family doctor (the Gillie report, by the Standing Medical Advisory Committee, 1963).

Although it is placed as the central channel of advice to the Ministry, and despite the importance of the subjects it has treated, the Council has an ill-defined role. It is not invariably consulted on major issues. The Ministry of Health is unlike the regional and local hospital committees in that its functions are diffuse; it does not operate through a central administrative committee to which a professional body might proffer continuous advice. The Council is also in competition with other channels of professional communication. The Joint Consultants Committee and the General Medical Services Committee, in particular, speak as the profession's own representatives in matters of hospital and GP policy. But in addition and of major importance, the Ministry has in many cases circumvented the Council in its search for answers to specific questions. As a result, many of the policy documents of the National Health Service have not been drawn up by the Central Health Services Council—perhaps because of the inflexibility of its membership or possibly because of the danger of overtaxing members (all of whom serve in an honorary capacity) to the detriment of their other activities.

Instead, there has been a growing tendency for the Minister of Health to appoint specialist bodies or committees of inquiry to consider each subject as it arises; and, more recently, to set up joint "working parties" of Ministry and professional representatives, such as the working party on the hospital medical staffing structure (Platt report, 1961). The Platt Committee included leading members of the Royal Colleges, the universities, and the Ministry's medical department, as well as those who regularly served on other professional bodies such as the General Medical Council, the Joint Consultants Committee, the Central Health Services Council, the BMA, and the Distinction Awards Committee. All were, however, appointed in their individual rather than their representative capacity.

With one or two exceptions, the working party or the committee of inquiry has had a greater role to play than special subcommittees of the Central Health Services Council. Indeed, it is remarkable how many important decisions affecting the NHS have been taken by such external committees. The Goodenough report and the Spens committees on medical and dental remuneration provided much of the essential framework for the hospital and specialist services. The Guillebaud Committee, chaired by an eminent economist, made a detailed report in 1956 on the cost of the NHS in the light of its expanding budget. Alarm over too many doctors led to the

Willink Committee's report in 1957; analysis of medical and dental incomes was referred to a Royal Commission (1957–60); maternity services were scrutinized by the Cranbrook Committee (1959); the development of hospital administration was the subject of the Lycett Green Committee (1963). The list can be extended to almost all aspects of NHS policy.

There appears to have been no formal distinction between subjects that are decided within the Ministry, with or without consultation with the Joint Consultants Committee and other professional bodies, those that go to the Central Health Services Council, and those that require the formation of a special advisory body or working party. It is a reasonable assumption that special committees are usually appointed when the subject is one of particular confusion, where it is surrounded by controversy that can effectively be allayed (or delayed) only by the appointment of a noncontroversial panel of experts, or where details need to be worked out in a cooperative venture. By being individually tailored for one specific purpose they may be able to consider in more detail the long-term policy questions affecting particular subjects or particular areas. Special committees are not bound to follow the stated policy of the Ministry, nor, of course, is the Minister in any way bound to accept their advice. But usually the advice of special committees and of the Central Health Services Council is accepted as it is submitted. It is, after all, not controversial, for how can the profession reject the considered finding of distinguished doctors on the committee—and how can the Ministry fail to put into effect such eminent advice? The committees are not merely advising; they are developing public policy.

This heavy reliance on outside advice promises to continue as the means of policy development. How efficient it is provides another question. There is a real danger that important decisions (and thus responsibility) may be shelved by the Ministry of Health in favor of outside discussion, and, as a result, basic planning techniques may remain undeveloped. The structure rests on an assumption that may no longer be valid: that busy practitioners, willing to give up part of their time for the public good, are in a better position to develop plans and programs than is a group of full-time doctors or civil servants. The lack of a cohesive plan for general practice is a prime example of the need for much more detailed development of alternative plans than has been customary in the past. It points to a failure not of the advisory machinery, whose responsibility is clearly to develop opinion, but to a lack of practical underpinning and even guidance of such opinion by expert planners in the Ministry of Health. In this sphere at least, an unfair responsibility may have been placed on the medical profession.

Group and Regional Advisory Machinery

Group and regional advisory committees, to conform with the group and regional structure of the National Hospital Service, were not set up by Act of Parliament; they have arisen in response to local demand. Each hospital group, representing a number of nonteaching hospitals with perhaps 1,000 beds, has a medical advisory committee (MAC) of consultants working in its constituent hospitals. Dependent on the size of the staff, the MAC may consist of all the consultants attached to the group, or their selected representatives. Because the majority of consultants are full-time hospital workers, there is a relatively small number of consultants in relation to the population. Thus even a large group of general and special hospitals, with some 2,000 hospital beds serving a population of 400,000 people or more, may have fewer than seventy consultants and SHMOs attached to it; and most hospital groups are much smaller. The group Medical Advisory Committee is thus reasonably compact and representative, and its opinions carry considerable weight. In the words of a BMA resolution: "The medical committee has always had direct access to the management committee, and usually a state of confidence and mutual respect has been present between them." The success of this system from the profession's point of view is indicated by the BMA's official distrust of a more formal medical administration at hospital level: "Consultants would view with disapproval a system by which administrative medical officers were created with a monopoly of medical administration and tendering of advice and all administrative responsibilities removed from clinicians." [6]

The Medical Advisory Committee considers questions raised by its own members or put to it by the Hospital Management Committee (HMC). These may concern questions of equipment, staffing, priorities in building or supplies programs, or drug costs; they include virtually anything in which professional advice is requested, in which the consultants are interested, or which the MAC discusses by tradition in one group or another. There are no set rules. The advisory committee usually meets in the interval between meetings of the management committees, so that its minutes and recommendations may go directly to the next HMC meeting and, if necessary, their policy recommendations may be forwarded promptly to the regional hospital board. Since there is usually no medical administrator or chief of service at hospital or group level, the medical committee acts also as the consultants' executive, and can exert considerable power. The MAC may or may not invite the hospital or group administrator to be present at its meetings. If it does not it can, if it so wishes, sidestep the administrator in two ways: first, by appealing directly to the HMC; second, by contacting medical administrators at the regional hospital board with whom consultants have a direct employment relationship.

The hospital management committee, which consists of lay volunteer members drawn from the community and (in a minority) the medical profession, is in no way bound to accept the advice of its medical advisory committee. But, in the words of one consultant interviewed, who was a member of both a MAC and a regional hospital board, "it is ill-advised not to do so." The relationships among the three groups attending HMC meetings make

6. BMA, *Members Handbook* (London, 1963), p. 101.

this almost a foregone conclusion. First, hospital administrators and representatives of the senior nursing staff attend the HMC by virtue of their position; they are not members but officers of the committee. The group administrator invariably acts as secretary to the committee; he reports and documents each item brought up for consideration. The second and largest group are the lay members. These are appointed to the committee by the regional hospital board on the advice of local organizations; but it is specifically understood that each member serves in his individual capacity as a private citizen and not as a representative of a public group. Nor, as in the days of the voluntary hospitals, are committee members major donors to the hospitals. They therefore exert little automatic local influence in the decisions they are called upon to make and thus may know little of the intricate details of hospital operation. As a result, a fairly typical pattern of organization is for the group secretary to work closely with the committee chairman and with the third and most powerful group: the two or three consultants who sit on the hospital management committee and uphold the MAC views, and who (by being employed by the regional board) are not subject in their employment relationship to the local hospital administration. Because of this pattern, consultants may exert considerable influence on the local operation of the hospital service.

The regional hospital board has its own medical advisory committee which serves a similar purpose at the regional level. The regional medical committee may consist of medical members of the regional hospital board, together with doctors co-opted by the board from a number of sources. There is no direct flow of communication between the regional and the group medical committees; nor, in turn, between the regional medical committees and the Central Health Services Council. Any decisions made by the hospital management committee on the advice of the medical staff go up through the administrative hierarchy to the regional hospital board, and only in cases of conflict between the group medical committees and the HMC does the MAC go directly to the regional board. More usually, when consultants wish to express disapproval of a HMC decision, a minute is incorporated in the HMC's minutes, which are routinely sent to the regional board's officers.

The administrative structure of the hospital service is thus surrounded with advisory machinery which intermeshes with administrative bodies at each level—group, regional, and national. The Ministry of Health's practice, particularly in the past, has been to rely on outside advice, sought and coordinated by a relatively large medical department; and to a large extent the same policy has been followed by the regional hospital boards and hospital management committees. The individual consultant may find himself involved in a plethora of committees whose sole function is to advise or organize local or national health services. He may be a member of the group and regional medical advisory committee, and of the HMC or the regional hospital board—excluding any special committees set up for particular purposes, such as maternity liaison committees between hospital and community obstetrical services, consultant appointments committees, or specialty subcommittees of the regional hospital board. One estimate of the committee work of consultants was:

> From a minimum of perhaps two or three committees a month through that of Chairmen and Secretaries of important hospital committees, who may have several a week, to busy medical members of Regional Boards and committees of the whole profession whose committees are not only more frequent but last longer, often for a whole day at a time.[7]

Some Effects of Professional Participation

The consultant was drawn into the administrative framework of the National Health Service to a greater extent than general practitioners. Consultants are part of the large hospital industry which, it was pointed out in 1955, was the third largest organization in the country, then employing nearly half a million people.[8] GP services, on the other hand, have never really been nationalized. Responsibility for general medical services in its area rests with the local executive council, which usually conforms to the local health authority area; it also arranges general dental services, and for paying NHS drug and optical bills. Like the hospital committees, the executive council is manned by voluntary members of the community. But unlike the regional hospital boards, executive councils are, as their name suggests, administrative rather than planning bodies. One chairman of an executive council, a dental practitioner who happened also to serve on a regional hospital board and a hospital management committee, admitted: "We are very much a stamping machine." The NHS Act stipulated that of the twenty-five members of the local executive council, seven should be appointed by the local medical committee, which acts as its medical advisory body. Any committee which the executive council felt to be representative of general medical practitioners in the area could be designated the local medical committee. This has meant that in many cases LMC members are the same persons who are active in the local divisions and branches of the BMA, a situation not equally true of consultant advisory committees, which exist for administrative rather than for local professional purposes. Local medical committees have a double role; they include functions that for consultants are divided between the NHS advisory committees and the completely separate structure of regional consultants and specialists committees that was set up by the BMA in the early years of the health service.

By being involved so closely in the administrative hierarchy, the medical profession, and particularly the consultant branch, has largely escaped the danger inherent in a national health system of becoming primarily a bar-

---

7. *Royal Commission; Minutes of Evidence*, p. 1098.
8. Acton Society Trust, *Hospitals and the State, Background and Blueprint*, p. 3.

gaining power on one side of the fence, wrangling for essentially selfish ends. How much the public image of a profession can be sullied by battles with the state was illustrated in the doctors' strike in Belgium in April 1964. Professions have been built up on the ideals of public service, integrity, and reliability; yet agreement between a monopoly employer and a monopoly employee group implies power politics, including the threat by employees of discontinuing their services. A balance of influence between the government and the profession rests on a degree of expertise and understanding, so that agreement may be reached at least with dignity.

If the profession is well organized and closely involved in administration and policy, it does not follow that increased government responsibility for medical services must weaken professional authority. Indeed, the reverse is equally likely to occur, for the greater the ambit of government, the greater is the government dependent on the goodwill, the advice, and the drive of the medical profession to make its services work. The professional authority of the consultant branch has been increased under the NHS, not only by streamlining the profession to speak with one voice but also in large part by its identification with the hospital service. This has meant that many vital planning decisions have been made quietly through a partnership between consultants and the Ministry of Health, or at a local level, which might otherwise have caused tensions between the administration and the profession. The staffing reports provide a useful example. When the profession felt that there were too many doctors in the country in the mid 1950s, the Minister of Health set up the joint Willink Committee to investigate the claim. The Platt Committee on hospital staffing met a similar need, as did the later Working Party on General Practice.

Specialization and developing interest in the provision of health services have increased the area for discussion between the medical profession and the public. The doctor is inevitably less socially independent than he was when his skills were less socially valuable. At the same time, the codification and extension of formal advice under the National Health Service strengthened professional influence on public opinion. Although there is more public interest in medical care than ever before, the medical profession has become more powerful. Moreover, the greater the organization of the profession, the greater, rather than less, may be the rights of individual practitioners. Instead of bureaucracy bringing with it stringent disciplinary and dismissal tactics, under the NHS it has become virtually impossible for a specialist to be dismissed from the hospital service save for flagrant violation of professional standards; and, if anything, the power of the specialist in relation to his employing board is stronger than before.

Instead of developing as an authoritarian bureaucracy, the Ministry of Health has shown itself to be remarkably restrained in its approach to health service policy and to be willing to use the advice of professional groups on all possible occasions. In some respects it has been almost forced to take the initiative—for example, with respect to hospital building plans, responsibility for numbers of doctors and for postgraduate education, and plans for the future of general practice. The overall Ministry of Health policy appears to have been to step in only where the professions, notably the medical profession, have been unable to develop acceptable policies of their own. This attitude has had two particularly interesting consequences. First, it has revealed the demand for central leadership by the government in certain vital areas—a demand that, with the publication of plans for hospitals and local health services and with investigations into general practice, is now being met. Second, it has developed, side by side with the medical advisory committees, working parties, and professional advisers, a stratified system of committees between the Ministry and the professional associations. This in turn has had a profound effect on the internal organization of the British Medical Association and on the role of the professional Colleges.

19

The British Medical Association and the Royal Colleges

By definition, a profession is a group practicing a common craft; it is usually identified by an association of members. The association attempts to raise the standards of competence by acting as a national interest group, through an examination system, or through nominations to a diploma; but it is also intimately affected by questions that touch upon members' livelihood or the practice of their skill. The relative importance of these two functions—regulation of standards and protection of interests—has a crucial effect on the association's structure. Usually a profession is governed by an oligarchy and represented by a democracy. The first, an exclusive body with competitive entry, dictates standards of skill and codes of behavior. The second is an open association with more material aspirations; it ensures the strength of the profession in agreements with outside bodies and may establish rules to protect each person in the profession from unfair practices by others. Here an advantage lies in an inclusive membership, for the greater the number of members, the larger the association's sphere of influence. The Royal Colleges represent the oligarchic function, the British Medical Association the democratic.

The establishment of a comprehensive state medical service challenged both the Colleges and the BMA to reconsider their positions in relation to their own membership and to the government. In so doing, their respective roles were blurred. The BMA as the chief democratic medical organization with the largest membership of doctors might be considered the natural consulting body for major health service decisions; membership at the end of 1964 surpassed 69,800,[1] and it was thought to include at least 80 per cent of general practitioners and 80 per cent of hospital doctors in Britain. But despite the modifications made in the BMA's basic organizational structure to accommodate special representative machinery for each major medical group, the BMA was not able to secure a monopoly representation of all National Health Service doctors. The Royal Colleges had been loath to relinquish their traditional leadership of the consultant branch. Indeed, under the NHS, through membership in such bodies as the Central Health

---

1. *Brit. Med. J.* Suppl. *i* (1965), 169.

Services Council, the Distinction Awards Committee, and special advisory committees, the College presidents extended their authority into a number of executive and policy-making fields. The creation in 1948 of the Joint Consultants Committee to speak for all consultants outside the BMA brought the Royal Colleges firmly into the political arena; and at the same time the existence of the Joint Committee created peculiar organizational difficulties within the BMA's own structure.

Structure of the British Medical Association

The basis of BMA membership, developed in the nineteenth century, is the local Division, often part of a larger branch. Members of the association automatically become members of the division and branch of the area in which they live, no matter to which section of the profession—hospital, general practice, or public health—they belong: "It is for the Division to form the link and to preserve the unity of the profession locally." [2] For a number of reasons the BMA Division tends to be dominated by general practitioners; GPs are by far the most numerous branch of practice. But, in addition, individual GPs working alone or in small partnerships may put more value on the activities of the Division than do consultants. The latter have the hospital or specialist associations as their institutional focus; public health doctors are too few in number to influence the Division as a whole.

The activities of the Division are grouped by the BMA under four heads: scientific, social, medicopolitical, and ethical. The Division, representing all branches of the profession, provides the means for carrying out locally the main objects of the BMA: "promotion of the medical and allied sciences and the maintenance of the honour and interests of the profession." Medical politics have engaged the Divisions as they have the central organization of the BMA. But two changes have affected the political position of the Division since the introduction of the National Health Service.

First, since more emphasis has been placed on negotiations at the national level, the scope of local politics has narrowed. The Division can exert pressure on executive councils, on local health authorities, or on hospital management committees, but many of the important questions must be taken to higher administrative levels. However much the Division may press for a new hospital, the hospital management committee can do little about it except to urge it on the regional hospital board. The regional board may add the request to its list of priorities, but the final decision will rest with the Ministry of Health, and the timing of the project will be the responsibility of the Treasury, from which the health service budget ultimately derives. Second, the local practitioner cannot haggle over rates of pay. Special centralized machinery has been extended or devised to deal with terms and conditions of service in the three main fields of medical practice—hospital, general, and public health—through specific negotiating machinery. As a result, major responsibility has been taken away from the local participants

2. BMA, *Members Handbook* (London, 1963), p. 20.

and has gravitated toward central organs of government. Because of this, professional influence has also moved upward. The branches and divisions are still important as internal pressure groups of the BMA and as two-way links between individual members and the central body but, as the National Health Service has become more centralized, so have the negotiating bodies.

One result was that the Divisions became apathetic to broad developments in medical practice. Lectures and discussions fulfilled their scientific and social needs and divisional committees forwarded ethical complaints to the head office of the BMA, but there was little impetus for experiment and reform in organization of medical facilities. Indeed, the BMA has warned Divisions to avoid discussions of controversial medicosociological issues, because of the "definite views, if not acute susceptibilities" of some members of the medical profession.[3] At the same time, the BMA structure continues to be based on a parliamentary system which, to be effective, relies on action being initiated within the Divisions. Apathy in the Divisions thus led to inertia in policy-making at BMA House, and to an increasing gap between the central negotiators and local constituents.

Nationally, the British Medical Association is governed by a representative body whose members are elected by "constituencies" composed of Divisions or groups of Divisions, or who are members of central BMA committees. The number of constituencies is limited to three hundred. The Representative Body meets annually and acts as the BMA's parliament, and special representative meetings may also be called to discuss matters of particular importance. The activities of officers and constituent or related committees must be ratified by the Representative Body, whose decisions become BMA policy. The central executive of the Association is the BMA Council, elected annually by the Representative Body; in turn the Council has a number of standing committees, including a private-practice committee and a committee on medical education and research. But the basic policy-making activity of the BMA has remained with the Representative Body— a democratic but not always efficient method of reaching major medical or political decisions.

Neither the Representative Body nor the BMA Council is a formal trade union. Discussions were held at the beginning of the National Health Service on the possibility of reorganizing the BMA so that at law it would be a trade union or a limited liability company—either of which would have had the advantage that the BMA could collect and disburse funds for political purposes and organize strike action. But the idea was not received enthusiastically and was rejected in 1949 in favor of a ghost organization, the British Medical Guild, the trustees of which are the members of the BMA Council. Thus the British Medical Guild and not the British Medical Association was concerned with mass resignations of practitioners from the National Health Service in 1957 and again in 1965. The difference is technical rather than real.

3. *BMA Calendar* 1964–65, p. 70.

Autonomous Committees of the BMA

Although the Representative Body is the core of the BMA, with responsibility for making its primary decisions, it has little direct contact with the Ministry of Health. Discussions with the Ministry are held by two other powerful bodies: the General Medical Services Committee for GPs and the Central Consultants and Specialists Committee for hospital staff. Both these committees and their constituents were set up by the BMA, and both are used as if they were part of the BMA; the GMSC, for example, is referred to in the BMA *Calendar* as "The Association's Organization for General Practitioners." Neither is, however, a subcommittee of the Representative Body or even formally part of the BMA. This has created an anomalous situation, founded partly on historical accident, in which the governing body of the BMA is not directly and formally responsible for major negotiations taken on behalf of either GPs or hospital staff.

The relationship between the BMA and the two sectional structures is shown in Figure 3. Members of the General Medical Services Committee are drawn primarily from the local medical committees, and regional consultants and specialists committees furnish members for the Central Consultants and Specialists Committee. Neither of these local committees has a formal connection with the BMA Division (or, indeed, with any part of the BMA) although there is overlapping membership. The three organizations exist in parallel, and there is no final authority to act as arbitrator in intraprofessional disputes.

The General Medical Services Committee is the direct descendant of the Insurance Acts Committee which was originally set up to deal with GP matters arising under the Health Insurance Act of 1911. Like its predecessor it deals directly with the Ministry of Health on all questions concerning general practice. The rejection by GPs of the Whitley bargaining structure for income decisions (Chapter 9) left the GMSC a wide authority. Besides being available for general consultation and advice, it negotiates on all matters of pay and conditions of service. The committee consists of the officers of the British Medical Association, six members appointed by the BMA's Representative Body, thirty-three practitioners elected from those nominated by local medical committees, and six from other bodies. Although the GMSC has strong ties with the central structure of the BMA, it is, at least in form, the national spokesman and bargaining agent of the local medical committees.

Representatives of the local medical committees meet annually at their national conference, to which the GMSC officially reports. As is the case with the BMA Representative Body, special meetings of the conference are called for matters of urgency. On such occasions it has become a common practice for the local medical committees to meet a few days before the Representative Body, each to hear reports from the same committees and to discuss a similar agenda.

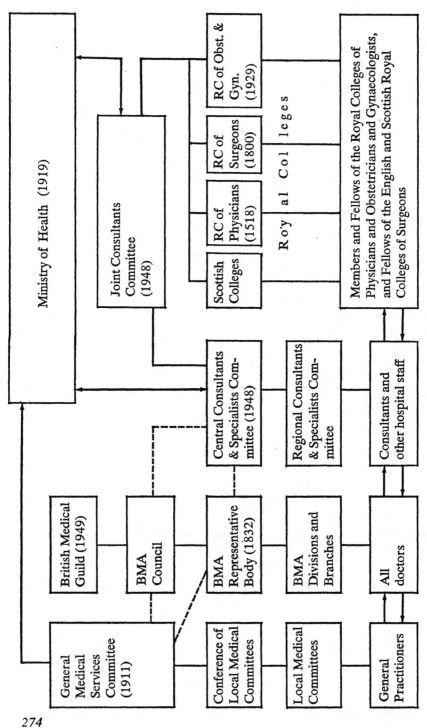

FIGURE 3. *Organization of the major medical professional bodies in relation to the Ministry of Health*

The supposed autonomy of the GMSC, illustrated in the fact that it is not restricted to BMA members, would indicate that the GMSC is not bound to follow BMA policy. But at the same time this very autonomy (together with that of the GMSC's sister committee for consultants) has to be confirmed each year by the BMA Representative Body. Confirmation is dependent, moreover, "on the understanding that no action be taken by either of these Committees which may prejudice the interests of other parts of the profession without full prior consultation with the interests concerned, and that their autonomous powers will be used so as to expedite the work of the Association." [4] Autonomy is thus partly a legal fiction. The GMSC acts as if it were a BMA committee, reports of its meetings being presented to, and defended at, BMA Council meetings. It follows rulings of the BMA Representative Body; and the reaction of general practitioners to unpopular GMSC policies is to attack the BMA. The chairman of the GMSC plays a strong platform role in the meetings of BMA representatives as well as in those of local medical committees. As is common among the committee structures of the medical profession, the same names recur from one committee to another, and this factor carries more weight than the formal separation of administration channels. Nevertheless, the potential for conflict remains in two parallel representative structures from local to national level —the one for GPs only (GMSC), the other for all doctors (the BMA).

While GPs were the only body of doctors involved in negotiations with the government, as they were before 1948, the conflict was latent. But the inclusion of hospital staff within the National Health Service made it imperative for the BMA to change its organization, either by abolishing the GMSC and strengthening divisional representation to ensure that specialists were adequately represented, or by creating a separate organization. It is usually easier to add to than to abolish; not surprisingly, the second method was chosen.[5] But the creation of a structure for specialist representation underlined the peculiar relationship already existing between the BMA and the GMSC. It was not clear whether the latter was the executive (and thus the servant) of the local medical committees, or bore a primary de facto responsibility to the BMA, or might pursue policies independently of either. The same confusion attached to the new consultant committee.

Regional consultants and specialists committees were set up to conform to the boundaries of the regional hospital areas; their national body, similar in purpose to the GMSC, is the Central Consultants and Specialists Committee. The organization of consultant services preordained, however, that the regional committees would not wield the same authority in relation to the administrative structure of the health service as that exerted by local medical committees.

The usual pattern is for the medical advisory committee of a hospital group to nominate representatives to the regional consultants and specialists

4. *Brit. Med. J.* Suppl. *i* (1963), 11.
5. See Chap. 6.

committees, where they may be joined by GP and public health service nominees. Thus the regional CSC represents consultants over the whole area. Unlike local medical committees, however, the regional consultants committee has no statutory function to provide advice. To the administration it is an outside body, and the potential for conflict between the regional CSC and the medical advisory committee of the regional hospital board is apparent. In at least one region (South-West Metropolitan) the regional CSC has insisted that it have actual representation on the medical advisory committee to the regional hospital board, and it now nominates six of the committee's members. But there is no set pattern, and the influence of the regional CSC on local hospital administration varies from one region to another. In parallel to the Conference of Local Medical Committees, the regional CSCs have what one consultant called "periodic jamborees," roughly every two years. But, possibly because there are fewer hospital regions than LMC areas, the need for such gatherings has been less pressing for consultants and specialists than for GPs.

Each regional consultants and specialists committee appoints two members to the Central Consultants and Specialists Committee. The central committee has a grand total of over eighty members and observers, including the officers of the BMA. This unwieldly body meets about five times a year. Its terms of reference are wide, and the committee acts as a kind of watchdog for hospital staffs.[6] Reflecting this function, its work is chiefly concerned with matters of status and employment. Typical activities in 1961 and 1962 were the consideration of recruitment to the profession, the income tax position of part-time consultants, the status of private practice, and medical examination of immigrants. On such topics the committee is free to negotiate directly with the Ministry of Health. The CCSC stands in similar relationship to the British Medical Association as does the General Medical Services Committee. It meets at BMA House and it reports to the BMA Council and Representative Body. It is also "autonomous," but its links with the BMA are strong.

Apart from differences in the statutory status and geographical breakdown of its constituent committees, the CCSC does, however, differ in one material aspect from its sister body for GPs: it does not have direct access to the Ministry on all questions of pay or of policy. The Whitley Committee for hospital staff, put into use at the beginning of the National Health Service (Chapter 9), has continued to operate; this committee rather than the CCSC discusses pay regulations with Ministry and other employer representatives. A more serious curtailment of the authority of the CCSC is the Joint Consultants Committee, established as a link between the CCSC and the Royal Colleges. The Joint Committee rather than the CCSC has become

6. "To consider and act in matters affecting those engaged in consultant and hospital practice, including matters arising under the National Health Service Acts or any Acts amending or consolidating the same and to watch the interests of all hospital medical staff in relation to those Acts." *Brit. Med. J.* Suppl. *i* (1963), 11–12.

the major spokesman for consultants and other hospital staff in consultations with the Ministry.

Thus the functions which for general practitioners are undertaken by the General Medical Services Committee are divided for hospital staffs among the Central Consultants and Specialists Committee, Medical Whitley Committee B, and the Joint Consultants Committee. The CCSC is the only one that has a direct link with the regional machinery, and perhaps for this reason it frequently acts as a trial ground for ideas. There is no formal distinction between matters discussed by one or the other committee. Generally, however, the Whitley Committee deals with pay details, the CCSC with administrative and policy problems, and the Joint Consultants Committee with questions that are important to the consultant branch as a whole.

The Joint Consultants Committee

Unlike the General Medical Services and the Central Consultants and Specialists Committees, the Joint Consultants Committee (JCC) has no link, formal or informal, with the BMA structure, and no local constituents; it is simply a joint body of CCSC and Royal College nominees. Originally the JCC consisted of eight members from the English Royal Colleges, three from the Scottish Colleges, and six from the CCSC. Representatives from the CCSC were thus outnumbered by what one consultant politician recently described as the "old established institutions . . . with comparatively small membership." [7] The JCC was not intended to cover the whole spectrum of specialist life. It included no university representatives, no representatives from specialties such as radiology that lay outside the purview of the older Colleges, and no representatives from the General Medical Council. The JCC was a compromise committee with a nice British flavor, which reflected the balance of influence in the consultant branch of the medical profession at the time. It included on the one hand senior representatives of three autocracies and, on the other, it drew from an "autonomous" committee of a democratic body (the BMA) which represented all hospital medical staff.

Over the years, complaints began to be heard from the more vociferous younger consultants in the BMA that their views were not sufficiently represented on the Joint Consultants Committee. The increase in the number of consultants after the inception of the National Health Service meant that there were more younger consultants than before; moreover, for the first time they were employed on equal terms with their seniors. In 1957, four to five of every ten consultants in the various specialties were under age 46.[8] Membership of the JCC, on the other hand, was of its very nature weighted in favor of the older age groups. Moreover, the JCC had shown itself to be a powerful negotiating as well as consultative body. It had advised consultants when to accept the terms of contracts offered under the NHS. Its influence over all fields of hospital practice was increasing, and by the 1960s it was

7. *Brit. Med. J.* Suppl. *ii* (1962), 47 (H. H. Langston).
8. Platt report, p. 12.

clearly established that the JCC was concerned with all policy questions, including the income differential between GPs and specialists.

Revised membership was approved by the JCC in 1962. The committee now consists of ten members appointed by the CCSC (an increase of four), eight members from the three English Royal Colleges and three from Scotland, two members from the British Dental Association, and an independent chairman.[9] But the committee remains oddly constituted. There are three members each from the English Royal Colleges of Physicians and Surgeons, but only two from the Royal College of Obstetricians and Gynaecologists and only one from each of the three Scottish Colleges. Proportional representation by specialty group would require one representative from the Royal College of Obstetricians to seven from the Surgeons and six from the Physicians; and in addition, one radiologist or radiotherapist and two pathologists. The JCC is a curiously instructive example of the operation of recognized interest groups. It shows in capsule form the organizational structure, though not the numerical composition, of the consultant branch of the medical profession. It suggests the battles and inheritances of the past and perhaps contains the seeds of discord for the future. For the present, increased representation of the Central Consultants and Specialists Committee on the Joint Consultants Committee has undoubtedly bound the two committees more closely together and thus lessened the likelihood for disagreement between them.

The Joint Consultants Committee is the single most influential committee of consultants in relation to the National Health Service—much more influential in terms of actual function than the Central Health Services Council or the British Medical Association. Its central position is shown in Figure 4. Through its membership the JCC has links with the whole of the committee structure surrounding ministerial decision. Formal representation extends to the Medical Whitley Council which negotiates conditions for hospital staff and to the Advisory Committee on Consultant Establishments which approves requests for new consultant and specialist posts. Members of the JCC can also be found—though not in their capacity as JCC members—on the Distinction Awards Committee and on the Central Health Services Council.

As the main channel of communication between the Ministry of Health and hospital staffs, the JCC negotiates a wide range of medical and organizational subjects. The report of the Platt Committee on medical staffing went before the JCC before any decisions were reached on principle. Recently, the Ministry has brought the following points, among others, to the committee for consultation: casualty and accident services; central sterile supply departments in hospitals; standardization of hospital medical records; the organization of X-ray departments; problems of communication among doctors, nurses, and patients; and progressive patient care. Moreover, the JCC expects to be consulted before any changes are made by the Ministry

9. *Brit. Med. J.* Suppl. *ii* (1962), 47.

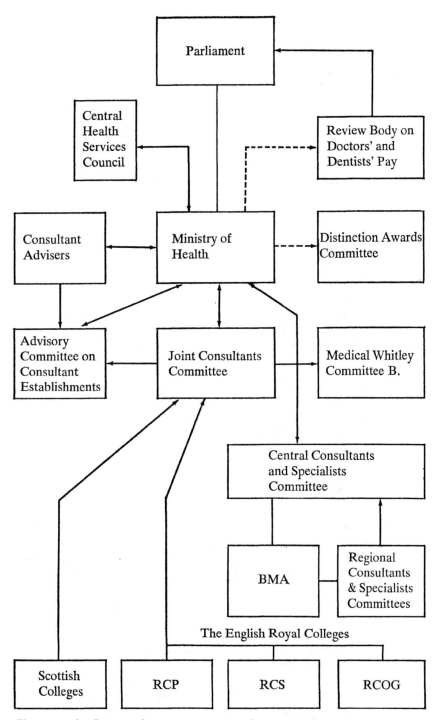

FIGURE 4. *Lines of communication between the Ministry of Health and consultants and specialists in England and Wales; Negotiating and advisory committees*

which will affect hospital medical staff, and any lapse is greeted with disfavor. This was the case with the hurried publication of the ten-year Hospital Plan in 1962:

> It has for years been understood that the Ministry will consult with the Joint Consultants Committee on any proposed changes that affect hospital medical staff before the changes are announced. It is regrettable to have to report that it has been necessary several times in recent years to remind the Ministry of this when circulars have been sent out without such prior consultation. There was no consultation with the profession before the publication of the Hospital Plans.[10]

Although it may discuss incomes, the JCC does not itself negotiate on matters of pay; it is, however, closely concerned with doctors' incomes. Two of its members sit as representatives on the profession's Joint Evidence Committee whose function it is to present the case for higher incomes to the Review Body on doctors' and dentists' pay. The JCC is also deeply concerned with the current question of a "proper differential" between generalist and specialist incomes. Collective bargaining on terms and conditions of service of hospital medical and dental staff is the function of the Medical Whitley Council's Committee B, which the establishment of the Standing Review Body on Doctors' and Dentists' Remuneration by no means made redundant. The Review Body outlines the pay structure, but the Whitley Council must fill it in and deal with a host of minor day-to-day problems arising out of the interpretation of existing terms of service. The staff side of Whitley Committee B is, however, the entire Joint Consultants Committee, with the addition of one member—the JCC's own secretary. The people are the same but the hats are different. Royal College representatives, albeit at two removes, are thus found sitting on one side of the bargaining table.

Interrelationships of the Professional Bodies

These interrelationships point up the pervasive influence of the Royal Colleges. They also indicate the close connections among the various specialist groups. The Central Consultants and Specialists Committee appoints an executive and twelve members, ten of whom sit on the Joint Consultants Committee. As members of the JCC they sit on the Whitley Committee; some also sit on the Joint Evidence Committee and the Advisory Committee on Consultant Establishments. Informally there are interrelationships with the councils of the Royal Colleges, the Ministry's consultant advisers, the formal negotiating machinery, and special advisory committees. Although the organization takes many forms, the actual people involved are few: possibly no more than fifty or sixty consultants who range over the vital areas of professional and thus administrative policy making.

The focus on the Joint Consultants Committee for hospital staff policy and the strong involvement of the Royal Colleges had an unfortunate effect

10. Ibid., p. 190.

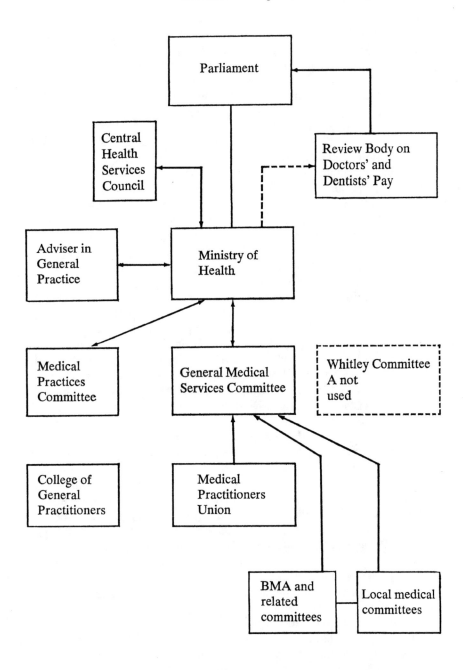

FIGURE 5. *Lines of communication between the Ministry of Health and general practitioners in England and Wales; Negotiating and advisory committees*

on the internal structure of the British Medical Association. The position of the BMA in relation to hospital and GP policy committees can be gauged by comparing Figures 4 and 5. Through the GMSC, regarded as its committee, the BMA retained a virtual monopoly of GP matters which it was not able to match for consultants and specialists. The professional bodies as they had developed under the NHS had built-in conflicts of interest. The BMA structure was particularly insecure. On the one hand there was the traditional integrated representative machinery from the local to national level; on the other there were two entirely separate structures dealing with sectional interests. The GP structure negotiated on behalf of general practitioners, the consultant structure on behalf of hospital staff.

Until the appointment of the Standing Review Body on Remuneration early in 1962, it was to the profession's advantage to develop sectional rather than integrated negotiating machinery. The GMSC on the one hand, and the CCSC and JCC on the other, developed an executive authority that was in many cases stronger than that of the combined Representative Body of the BMA or the BMA Council. BMA representatives from the Divisions were bypassed; and typically, when the Review Body requested a unified pay claim for the profession at large, this was forthcoming not from the body of the BMA but from a coalition of the major sectional protagonists. Angry letters to the *British Medical Journal* on the position of general practice in 1963–64 testified to the sudden realization among many general practitioners of their lack of knowledge of what was being done on their behalf: "At the periphery we feel naked and abandoned despite having two channels of communication." [11] Indeed, it was because there were two such channels —the Divisions and Representative Body on the one hand and the sectional machinery on the other—that there was not always clear organizational communication between the representatives and the represented.

This was not the only outcome of the separate machinery for consultants and general practitioners. Unhappily, the BMA structure for hospital staff modified the old status struggle between GPs and specialists, by bringing the potential conflict between the two branches within the BMA itself. The BMA became an uneasy triumvirate: in the center was its old established Representative Body, drawn from all spheres of medical practice, but primarily GPs; and at each side was a powerful sectional interest with direct negotiating rights with the Ministry of Health. The General Medical Services Committee had a long and successful tradition of representing GP interests. The Central Consultants and Specialists Committee was also proving its mettle, although many of the most important decisions were referred outside the BMA structure to the Joint Consultants Committee.

The two major disadvantages of the existing system are complexity and lack of a clear channel of responsibility. The complexity needs no explanation. The same topics are discussed by the local medical committees at their conference and by the GMSC, by the BMA Divisions and by their repre-

11. *ii* (1963), 1197 (E. Anthony).

sentatives at meetings of the Representative Body, by the BMA Council, and by the regional and national specialist committees. For most questions this plethora of committees is immaterial, but major difficulties arise where consultants and GPs hold divergent views. This potential was generated not only by the existence of the National Health Service but also by the much older question of the relationship between the Royal Colleges and the BMA and of consultants and general practice.

The Royal Colleges, as elites, have been able to dictate to the profession as experts in certain fields of medical policy, particularly in the field of education and training. By being examining bodies the Colleges have exercised direct and indirect control over professional standards. They also developed their own canons of behavior. Their function is largely to advance the profession's prestige; even the desire to increase the educational potential of the profession is motivated by the general social and economic advancement of all its members. Thus from its role as an educational institution, the professional association easily moves into the areas of professional behavior and professional status.

Traditionally, the Royal Colleges did not concern themselves with the incomes of their members, although there was nothing to prevent them from doing so. Other professions did not so limit themselves; the Law Society, which is also a professional examining and regulating body, recommends fees for standard procedures undertaken by solicitors, and the Royal Institute of British Architects issue a scale of fees for architects. But the Royal Medical Colleges were able to remain aloof from questions of payment, since by raising the status of one section of the profession, and by keeping this section relatively small, the Colleges automatically affected the professional incomes of their members. Fellows of the Colleges have always earned more than the average members of the medical profession, first because their patients came from the richest strata of society, and later because of their professional—particularly specialized—competence.

The existence of a National Health Service raised the problem of income determination as well as the possibility of exerting influence in the field of general administrative policy. The interests of the Colleges and the British Medical Association inevitably overlapped. Both felt they had a mandate to speak for the consultant branch of the profession: the Colleges as its leaders, the BMA as its representative. A number of questions inevitably arose, crystallized in the various pay disputes between the government and the medical profession, when effective representation was of primary importance. If the GMSC represented general practitioners and the JCC hospital doctors, did the Representative Body of the BMA still have a valid claim to represent the *profession?* The degree of autonomy of the General Medical Service Committee and the Central Consultants and Specialists Committee also needed clarification. Which line, for example, ought the GMSC to follow, if the local medical committees and BMA representatives recommended different courses of action?

There was always the possibility that the relationship between the BMA and its "autonomous" bodies—the GMSC and CCSC—might be formalized by changing the BMA structure. But there were dangers as well as benefits in such a move, because of the peculiar position of the Joint Consultants Committee. Thus the GMSC and CCSC might be reconstituted formally as subcommittees of the BMA Council, but this might have the concomitant disadvantage of reducing the stature of the General Medical Services Committee in relation to the Joint Consultants Committee. The latter, being genuinely autonomous, would remain outside the BMA. This move might only emphasize more strongly the BMA's failure to bring consultants within its monopoly, and penalize GP negotiation in relation to that of consultants. The BMA might be strengthened if the Joint Consultants Committee excluded all matters concerning pay and conditions of service, leaving such trade union functions to BMA machinery. In essence, therefore, the structural problems surrounding the BMA hinge on the role and function of the JCC; and this in turn relies in large part on the expectations of the Royal Colleges. So far the respective positions of the democratic inclusive organization and the exclusive elite have not been openly discussed by the professional bodies themselves.

Taken together, the impact of the professional bodies on the National Health Service has been profound. Doctors have established an independent pay review system and representation on all central administrative bodies, including those that decide geographical distribution of doctors, and the profession expects that no major decision will be taken by the government without adequate consultation. If there is a general lesson in this history, it is that it is wise for the professional association whose members come under public control to accept a greater public responsibility. Its overall influence may otherwise be diminished, and professional advice may be sought by the government from bodies set up by the government, such as the Central Health Services Council, created by Act of Parliament to advise the Ministry of Health. The GMSC and Joint Consultants Committee, set up by the profession, are much more powerful advisory bodies since each has the direct support of the profession. A government may override a weak, disoriented profession. It will have difficulties when faced by a compact, united group with practical organizational policies of its own. Indeed, when the aims of government and profession are made to coincide, the influence of the profession may be considerably strengthened. The Royal Colleges provide a specific illustration. By accepting involvement, they have increased their sphere of influence in shaping public policy. As a result, the Colleges have expanded their role from that of educational and ethical bodies to one which extends over social as well as strictly professional issues. Many of the problems besetting the English professional associations of medicine have been not of authority in relation to the government but of their own interrelationships.

Tension between the government and the profession has centered on doctors' incomes and on matters in which the profession itself has no effective policy to suggest. On most other questions there appears to have been a reasonable equanimity between government and profession. Indeed, it is arguable that the pendulum has swung too far in the direction of professional influence. In contrast, the consumer's voice has been seldom heard, and the question remains of what should be the proper balance between professional influence and public responsibility in a publicly supported service. Reliance on the traditional structures of the profession has also affected health service development; the dichotomy of the medical profession, reflected in the dichotomy of Ministry of Health and other official bodies, has obscured consideration of the total sum of health and welfare services by both the profession and the government.

20

Professional Differences and Financial Differentials 1962–1964

The dispute within the medical profession over the appropriate income ratio between consultants and general practitioners in the early 1960s provided a focus for a number of the major problems besetting medical practice. The first was the structure of the British Medical Association and its related bodies, subjected to the stress of having to issue a statement on medical incomes. The old status differences between general practitioners and consultants were resurrected, and the potential for conflict in the professional structure was realized. A second primary cause for concern to general practitioners was the future of the capitation system and the need to unravel the increased complexities of payment from the "central pool." Third, and closely interwoven with discontent over the capitation system, was the demand of GPs for a positive commitment as to their future role in a specialized medical system. Finally, there was the fundamental question of the appropriate balance of manpower between consultant and general practice in the National Health Service of the future.

The search for an acceptable solution to determining medical incomes under the National Health Service had ended in the establishment of a Standing Review Body, independent of the Ministry of Health and of the professional groups.[1] The Review Body was appointed by and was responsible to the Prime Minister, and it was intended that it should make recommendations on income levels every three years. As the period covered by the Royal Commission's income proposals (1960–63) progressed, the potential of an independent pay review system began to be appreciated. At its annual representative meeting in 1961, the BMA expressed "grave disquiet" at the government's delay in setting up the new group, and it was not until the first quarter of 1962 that the Standing Review Body was actually appointed.

Lord Kindersley, a City financier, and an Honorary Fellow of the Royal College of Surgeons for his interest in that body, was announced as the Review Body's chairman. His task was "To advise the Prime Minister on the remuneration of doctors and dentists taking any part in the National

1. See Chap. 9.

Health Service." Why the Body should be made responsible to the Prime Minister and not to the Minister of Health was not entirely clear. Lord Moran had suggested this as a parallel to the Civil Service procedure, but it was without parallel in the history of salary negotiations of a particular profession. As expected by the profession, none of the seven committee members was medically qualified.[2] But the membership was sufficiently elevated to fulfill the terms of the Pilkington Commission's resolution that its recommendation be of such weight and authority that "the Government will be able, and indeed feel bound, to accept them." [3]

The Review Body signified its wish for a single document or claim on behalf of the whole profession, rather than separate cases for GPs and consultants. The BMA accepted this advice; its Council declared in April 1962 that "it considers it vitally important that the profession shall speak with one voice." [4] This was not an easy task in view of the profession's separate representative and negotiating machinery. Almost inevitably in these circumstances, the approach to the Review Body was to be invested with the deeper problems of the professional rift: the need, because of increased specialization, to restate and perhaps reorganize the relative functions of the two branches of practice; the need, too, to set a value on the functions of each branch. By demanding a combined approach, the Review Body forced the profession itself to set monetary values on each branch in terms of the other. The question of the appropriate differential between consultant and GP incomes was to be raised with increasing bitterness through the unwieldy structures of the profession from 1962 on. It became clear that this was not a subject the medical profession alone could solve; and the first institution to suffer was the BMA.

The initial moves of the profession in relation to the Review Body were harmonious. A small committee was set up, which included representatives of each major interest group: the chairman of BMA Council, the chairman of the General Medical Services Committee, the chairman and one other member of the Joint Consultants Committee. It happened that only one of these representatives was a general practitioner (the GMSC chairman). Another GP, the chairman of the Conference of Local Medical Committees, was added to strike a better balance, but consultants still outnumbered GPs on the committee by three to two, a source of concern to GPs in the coming debates, since this committee was to be the only direct professional link with the Standing Review Body.

At the Annual Representative Meeting of the BMA in Belfast in 1962 the question of the proper "differential" between consultant and GP pay

2. See *Brit. Med. J.* Suppl. *i* (1962), 151. The names of the six other members of the seven-man Review Body were announced in March 1962. They included an eminent lawyer, an actuary, two university professors, a banker, and the chairman of an investment corporation.

3. *Royal Commission on Doctors' and Dentists' Remuneration; Report,* p. 147.

4. *Brit. Med. J.* Suppl. *i* (1962), 151.

was publicly raised for the first time as the focus of GPs' resentment of their inferior status. The resolution (from the Sunderland Division), incorporated into the meeting's agenda, was somewhat embarrassing to BMA leadership. The Joint Evidence Committee was naturally anxious to preserve professional unity, for only with a unified profession could the joint memorandum be prepared. Attempts to placate GPs would risk antagonizing hospital staffs, and the BMA was not prepared to champion the GP against the rest of the profession at a time when an apparently favorable income machinery had finally been set in motion. The chairman of the BMA Council reminded the representatives that the Review Body "if treated properly" would be of great benefit to the profession. The inference was not that it would be uninterested in the differential question; indeed, in a letter to the profession it had specifically left open future discussions of remuneration generally, of particular aspects of remuneration, and of "the structure of the system." [5] Any immediate discussion within the profession on income relativities might, however, hold up the general increases in pay then being discussed.

The Representative Body agreed, on Chairman of Council's suggestion, that two memoranda be prepared. The first would make out a claim for general increases which could go forward without delay. The second—which would also have to be agreed on by the whole profession—would deal with differentials and with the pay structure of general practice. The wisdom of this decision was immediately apparent. The Joint Evidence Committee completed the first memorandum by August 1962—well before the end of the proposed pay review period. Its contents were secret, but it was generally known to contain no reference to differential incomes. The second memorandum was, however, to raise long and serious questions, not only of the status differential but of the method of payment of general practitioners.

The professional body responsible for making primary suggestions on the GP pay structure was the "autonomous" General Medical Services Committee. In February 1963 the GMSC spent a day discussing the pay structure in general practice, thus producing, its chairman remarked, one of the best debates he had ever heard in that committee.[6] Unfortunately, however, the debate produced no clear-cut policy. One problem was that it was not certain how far the growing discontent in general practice was related to money and how far to other factors. "We know that the feeling throughout the country is that something is wrong," said one member. "No one can pinpoint it, and I believe it is because our present system does not remunerate general practitioners for the work that is done." Others were not so sure; but none had a generally acceptable alternative.

The pool system of payment had been complicated by the proposals of the Royal Commission on Doctors' and Dentists' Remuneration. It was further threatened by a recommendation by the Platt Committee on hospital staffing that there should be increased GP participation in hospital work.

5. *Brit. Med. J.* Suppl. *ii* (1962), 22–23.
6. *Brit. Med. J.* Suppl. *i* (1963), 62.

The size of the global pool was determined according to the income thought desirable for the average GP. If a greater proportion of the pool were devoted to hospital work, the amount available for capitation fees would be correspondingly less; there might eventually be a substantial built-in bias against those GPs who concentrated all their energies on their general practice.

If the pool system could be related solely to capitation payments, the GP would lose the safeguard of having a guaranteed national average income to cover all official sources; and this he had come to see as a positive rather than a negative force. The capitation system had become a form of salaried service in a different guise, and the GMSC had become accustomed to negotiating for an average annual income rather than an average fee scale. The GMSC was not at this stage prepared either to reorganize the existing system as a form of salary or to recommend a completely new start: these possibilities were to come much later, after the committee had suffered the tribulations which followed this lack of decision. It expressed its disapproval but it made no changes. A golden opportunity for leadership was thereby lost.

Fourteen Per Cent

The Standing Review Body made its first report in March 1963 and, as expected, it did not take pay differential questions into account. The incomes of GPs, hospital doctors and medical administrators should, it was recommended, receive an across-the-board increase of 14 per cent effective from April 1963, with the understanding that there be no further increase for three years.[7] These recommendations were received with equanimity by the medical profession. The chairman of the BMA Council thought that the profession "had received no more than justice," [8] and the Ministry of Health quickly accepted the recommendation in principle. As *The Economist* pointed out at the time, it was a "pleasant novelty that both Government and profession have this week accepted the review body's recommendations without argument".[9]

But the contentment that greeted the 14 per cent announcement was short-lived. All over the country, GPs worked out their 14 per cent increase in terms of their previous year's income, oblivious of the intricacies of the central pool system which the GMSC had just voted on their behalf to retain. Consultants would receive the full 14 per cent increase on all their NHS income, including distinction awards. This was merely a question of calculating new salary and related rates. General practitioners had to await the results of long calculations of the pool's finances made by a joint working party of the GMSC and the Ministry of Health. As the weeks went by they became progressively more uneasy, as many for the first time began to

7. The Review Body's recommendations were contained in a letter addressed to the Prime Minister. See *Brit. Med. J.* Suppl. *i* (1963), 131–33.

8. Ibid., p. 101.

9. March 30, 1963, p. 1227. And see Rosemary Stevens, *New Society 37* (1963), 15.

comprehend the ramifications of the global pool. There were two important factors. First, although the agreed net income of the average GP was to be increased by 14 per cent (from £2,425 to £2,765), his gross income would not increase by this amount. At least one third of the ordinary GP's total income went on expenses, which were not to receive the same boost. Thus the 14 per cent applied only to part of his income. The sum involved was not large, but the principle assumed enormous importance in the eyes of individuals. Second, and of greater importance, it was found that increased fee scales had already overdrawn the pool. GPs had been receiving overall a greater amount than that allowed for their average income. Thus a proportion of the 14 per cent increase (£2.7 million out of a total of £7.6 million) had already been paid out. Another £0.8 million had to be left in the global pool in respect of increased earnings from other sources (e.g. hospital work). This left only £4.1 million to be distributed through raised capitation and other general medical fees: the individual GP would receive no more than a 7 or 8 per cent increase in his net pay, and only 5 or 6 per cent increase in relation to his gross income, including expenses.[10] To the average GP it seemed that the consultant had received more from the Review Body than he had. General practitioners were already sensitive about their relative status, and the results of the award seemed a further blow. What made it worse that this was not the fault of the Review Body or of the government, but of the pool system—and the calculations, being logical in terms of the system, had been agreed to by the GPs' own nominees on the joint working party. Thus the growing resentment of GPs was frustrated by the lack of any villain but their own leaders.

The annual meeting of BMA representatives in July 1963 provided the occasion for a clash between two views that had been apparent in embryonic form the year before: the need to maintain organizational unity in the approach to the Review Body, and the feeling among the GPs that their incomes should be raised in relation to consultant incomes. Pressure to increase GP incomes had intensified in the interim. Moreover, although it was assumed that a second memorandum would be submitted to the Review Body on the differential question, there was some difference of opinion as to what the Review Body was prepared to do about the differential in the period 1963–66. This period was covered by the 14 per cent increase the Review Body had just made. A second pay raise for GPs within the three-year period might set a dangerous precedent for future breaking of long-term agreements and endanger this method of income decision.

The representatives from the BMA branches and divisions, the majority of whom were general practitioners, gathered in Oxford for their parliamen-

10. The gross annual pay of the average GP in 1960–61 (the latest data available at that time) was given as £3,750. The average increase under the Review Body was approximately £180. See *Brit. Med. J.* Suppl. *i* (1963) 266–69, and *The Guardian*, July 2, 1963, "Family Doctors Up in Arms."

tary meeting, filled with a spirit of righteous but baffled indignation. Already there was talk of independent action. The Chairman of Council, a consultant, warned representatives that sectional interests would not do better by themselves. The BMA must speak with one voice, not two or three "or even a multiplicity of voices and in discordant tones"; and he urged the Representative Body not to throw away "in a moment of exasperation" all the advantages which had been built up by the BMA over many years. This theme was continued by the chairman of the Central Consultants and Specialists Committee. He told the BMA representatives that the Joint Consultants Committee (to which he and the majority of CCSC members belonged) was quite prepared to examine the differential question once they were given a statement of the GPs' case. He too urged the importance of maintaining the unity of the profession, and he ended on a note of warning that emphasized the formal autonomy of the consultant committees. "We, the consultants, are in your hands. . . . After all, we have negotiated on matters of salary through the Joint Consultants Committee, and you can drive us to the stage where we can go away from this body." This threat was real; the complete independence of the Joint Consultants Committee from the BMA was to be one of the stumbling blocks in internal BMA agreement and in rising GP hostility.

The talk of unity appeared to be successful. The chairman of the BMA Council moved that the Representative Body should instruct Council to ensure that discussions on the differential (and this very word was used) between the GP and the consultant committees should proceed "with the greatest possible speed" so that a suitable case could be presented to the Review Body.[11] The motion was carried; it thus automatically became BMA policy.

The all-inclusive agenda system of a representative meeting meant, however, that this motion was not the only one relevant to the differential incomes on which representatives had to vote. Dr. Ivor Jones, a prominent GP leader in the differential debates, voicing a motion from Sunderland, asked the representatives to take a stronger line to reaffirm "the urgent need to upgrade the financial status of family doctors," by requesting the BMA Council to place the matter before the Review Body "at an early date." This motion brought the differential question into the open; for so far, although consultants had expressed a willingness to discuss the GPs' case, they had not committed themselves to supporting higher GP incomes. The CCSC chairman thus objected to the motion. The debate was heated and confused and there were occasional references to historical themes. One consultant was reported in the national (but not in the medical) press as supporting a higher income for consultants "because of the difference in the manner of living."[12] The chairman of the BMA Council endeavored to lessen the effect of the differential motion by asking the meeting to refer it to

11. *Brit. Med. J.* Suppl. *ii* (1963), 30–35.
12. *Guardian*, July 11, 1963, "Need to Upgrade the 'Finance Status' of GPs."

the Council instead of passing it as BMA policy. But the representatives were not to be stilled. Dr. Jones' motion was carried by an overwhelming majority.

Thus the representatives passed two potentially conflicting motions—one affirming the continuance of joint discussions and a joint approach to the Review Body on the differential question (sponsored by the Chairman of Council) and one on presenting the GPs' case to the Review Body (sponsored by Dr. Jones). The latter could be interpreted as an instruction to prepare an independent case for GPs which would not have to be approved by the consultant branch. The BMA Council, in a special statement issued at the end of the meeting, interpreted the two resolutions together: namely as an instruction to prepare a case on behalf of GPs as part of the evidence to be presented to the Review Body by the whole profession—after adequate consultation with all interests involved.[13] Professional unity was to come before sectional interest.

But this interpretation, however fair, unleashed a flood of protest from general practitioners, which found expression in vehement letters to the medical press. To some it seemed that the BMA, traditionally considered the bulwark of general practice, had lost interest in the problems of the average practitioner. Two rural GPs from Huntingdon cried:

> We write to you in despair. Can we believe that the BMA is really interested in our welfare? Can we believe that the BMA really means us to improve our standard of practice? Can we believe that the BMA really has our interests at heart when it negotiates within the Ministry? [14]

Unhappily the Annual Representative Meeting fanned a flame of discord that was already there. As one writer complained, legitimate criticism of the Review Body had become "misdirected into argument between the spokesmen of one section of the profession and another." [15]

The clumsiness of the BMA structure was now apparent. Consultants could, if they wished, remain aloof in the Joint Consultants Committee. The meaning of motions passed by the Representative Body was subject to doubt. The *British Medical Journal* commented:

> During the passing years there has grown up a feeling that so far as GP matters are concerned the GMSC is more powerful than the Council of the BMA and the Annual Conference of Representatives of Local Medical Committees—the old panel conference—more powerful than the Representative Body. The BMA's own central Council and Annual Representative Meeting have from time to time, rightly or wrongly, felt as if they were rubber-stamping mechanisms for these powerful and independent general-practitioner bodies.[16]

13. *Brit. Med. J.* Suppl. *ii* (1963), 62.
14. Ibid. (P. M. Morris, J. K. Paterson).
15. Ibid., p. 101 (R. L. Luffingham).
16. *Brit. Med. J. ii* (1963), 453–56.

Similarly, the consultants were determined not to let their destinies be settled or diverted by a majority vote of the BMA's Representative Body. The ordinary BMA representative, whether GP or consultant, was thus becoming less powerful. The BMA was moving from a democratic body governed by a parliament of members elected from constituencies to an organization dominated from the top by two autocratic interest groups which were not formally part of the BMA structure. Each of these factors contributed to the frustrations of the representative meeting in July 1963. The GMSC was not providing the vigorous militancy that many GPs, awaking from fifteen years of political torpor, now demanded. The GP was in an odd kind of limbo, and his reaction was to attack the BMA.

Confusion in General Practice

On the Review Body's award of 1963 was hung the discontent of general practice. There was no clear plan of action that might remove this discontent. The BMA was committed to the capitation system of payment, but it was this system that had given general practitioners less than they considered their due—particularly in relation to consultant incomes. On the more important long-term future for general practice the BMA was silent. It had no forward planning team, and still relied on policy being generated from the increasingly confused representative meetings. The College of General Practitioners appeared reluctant to formulate a planning blueprint and even more reluctant to become involved in a dispute over pay. The Medical Practitioners' Union (MPU) was the most important of the other professional associations and was actively interested in pay. After the 14 per cent award, the MPU instituted protest meetings throughout the country, thereby achieving, according to its secretary, a "measure of prestige and influence which it had not known before." [17] But the MPU, with under five thousand members, was relatively small. It had scarcely grown in size since the 1930s, and it was criticized by many doctors for its "left-wing" tendencies.[18] There was thus no constructive channel into which GPs' burgeoning political energies could be diverted. Instead of leadership from the center, there was increasing pressure from the periphery.

In August 1963, the weekly newssheet *Pulse* [19] made specific references to the Oxford meeting and to the BMA and asked GPs whether they would like to form an independent association. It ran articles, sponsored a questionnaire, and elicited considerable support for such a move. In October 1963 the General Practitioners' Association (GPA) was formed through this

17. *Economist,* Jan. 30, 1965, p. 401 (P. Sidney Greaves).
18. *Guardian,* Sept. 28, 1963.
19. *Pulse* was founded by a drug firm, Bayer Products. It became officially independent in November 1961, but Bayer continued to use it liberally for advertising its products, thus supporting its operation. The newssheet is still largely an advertising vehicle, sent free each week to every GP in the country. This commercial association led to some criticism by the MPU and others when *Pulse* began to champion the GP's cause. See *Pulse,* Sept. 14, 1963, p. 1.

source to provide the leadership the BMA was alleged to have lost. The GPA proposed to appoint a professional negotiator on a "top salary" and to call in management consultants to work out a system of remuneration in general practice. Not surprisingly, the new association was opposed by the BMA, whose strength chiefly depended on GP support. The *British Medical Journal* pointed out that the BMA was an "easy target for the discontented" and warned that there was more at stake than pay alone.[20] But the more militant attitude of the GPA appealed to those who felt that neither the BMA nor other representative bodies had satisfactorily provided leadership. In essence therefore the foundation of the GPA was a reflection of inadequacy. The BMA had, in the words of its own organ the *British Medical Journal,* "lost the initiative in strategy."[21]

While the new association was being discussed, the official Gillie report on the future of general practice—the fruit of two years' deliberation—appeared, in October 1963. As a publication of the Central Health Services Council, it represented the best professional advice available to the Minister of Health; but it was a planning disappointment. It contained few details of staffing and none of buildings or of future needs in general practice, and it laid down principles that were so general that they merely reflected a current opinion that would have held good any time in the previous twenty years. Nor did it discuss the relativities of general and specialist practice that were at the root of the differential dispute.

In the absence of other solutions, the onus for action rested on the Ministry of Health. But the Ministry was little better prepared than the professional bodies. It had announced in August an increase in group practice loans;[22] but on long-term issues the Ministry was silent. It was evident that in this, as in other fields, the Ministry would be forced to take a stronger planning initiative, both to safeguard general practice and to reinforce the professional associations whose strength was essential to running the health service.

Meanwhile, the General Medical Services Committee was fully employed in composing a single memorandum on pay structure, agreeable to the whole medical profession, which could be presented to the Review Body on Doctors' and Dentists' Remuneration. This memorandum had to pass both the General Medical Services Committee and the Joint Consultants Committee, and also be approved by another meeting of BMA representatives. With tempers as they were, its chances of success were small. One informal meeting was held between the GMSC and the JCC in the summer of 1963, the object being "to try to avoid dissension and to get a preliminary understand-

20. *ii* (1963), 945–46.
21. *i* (1964), 852.
22. Group practice loans were increased by £500 to £2,500 per doctor, or £3,000 in areas of exceptionally high costs. In addition the number of loans approved was increased from 59 in 1962 to 95 in 1963. Ministry of Health, *Annual Report for 1963,* pp. 8, 71.

ing of points of view," [23] and in September the GMSC formally decided that a case should be made for increased GP remuneration.

But the GMSC had as yet no strategy, nor was it assured of consultant cooperation. Its BMA counterpart, the Central Consultants and Specialists Committee, quickly announced that it would not deter GPs from presenting an independent case to the Review Body, but at the same time it would feel free to ask the Joint Consultants Committee to approach the Review Body for similar concessions on behalf of hospital staff.[24] The potential rifts in professional organizations were being realized. Although there were indications that consultants wished to discontinue discussing income relativity, GMSC members resolved to continue: "We want the differential improved whether consultants agree or not." [25]

Both sides possibly realized the destructive qualities in such arguments, for this dispute was evidently resolved behind the scenes. The General Medical Services Committee decided to widen its scope of inquiry to the broader problems of general practice, and to prepare a draft report on remuneration. The CCSC stressed that consultants did not wish to be obstructive or to employ delaying tactics, and BMA Council agreed in a statement in November 1963 to reassure GPs that everything possible was being done on their behalf.[26] The GMSC had interpreted its position as a policy maker rather than an income bargainer, and as part of the total BMA complex than as executive of the increasingly militant local medical committees.

By the end of November 1963 the General Medical Services Committee had prepared a draft of the second memorandum to be presented to the Review Body (the first having elicited the 14 per cent rise). The memorandum consisted of two main themes: the case for upgrading general practice on its own merits, and the differential between consultant and GP incomes. After long debate, the GMSC had decided to delete much of the material in the document referring specifically to the differential and to consultant earnings. The success of this decision was apparent when the revised document was shown to the CCSC executive a few days later. The atmosphere of this meeting was reportedly "warmer and more friendly than the series of meeting we had in the last session." Some conciliatory changes were suggested and carried out, and in December the CCSC resolved unanimously to give its "strongest support" to the GPs' case: this was endorsed by the planning committee of the Joint Consultants Committee.[27] Unity was thus achieved among the national committees; but the memorandum had yet to pass the critical scrutiny of a special conference of local medical committees (the GMSC's constituents) and a BMA representative meeting. These represented the new militancy of the ordinary GP, from whose ranks the

23. *Brit. Med. J.* Suppl. *ii* (1963), 163 (H. Langston).
24. Ibid., pp. 129, 133–34.
25. Ibid., pp. 151–52.
26. Ibid., pp. 161–63.
27. Ibid., pp. 196, 199.

General Practitioners' Association was recruiting its members. As the GMSC stressed in its memorandum, "Those who have had long experience of representing the interests of general practitioners cannot remember a time when dissatisfaction was so widespread, vehement or vociferous." [28]

The memorandum produced by the General Medical Services Committee called for changes that would result in an increased National Health Service budget of £18 million a year. Two measures were proposed. First, it was suggested that all items except payment for general medical (GP) services should be excluded from the pool calculations. Thus the average net income decided nationally would relate only to the individual's work as a GP; it would no longer include hospital and other work. This meant that the individual doctor with an average list would be assured of the average agreed net income, plus any extra work he might wish to do. Second, it was proposed that extra payments be made to GPs for seniority and experience, to combat a falling income concomitant with increasing age and decreasing work. These proposals would bring the pool system into line with other forms of salaried service.

At the beginning of January 1964 the Review Body met the profession's representatives, once more united, and the Review Body agreed to consider the case for an increase in GPs' pay.[29] A notable milestone had been reached, for the differential was to be subjected to independent scrutiny. A new era for general practice might result. Moreover, the unwieldy machinery of the BMA and the Joint Consultants Committee by sheer determination had been made to work.

The herculean effort involved might have won the GMSC the united support of the whole profession. But the GP discontent was due not only to income; GPs were involved in a kind of chain-reaction criticism of their professional leadership, which was continually growing in volume and vituperation. One correspondent, commenting on the personal message the Chairman of Council of the BMA had sent to each GP at the end of December, begging for his support, said one of his colleagues "laughed cynically and the other remarked that it might have been signed 'Rip Van Winkle' "; both, he noted, were BMA members of long standing.[30] The same viewpoint was echoed again and again in the journals: "The ordinary rank and file GP tends to feel that his views are not represented centrally." [31] Of much greater glamor was a petition to Parliament organized by the General Practitioners' Association on behalf of more than 6,000 GPs, of the total of about 22,000.[32] The Humble Petition, couched in Parliamentary gothic, ("Sheweth that their present terms of service in general are of an inequitable and oppressive nature . . .") was an effective public relations

28. *Brit. Med. J.* Suppl. *i* (1964), 17.
29. *The Times*, Jan. 3, 1964.
30. *Brit. Med. J.* Suppl. *i* (1964), 6 (R. C. McLaren).
31. *Brit. Med. J.* Suppl. *ii* (1963), 1123 (Bruce Cardew).
32. *Brit. Med. J. i* (1964), 250.

device and a sign that the GPA was fulfilling its promise of immediate action. The BMA had moved too late and its image was blemished.

It was not at all clear what the average general practitioner would put in place of the memorandum, although gratuitous advice on all major issues flowed freely into the medical journals. One issue of the *British Medical Journal* elicited 30,000 words in correspondence—enough, commented the editors, to make a small paperbacked book:

> Hardly one of the writers had a good word to say about existing terms and conditions of service, about the NHS, about consultants, about the committee (the GMSC) which represents the GPs in the NHS, or about the BMA and its officers.[33]

Despite these outpourings, GPs continued to work as usual. Many may have given the pay question little thought; and many, if not most, were content with their work and considered it a rewarding occupation. Many of those who wrote to the journals did so with practical suggestions; and those who wrote with adverse criticism probably formed a biased sample. Officials of the General Practitioners' Association, who had called in a firm of business consultants, later said they had been "stimulated and heartened at all times by an 'esprit de corps'—the common bond of facing the same problems together and of sharing an honest desire to try to build a solid foundation for the future of general practice as we see it." [34] At the same time, GPs were showing their enthusiasm for better postgraduate facilities and hospital connections in many parts of the country by joining with local consultants to build combined clubs or centers. The hurricane center of this part of the dispute was the BMA.

Despite its memorandum, the BMA—or rather the General Medical Service Committee, treated as a BMA committee—had not provided dynamic leadership on any of the underlying issues involved. It had not faced the real question of status relativities between general and specialist practice; indeed it had deliberately avoided raising them. It had not developed a practical master plan for the future development of the two branches of practice. It had not come to terms with the capitation system, merely suggesting some further modifications. The dispute had revealed the unsatisfactory organization of the profession. Finally, the BMA had committed, in the eyes of its members, the worst crime of all: it had lost their confidence. The special meetings of local medical committees and BMA representatives scheduled for March 1964 promised to be stormy.

The Ministry Intervenes

During these debates on the differential within the profession, the Ministry of Health had been discussing a number of pressing organizational

---

33. Ibid., p. 447.
34. General Practitioners' Association, *The GPA Report*, Part 1, p. vii.

problems, including new ways of paying GP expenses, with the profession's representatives. The time had come for more direct Ministry intervention. In February 1964 the Minister of Health (Anthony Barber) invited the chairmen of the BMA Council and the GMSC to a top-level meeting which was attended by senior medical and administrative officials from the Ministry. A "full and frank discussion" ensued, the details of which are unavailable, but the results of which were immediate. The Minister, in an open letter to the BMA published the same week, voiced his concern about the discontent of general practitioners and invited the profession to form a new working party to deal with problems of general practice.[35] It was announced that the Ministry's Permanent Secretary (chief administrator) Sir Bruce Fraser, would be the chairman of this body, which would thus (since he would hardly agree to recommendations that could not be fulfilled) carry considerable practical weight. This statement illustrated the acceptance by the Ministry of a tighter and more positive planning authority for general practice, as it had already accepted a more dynamic attitude toward national hospital planning.

The Fraser working party was not to be concerned with remuneration, but a second and almost simultaneous official announcement broached this problem. The Standing Review Body told the profession that it had asked the Ministry of Health, from which it is technically independent, for statistics on the career earnings of general practitioners and hospital doctors. This was prima facie evidence of a desire to compare the two sets of data in preparation for consideration of the differential claim. Both these moves were warmly welcomed by the BMA Council, although the GMSC was less sanguine.[36]

The effects of these two announcements had made little impact by the time of the Conference of Local Medical Committees, which was attended by some three hundred GPs from all over the country, to consider the GP pay memorandum drawn up by the General Medical Services Committee. Local medical committees wanted a stronger case made out for GPs, and more vehement representatives. Only fifteen groups, mainly from the south and west of Britain, were reportedly willing to express unqualified approval and support of the memorandum.[37] The conference was dominated from the floor—participants were at times loudly critical of what the GMSC has done on their behalf. The precipitating resolution demanded the inclusion in the Joint Evidence Committee of a doctor other than those selected by the General Medical Services Committee and BMA Council, namely Dr. Ivor Jones, whom a growing number of GPs had marked as the leader of their cause for greater recognition. After the meeting, the chairman of the GMSC (Dr. A. B. Davies) resigned from his position.

This resignation came at the peak of the dispute. The special meeting of

35. *Brit. Med. J.* Suppl. *i* (1964), 55; *The Times,* Feb. 21, 1964.
36. See *Brit. Med. J.* Suppl. *i* (1964), 55–58, 63–64.
37. *The Times,* March 13, 1964.

BMA representatives held later the same month was more reasonable in tone. The new GMSC chairman (Dr. J. C. Cameron) faced the issues squarely: deep discontent with the terms of service in the National Health Service, a loss of confidence in BMA leadership, and dissatisfaction with the structure of the pool system. He welcomed the Fraser Committee as one of the greatest opportunities since 1948 to answer the first difficulty, accepted the fact that there had been a loss of confidence in the BMA and pledged better communication, and spoke of the pay differential dispute as a historical factor, now that the Review Body had asked for figures of comparable earnings.[38] The BMA representatives voted for much the same amendments in the memorandum that the local medical committees had, thus restoring references to the differential; and they voted for Dr. Jones as an extra member of the Joint Evidence Committee.

The changes made in the GP pay memorandum during the two March meetings meant that the memorandum had to be sent back to the sectional committees for their approval. This time the progress was relatively smooth. Instead of insisting that the offending paragraphs supporting a reduced differential between GP and consultant incomes (originally in the memorandum, taken out by the GMSC to mollify consultants, but restored by the representatives), the consultant bodies ingeniously resolved to add a statement of their own, which might offset them. Reading this, the usually staid *Times* acidly remarked:

> It needs no prophet to foretell that when GPs in the country read the consultants' addendum, which lays emphasis on the special discipline and vocational drive of potential consultants, the reaction will be sharp. . . . This wrangling over wording continues to be of obsessive interest to the activists in the profession as a means of safeguarding the status of individual branches of medicine.[39]

But the statement was accepted by the GMSC and the BMA Council; the memorandum was finally complete. At the beginning of May 1964, for a second time but at considerable emotional cost, unity was achieved. There was one revised memorandum, agreed to by all, which could be offered to the Review Body on Doctors' and Dentists' Remuneration.

The wider problems remained. The organizational structure of the profession was still divisive; the pool and capitation system had to be reappraised; the *real* questions of relativities had to be tackled, so that the reasons for relatively higher and lower incomes would be clearly understood by all; and this implied a clear and detailed statement on the future of general practice. Two major events had emerged from the almost two-year dispute over the GP differential. One was the loss of leadership by the BMA and its related committees—disturbing because there was no body of similar status

---

38. *Brit. Med. J. i* (1964), 851–52 and Suppl. *i* (1964), 115–28.
39. May 22, 1964, "Behind the Unity."

to step into its place. The second event was the appearance on the scene of the Ministry of Health. It was becoming clear that if the profession could not solve its own difficulties the Ministry of Health would have to help. This would mean a much stronger Ministry line on GP policy than it had been accustomed to take in the past. It was in the interest of the profession as well as of the general public that one body or the other should develop positive planning norms. So far such norms had been sadly lacking.

Meanwhile the Review Body on Doctors' and Dentists' Remuneration had to consider whether general practitioners were worth an extra £18 million in terms of the arguments used by the profession.

2 I

Arbitration of Incomes: Substitute for Planning?

In presenting a memorandum concerned solely with general practitioner pay, the medical profession asked the Standing Review Body on Doctors' and Dentists' Remuneration to adjudicate on the relative values of general and specialist practice, a question which the Royal Commission had carefully avoided, and on which the profession had been unable to agree. It was doubtful whether this small group would be able to make a satisfactory judgment when neither the profession nor the Ministry had a clear-cut plan for the future development of general practice in relation to the other specialties. It is not known what took place behind the closed doors of the conferences in the nine months before the Review Body reported on GP incomes in February 1965, but all concerned could hardly have been unaware of the wide significance of their decisions.

The Review Body has no pay research unit, nor any connection with government agencies interested in general income levels. The Conservative Government had set up a National Incomes Commission in 1962, but the Review Body was specifically excluded from its jurisdiction, together with the nationalized industries and the higher civil service.[1] Later the Labour Government (elected in October 1964) inferred that it would not refer medical awards to its National Board for Prices and Incomes. In theory the Review Body (whose membership survived the change in government) was in no way bound to observe any national incomes policy. The 3 to 3.5 per cent increase in incomes per year was therefore irrelevant to consideration of the GPs' claim for a 32 per cent pay rise in 1964, when they had been given a 14 per cent increase only the year before. The Review Body was expected to bear the brunt of any decision it felt was justified. Seven eminent bankers, businessmen, and professors, serving voluntarily, were being asked to decide, with few guidelines, a major question of medical practice.

Their task was not made easier by the tradition of the Franks Committee for higher civil servants, on which the Review Body was modeled. The Franks Committee approach was one of informal private discussion among

1. See Cmnd. 1844 (HMSO, 1962) paragraph 4; and, for the guidelines set up by the N.I.C., Cmnd. 1994 (HMSO, 1963), p. 9.

the various participants on the basis of written statements of their position which might not even include requested income figures; no evidence was published, nor did the committee feel the need to justify its decisions in any detail. The Review Body (whose secretary, from the Cabinet Office, was also secretary to the Franks Committee) began along similar lines. Its 14 per cent award of 1963 had been announced in a short letter from its chairman to the Prime Minister; neither the evidence taken nor any details of the decision were divulged.

With the growing anxiety in general practice, culminating in the memorandum on GP incomes, a new role was forced on the Review Body. GPs made a specific pay claim, publicized for many months in the medical and national press, on which the committee was asked to adjudicate. Since the Ministry of Health did not at that time release its evidence for publication, it would be impossible to gauge what compromises the Review Body was making. Only the profession's claim could be measured against the ultimate award, and only the degree of professional (not Ministry) failure assessed. This added to the general difficulties awaiting the award—for the future authority of the British Medical Association in relation to the profession rested on the Commission's taking a favorable view of its claims.

In the interim period before the Review Body reported, the underlying issues continued to be discussed, and the unrest among general practitioners continued unabated. Dissatisfaction with the pool payment system increased, in respect both to its complexities and to the built-in concept of a fixed average net income. The GP, it was now appreciated, had all the disadvantages of salaried service, in that he could not state his own fees and had to comply with national regulations, yet none of the advantages. He had sought to be free but had found he had, if anything, less freedom and far fewer fringe benefits than the salaried consultant. Each improvement in general practice conditions had meant greater central supervision of general practice. A new system of expense reimbursement was being considered, but this, too, if made more equitable (so that the GP who spent more on staff and facilities received more expense money) would mean that quality controls would have to be introduced, and that the GP service would become more dependent on the Ministry of Health. Many GPs were becoming aware of the arguments in favor of a salaried service, or at least of reconsidering the whole basis of GP payments.[2]

2. One BMA Division had moved unsuccessfully at the representative meeting in March 1964 that the BMA Council devise a scheme for a salaried service for discussion and approval. The first GPA report (May 1964) recommended either a variable salary or capitation fees together with extra item-of-service payments, although a ballot of members showed stronger support for the second method. In July 1964 the Junior Members' Forum of the BMA asked for a thorough consideration of partial (voluntary) salaried service. An inquiry of GPs in Lancashire revealed 35% in favor of a salaried service, 43% against, and 22% unknown. A subcommittee of the Birmingham Executive Council recommended the appointment of salaried GPs in selected areas as a pilot study. *Brit. Med. J.* Suppl. *i* (1964), 127; *ii* (1964), 139;

Meanwhile, the joint working party on general practice, staffed by professional and Ministry members, was attempting to suggest specific improvements in the GP's position which could be attained through Ministry action. Its first report, issued as a series of commentaries (July 1964), discussed the distribution of doctors (for example, through a higher capitation fee in underdoctored areas); the provision of deputies during doctors' absences; the employment of secretaries, receptionists, and nurses; and educating the public in not abusing the doctor's time.[3] Concurrently the General Medical Services Committee was discussing the GP expense system with the Ministry of Health, and in the autumn of 1964 the Minister of Health announced that he was considering introducing a scheme for direct reimbursement to GPs for part of the salary of whole-time nonmedical assistants employed by them. If this went through, the expense system would have two components: an average sum and a specific payment. The new scheme might act as an incentive for GPs to employ nurses, receptionists, or secretaries and thus increase the efficiency of their practices.[4] It had, however, one serious drawback, once again concerning the pool payment system. Money for the direct reimbursement scheme would be diverted from the global pool. As a whole doctors would get no more, but the money would be redistributed in a slightly different way; many GPs would in fact receive less. In the explosive situation already existing in general practice, this suggestion was not likely to find favor.

These developments marked changes in the attitudes of both the medical profession and the Ministry of Health. The profession had entered the National Health Service firmly opposed to any "fixed element" (with its undertones of salaried payment) in their income, and committed to a capitation system administered through a central income pool. Each attempted improvement in GP payment had been built around these two concepts. By the 1960s, however, the battles between the BMA and the government at the introduction of the NHS had faded into history. The fear of GP dependence on the state had been replaced by demands that the state should take more responsibility for GP work by reducing work loads, introducing fringe benefits, and limiting the GP's ordinary duties to those undertaken during a normal working week. There was now a growing demand for a completely new look at the whole GP payment system.

The Ministry of Health had accepted a stronger guiding role for general practice. Clearly it would have to offer increasingly detailed technical assistance to the Review Body through memoranda setting out the implications

---

The GPA Report, Part One (London, 1964) p. 34; *Brit. Med. J. ii* (1964), 635 (R. M. Franklin); *The Times,* Dec. 24, 1964, p. 6.

3. *Brit. Med. J. ii* (1964), 113–14.

4. Under the proposals the GP would be reimbursed for half to two thirds of the salary of a whole-time assistant, dependent on the annual salary given—the higher salary, the less the reimbursement. Income tax relief would bring the real reimbursement to between 65 and 77%. *Brit. Med. J. ii* (1964), 463; Suppl. *ii,* 121.

for general practice of each suggested alternative. Payment was not merely a question of broad income levels. It could be manipulated to encourage doctors to enter different professional fields or geographical locations, to reward the outstanding or the better educated, or to favor certain types of practice (e.g. group practice) over others. This had of course always been true. But the shortage of general practitioners, together with the changing attitudes of practitioners themselves, emphasized the potential of income as an instrument for planning, to be used by government and profession alike.

The government changed before the Review Body had reported and before decisions had been made on GP conditions of service. General elections of October 1964 put a Labour Government into power—the first since 1951. It was not initially clear whether this would make any difference in health service decisions other than those (such as the abolition of the small prescription charge) to which the Labour Party had been committed in its election manifestos, and both the Joint Evidence Committee and the BMA issued statements in December 1964 affirming their complete confidence in the Review Body machinery.[5] This was followed in January 1965 by a letter from the new Minister of Health (Kenneth Robinson) to GPs, assuring them of his deep concern over the future of general practice and accepting the continuance of the Review Body and the working party on general practice. The Minister also announced his intention of setting up a fairer system of meeting practice expenses, more group practice, better premises, an increasing number of GPs and other staff, better educational opportunities, and a pattern of medical care "in which the family doctor must be the central figure." [6] The tone was friendly, but the Labour Government had a tiny majority and a straitened national budget. It was committed to the large-scale development of hospitals initiated under the Conservatives' hospital plan of 1962, and it was uncertain whether it would be prepared to initiate changes in policy that would require large financial investment.

The new government was also unlikely to be aided by the divisive structures of the medical profession, whose tensions became more apparent the longer the Review Body's decision was delayed. The BMA did not appear to provide a unified forum of opinion and had no plan for the GPs' future other than the memorandum submitted to the Review Body. The General Practitioners' Association (GPA) and Medical Practitioners' Union (MPU) continued to be small, the first with about four thousand, the second with five thousand members, although both were active. The second GPA report, December 1964, made recommendations based on job evaluations by business consultants of the relative work done by consultants and GPs—the first time this had been done. The conclusions suggested a differential of about 10 per cent, as compared with an actual noted difference of 40 per cent.[7] The

5. *Brit. Med. J.* Suppl. *i* (1965), 3.
6. Ibid., p. 10.
7. Consultants were given 147 points and GPs 133 out of a possible total of 165.

GPA proposals for GP incomes, forwarded to the Review Body, were based on this observation.

The MPU was harassed in the last few months of 1964 by claims that several of its council members were communists.[8] As a result, the Union received a great amount of adverse publicity. But at the same time it produced its own ten-point plan for general practice, which included abolition of the central pool, introduction of voluntary salaried service for GPs, the provision of efficient premises and adequate supporting staff, and the end of a twenty-four-hour responsibility for patients, without extra pay: all points later adopted by the BMA and all indicative of the new look in GP attitudes.

There was also continuing GP militancy. In January 1965, while the profession was still awaiting the results of its claim to the Review Body, the MPU announced that it would ask family doctors whether they would be prepared as a last resort to withdraw from the National Health Service. "Rather than accept second-rate standards," stated the MPU secretary in a letter circulated to GPs and Members of Parliament, "doctors will rebel." [9] It was suggested that GPs would retain on their NHS lists only the old and the young, and those sick or chronically ill; other members of the population would be seen only as private patients. The idea of some kind of strike or withdrawal began to take root. Already a group of sixty GPs in Birmingham, the "Birmingham Action Group," had agreed among themselves that resignation from the NHS was the only step "which could save the family-doctor service from permanent collapse." [10] The MPU's plan was denounced by the General Medical Services Committee by thirty-four votes to eleven. Never at any time, said one member, had there been any desire on the part of the GMS Committee, or indeed on the part of the profession generally, to take "such irresponsible action as had been taken by the MPU in the last

---

The validity of this ratio clearly depends on the appropriate selection of factors and the views of the evaluators. For example, the mental–technical requirement for keeping up to date was rated higher for consultants than for GPs, and job satisfaction was rated higher for GPs than consultants; another committee might not have agreed with these conclusions. Nevertheless, the method was promising, and it at least widened discussion of medical practice from vague statements to the concrete and quantitative field of business techniques. General Practitioners' Association, *The G.P.A. Report, Part Two; Doctors' Remuneration* (GPA, London, 1964).

8. During the altercation among MPU members, the president and treasurer of the union were deposed, only to be later restored to their positions by the council on the grounds that the circumstances of their removal were not technically correct; but the decision to reinstate them was not unanimous; 7 of the council's 36 members promptly resigned. The MPU did not deny it had communist council members, observed that such charges could have been made at any time within the past 15 years, and set up an inquiry to examine the whole issue. *Medical World Newsletter,* Dec. 1964.

9. *The Times,* Jan. 11, 1965, p. 6; Jan. 12, p. 6; Jan. 18, p. 6. It was suggested in at least one journal that the proposed withdrawal might be communist inspired (*Economist,* Jan. 23, 1965).

10. *Brit. Med. J. ii* (1964), 1600 (G.D.H. McQuitty).

few days.[11] It was not long, however, before the GMSC was to borrow the MPU's tactics.

The government was faced with a difficult situation. *The Times* pointed out that the Review Body had an unenviable task: "In purely economic terms the family doctors' case is thin." [12] It was clear that wider issues were at stake than pay levels, but these wide issues could not be settled overnight. Nor was there any clear opinion of what a new structure should be. Observations collated by the BMA from its Divisions and from local medical committees on suggestions for improving general practice revealed little that was new. There was general support for a system of direct reimbursement of practice expenses, but not for its consequences. The large number of GPs whose expenses were low would lose in net income unless such a scheme were introduced at the same time that extra money was injected into the central pool. This could be done, as the *Lancet* had suggested several months before, at the time of the Review Body's award; but such a suggestion had not been included in the profession's memorandum, on which all the hopes of the BMA hung.[13] Finally, although it was suggested that the pool system be abolished, there was no clear preference as to the kind of payment—capitation, fee-for-service, or salary—to replace it. The weight of all these problems was, somewhat unfairly, being placed on the Standing Review Body. If it did not report favorably, there was growing danger of a GP strike. On February 7, 1965, the day before the Review Body's decisions were published, the MPU announced that 4,000 GPs out of 5,500 who had replied to its questionnaire would be in favor of "some sort of sanction" if talks with the government broke down.[14]

The Review Body Reports

The Joint Evidence Committee of the medical profession had made four major requests of the Review Body. The first was that the pool system be modified to exclude all income except capitation fees and the "loading" or weighting factors attached to them, instead of including income from all official sources. The second was that expenses be paid through the pool in relation to all expenses of a general practice, not merely those incurred in the duties performed for capitation fees. Third, on the basis that incomes for general practitioner services had been too low since 1948, a claim was made for an extra £13 million; this would give the average GP a net income of £2,765 per year from capitation fees alone instead of from all official sources (including hospital work and so on). Finally, the profession had asked for an extra £5 million to set up a system of awards for seniority and experience. Together, these recommendations formed a curious mixture. There was a desire to return to a realistic capitation fee—realistic, that is, in

11. *Brit. Med. J.* Suppl. i (1965), 34–36.
12. Jan. 20, 1965, p. 11.
13. *Brit. Med. J. i* (1965), 265, and Suppl. i (1965), 27; *Lancet ii* (1964), 395.
14. *The Times*, Feb. 8, 1965, p. 10.

terms of the service actually given. At the same time there was, in the proposals for seniority payments and reimbursement of expenses, a further move toward a salaried service.

The Standing Review Body, whose report was simultaneously published and announced as accepted by the government on February 8, 1965, satisfied the profession on none of these points.[15] It did not agree with the profession that GP remuneration had been seriously inadequate since 1948. Although it accepted the profession's view that payments made to GPs by hospitals, local authorities, and government departments should no longer be included in the global pool, it rejected the proposal that other Executive Council fees, such as maternity medical fees, should also be excluded. The average net income under the new pool would be £2,775. This, the Review Body estimated, would be the equivalent of a net £3,000 from all official sources; and it would represent an average increase of just under 10 per cent in respect to Executive Council services only. The new arrangements would increase the amount in the pool by about £5.5 million, instead of the £13 million requested by the profession. Seniority payments (for which the profession had claimed another £5 million) were rejected on the grounds that it would be "particularly difficult to introduce such a concept into a profession where the relationship is one of professional contract rather than of salaried employment," and that in any case it would prefer awards for merit rather than for seniority. The profession had asked for a total of £18 million (although the Review Body estimated the cost of its demands as nearer £20 million); it was offered £5.5 million, with the possibility of more through a future scheme of merit awards.

As a final blow to the profession, this increase was not to be applied across the board. The Review Body had taken a broad view of its role. It had considered the structure of GP payments as well as their overall levels, and had not limited itself to arbitrating on the profession's claim alone. To the Review Body (and probably also the Ministry of Health whose views were undisclosed) the award, which was not linked with demands for consultant increases, provided a golden opportunity to introduce the scheme for direct reimbursement of certain GP practice expenses. About three quarters of the £5.5 million would be assigned to new expense schemes; the remainder would be paid as extra capitation fees. This would mean an uneven distribution of the pay increase. In terms of concrete examples, issued promptly by the Ministry of Health, the average GP with no assistants would receive an increase of only 2.5 per cent, but the average GP with one full-time and one part-time assistant in approved categories would receive as much as 22 per cent. The award was thus being used not to increase the level of the average GP's net income, but to redistribute gross incomes.

However sensible these suggestions, and however applicable to the long-term prosperity of general practice, the award expressed a flat rejection of

15. *Review Body on Doctors' and Dentists' Remuneration, Third, Fourth and Fifth Reports,* Cmnd. 2585 (HMSO, 1965).

the profession's joint memorandum. The General Medical Services Committee received a further blow to its prestige; the very basis of its case—the continued underpayment of general practitioners—had been rejected. The reaction of the professional bodies to the award was thus immediate and adverse. The BMA sent a letter to all GPs expressing the disappointment of the Joint Evidence Committee. It spoke derogatorily of the increase in the capitation fee as only one penny per consultation; and it observed that the award represented "no encouragement to family doctors to remain in this country." [16] This was followed by a statement to all GPs from the General Medical Services Committee, in which they were asked to consider in detail the facts and possible implications of the award before emergency meetings later in February. The General Practitioners' Association announced that it would send a letter to all doctors asking them to resign from the National Health Service. The Medical Practitioners' Union, after a long committee meeting, decided to advise GPs to end their contracts with the government and withdraw from the National Health Service unless the government negotiated on an entirely new basis within the next three months. It further stated that if the GMSC did not support this view, the MPU would continue alone. Meanwhile, local medical committees in various parts of the country were meeting to consider resigning from the NHS.[17] The BMA, sensitive of previous criticism of its failure to represent the "periphery," was forced to take a stronger position than it might otherwise have done.

As before, the difficulty was to find the villain. The Review Body had been welcomed by the profession; its recommendations had been accepted in full by the government. Consultants, who were not concerned in the latest award, were particularly interested in retaining the Review Body. If this method of income determination were to be continued in the future, the profession could not reject the report outright. On the other hand, if the GMSC accepted the award without demur, as it had accepted the 14 per cent award in 1963, the GMSC itself, in the opinion of the BMA secretary, would not last 24 hours.[18]

The primary reaction of the GMSC was to demand that the whole of the £5.5 million should be "immediately and unconditionally" credited to the pool in respect of capitation fees—even though it had previously supported the introduction of a new scheme for reimbursing expenses.[19] The GMSC also steered discussion away from the award by indicting the pool system of payment as the root of the GPs' problems, and recommended that the pro-

16. *Brit. Med. J.* Suppl. *i* (1965), 48–49.

17. See *The GMS Voice*, no. 4, Feb. 1965; *The Times*, Feb. 10, 11, 1965.

18. *Brit. Med. J.* Suppl. *i* (1965), 56.

19. Agreement had been delayed for two main reasons: discussions on how far doctors' dependents (particularly wives) might be included, and how to begin the scheme without prejudicing certain doctors' incomes at the time of changeover. The Review Body award would have answered the second question, in that every GP would have received some increase, even though some would get much more than others.

fession's representatives initiate immediate discussions with the Ministry to establish an entirely new form of contract of service. Both the MPU and local GP groups had spoken of withdrawal of services if certain demands were not met. The GMSC, anxious to retrieve a position of leadership, adopted the same policy, resolving to put withdrawal machinery into motion through the BMA's own body, the British Medical Guild; but the BMA was careful to cushion the effect of its decision in the public press. The threat of withdrawal, it was emphasized, was not intended to sabotage the National Health Service but as a lever at the bargaining table; withdrawal did not mean a "strike" against patients—merely the return to private practice. Hospital staffs were unaffected; their incomes were not in dispute, and there was no suggestion of withdrawal in sympathy. The Central Consultants and Specialists Committee, however, joined the MPU and the GPA in giving the GMSC their support; and there was reluctant agreement from the BMA Council.

By no means were all general practitioners in favor of withdrawal or even displeased with the Review Body's award; one GP who wrote to *The Times* claimed that "a few more of us are willing to accept the Review Body's awards than is generally supposed," and urged the Minister of Health, who had stated that no changes were intended in the award, to have the courage of his convictions.[20] GPs with good premises and several supporting staff would have received increases of both 14 per cent and over 20 per cent in just over two years. But these were not the most vociferous. The situation, as before, released a flood of indignation and protests which ranged over all aspects of general practice. By this time, the GMSC was not merely claiming that the Review Body had given GPs too little: it was claiming a new type of contract—a matter which had not even been put to the Review Body by the profession. Indeed, there would have been an even greater outcry if the Review Body had changed the whole income basis of practice, which was what the GMSC was now suggesting ought to be done.

Both the profession and the Ministry were in a curious position. The GMSC had announced the possibility of withdrawal, a popular move with local medical committees, yet it had no blueprint on which to negotiate a new contract. The Minister of Health (Mr. Robinson) was not formally responsible for the views of the Review Body, although it was entirely possible, even probable, that the Review Body's report reflected the opinion of the Ministry—the contents of the Ministry memorandum on the claim had not been made public. Expressing his willingness to discuss methods of remuneration and the reconstruction of general practice, the Minister put responsibility for the "turbulence which is now being exhibited" squarely on the profession, and spoke of the "competition in militancy between various warring factions." [21] Thus there was a danger of deadlock. On the one hand there were threats to resign, but on the other there was no villain and no

20. See *The Times*, Feb. 13, 1965, p. 6; Feb. 16, 1965, p. 23 (J.H.S. Hopkins).
21. Ibid., Feb. 18, 1965, p. 9.

alternative plan. Both sides were similarly concerned to improve general practice, to remove GP discontent, and to restore the authority of the BMA, without which there was a danger of organizational anarchy among general practitioners.

One question for immediate resolution was whether the £5.5 million, which GPs had no intention of foregoing, could be given wholly in the form of capitation fees. After discussions, called for at the request of the BMA, between the Minister of Health and his chief civil servants and leaders of the medical profession, it was agreed to ask the Review Body to "clarify" certain aspects of its report. Fortunately, the body was due to meet on February 25, although not, it was stressed, at the instigation of the Minister. It was agreed to defer further discussions until after that meeting. Meanwhile the GMSC appointed four of its members, together with the secretary and deputy secretary of the BMA, to draft the outlines of a new contract of service. There were various possibilities. The pool could be retained but with further alterrations to it, or it could be abolished in favor of a completely new system or choice of systems, with or without capitation fees. Suggestions might be made for reducing the work load, limiting the GP's responsibility, and paying his expenses. The GP might even be incorporated into the hospital staffing structure. It was more likely, however—from the need for immediate action as well as from the lack of existing plans—that the contract would stem from ideas that had been germinating in different professional groups in previous months, than indicate a complete departure from the existing system.

Meanwhile the completed (but undated) resignation forms from GPs began to pour into BMA House; by February 24, 1965, there were almost 4,800 and by March 1 almost 9,500, with the number increasing day by day.[22] It was recommended that the resignations, held for future action by the British Medical Guild, would be handed to executive councils on April 1, to go into effect on July 1, unless the dispute were settled. Final decisions would, however, be taken by another series of special meetings of the Conference of Local Medical Committees and the BMA Representative Body, called for March 24. The Review Body met and, as the BMA had hoped, stated (although registering protest) that it would not insist on making payment of expenses a part of the award; the £5.5 million would be added to the pool unconditionally. This part of the battle could be seen as a victory for the profession. By now, however, long-term issues were at stake.

A Charter for Family Doctors

The BMA published its "Charter for the Family Doctor Service" on March 8, 1965. Publication was reached, in comparison with the BMA's earlier activities, with remarkable speed and it bore some of the marks of hurried creation.[23] In a busy weekend the GMSC had succeeded in produc-

22. Ibid., Feb. 20, 1965, p. 10; Feb. 22, p. 6; Feb. 25, p. 12; March 2, p. 12.
23. *Brit. Med. J.* Suppl. *i* (1965), 89–91.

ing a concrete plan: the first major contribution on general practice from the BMA for some fifteen years. Its kernel, borrowing the previous suggestions of the Medical Practitioners' Union, was a proposed revision of the pool system of payment, together with a claim for limited liability by GPs for NHS work. It was suggested that the GPs' contractual obligation with the National Health Service be related to a specified working day, a 5.5-day week, and a working year which provided six weeks of vacation; and it was also suggested that GP principals should not be held professionally responsible for the work of their assistants. "The onus of making arrangements for out-of-hours medical attention," stated the Charter, "must rest on the Government." This was a sad comment on the failure of voluntary group practice to provide, as some practices had done, efficient off-duty rotas, appointments systems, and other labor-saving devices within a purely professional environment. Moreover, if established, this system would put GPs much farther into a salaried pattern, even if not technically on salary, than were salaried consultants. Even part-time consultants were expected as part of their NHS contracts to be individually and continuously responsible for their own patients at all hours of the day and night and to be responsible for work performed under their direction by junior medical staff.

Despite these similarities to salaried service, the GP charter urged that the basis of payment be more closely related to private practice. The existing capitation system was merely a device for determining differential incomes, according to list size and in relation to a nationally negotiated average income. GPs now requested a capitation fee which would compare with fees given for medical visits outside the NHS; three government agreements were given as evidence that might be used as the basis to recalculate the fee. This new fee would be multiplied by the total NHS population and paid to the GP as income in the form chosen by the profession. In other words, GPs wished to return to a method of payment according to the number of patients instead of according to the number of doctors—the concept on which the pool had been based since the Danckwerts award of 1952. Since the population was now increasing faster than the number of GPs, the suggestion was clearly advantageous. GPs were claiming the best of both worlds: first, the Minister of Health's twenty-four-hour responsibility for providing a GP service and, second, a method of payment based on an increasing work load.

Claims were also made in the charter for the reimbursement of expenses for assistants directly and in full (another parallel to salaried service) and for reimbursement for maintenance of practice premises. The establishment of an independent corporation financed from public sources was recommended, to lend money to GPs for purchasing or improving premises and equipment and to acquire buildings for lease or sale. Comments were also made on the need to reduce the amount of certification of sickness for employment and other purposes, on the need to overhaul the GP disciplinary machinery, on prompt payment of the compensation due for practices taken over in 1948, and on the need to reduce the maximum list size. Finally, groups of GPs should, it was suggested, be given a choice of payment—by capitation fee, item of service, or some form of salary—although the financial basis for each type would be the same. The BMA estimated that the proposals would cost between £30 and £35 million—a total revised by the Ministry to over £40 million; and that sum would be in addition to the £5.5 million just granted by the Review Body. The profession had asked the Review Body for £18 million; it now claimed two and a half times this amount. "How many other unions," commented *The Times,* "can boast of having gone to arbitration, been disappointed, had the arbitrators obligingly change their recommendations, and finally had expenditure suggested on a scale far more lavish than the originally rejected claim?" [24]

Concentration on the demands of general practitioners, and the growing militancy of certain sections of the profession, had obscured wider questions on the relative place of general practice in a comprehensive medical service. Again, general practice was being regarded by itself instead of as a section of one profession. Specialists were not involved in this dispute. They shared neither the GP's problems nor his anxiety. Once more the traditional division of the profession was a stumbling block. The profession's new charter was for GPs only: it concentrated on GP pay instead of the basic problems of training and organization. Whatever the justification for a further rise in net income of about 60 per cent, the problems of recasting the capitation system, as it had been built up under seventeen years of the National Health Service, would require lengthy negotiations. The Review Body had already acceded to the profession's request to consider GP incomes separately from those of other medical practitioners, within the three-year period covered by the 14 per cent award. The next general review of medical incomes was due in the spring of 1966; it was doubtful whether negotiations on a new GP contract could be completed before that time. The charter's terms were vague. They would not provide the immediate answer to the threat of withdrawal. The Minister of Health expressed himself willing to discuss the charter, but he emphasized that the pricing of any new contract—the amounts to be paid—had to be left to the Review Body. Time was short; by March 17, 1965, the British Medical Guild had received 16,500 potential resignations from GPs, with the intention that these should be handed in on April 1.

The GMSC had to decide what advice it would give to its constituents—the Conference of Local Medical Committees—who were scheduled to meet on March 24. There were three choices: withdrawal of the threat of resignation, continuance with plans for notice of resignation on April 1, or a deferment of notice. The first might weaken the GMSC's position. The second would mean that negotiations would cease, just when the Minister had agreed to discuss alternative methods of remuneration, a separately financed public corporation for providing practice expenses, and other matters in the charter. The GMSC thus decided, with only one dissent, to recom-

24. March 9, 1965, p. 13.

mend the third alternative to the local medical committees, namely that resignations not be handed in until the beginning of July, to take effect in October. BMA Council agreed, and a report to this effect was sent out promptly to all GPs.[25] The General Practitioners' Association, still militant, spoke of the decision to defer the resignations as a "shattering blow." [26] But the seven hundred doctors who met both jointly and separately as representatives of local medical committees and members of the Representative Body of the BMA overwhelmingly accepted their leaders' advice.[27] For the next few months the threat of withdrawal loomed only as a paper tiger.

The situation was now concerned with a long-term and a short-term issue. The Minister had estimated that negotiations on the charter would not be completed before April 1966. The profession was being asked to defer resignations only until July 1965. For this short interval the GMSC specified certain conditions, partly designed to test the Minister's intentions toward the profession. Thus the Minister was asked to promise amending legislation to provide an independent corporation for practice expenses, to make "positive and unequivocal assurances" of additional finance for the employment of assistants and the reduction of the burden of certification, and to agree to other major concessions such as the abolition of the pool and the allowance of alternative payment schemes.[28] Negotiations proceeded on these subjects, and the first joint report from the negotiators appeared early in June 1965, shortly before the professional bodies were to meet again to determine whether to resign.

The first joint report indicated considerable progress in the charter discussions. The government undertook to introduce legislation for a finance corporation to make loans to general practitioners, agreed to set up a scheme for partial reimbursement of the salaries of selected staff, and arranged to relax National Insurance regulations for compulsory certification in respect of sickness and injury benefit claims.[29] Preliminary agreement had also been reached on making GPs' deputies responsible for their own actions, and on the need for additional incentives in underdoctored areas. There was no guarantee that average GP incomes would be increased, even if these new schemes were introduced, for the Minister would make no commitment on the question of pricing. A curious position had been reached; direct bargaining with the Ministry was once more favored over independent arbitration. Pricing, the Minister urged, was for the Review Body, to whom further representations would have to be made—and which had categorically stated that GP incomes were not too low.

25. *Brit. Med. J.* Suppl. *i* (1965), 104–10; *The GMS Voice,* March 18, 1965.
26. *The Times,* March 20, 1965, p. 8.
27. *Brit. Med. J.* Suppl. *i* (1965), 113–27.
28. Ibid., p. 103.
29. BMA, *Remuneration and Terms of Conditions of Service of General Practitioners in the National Health Service. Joint Report with the Minister upon the Charter for the Family Doctor Service* (June 2, 1965).

Although there was some doubt about how far these agreements represented adequate concessions by the government (the MPU, for example, asked for their rejection) both the Conference of Local Medical Committees (on June 16) and the Representative Body (on June 23) resolved that negotiations should continue, and that the undated resignations held by the British Medical Guild be reserved until negotiations were completed.[30] This decision appeared to offer the GMSC time to continue discussions with the Ministry and for both sides to develop detailed policies to replace piecemeal negotiations on unrelated topics such as had taken place so far. A grand design for general practice was still in the future.

The General Medical Services Committee was, however, almost immediately faced by unexpected difficulties. The BMA annual representative meeting was scheduled to begin on July 8, and a large number of items connected with the GP charter was already included in its agenda, which was not consolidated or controlled at BMA House. At the meeting in Swansea, a representative moved (as one of over four hundred agenda items) that one method of remuneration to be included in the charter ought to be payment by the patient of fees for items of service.[31] This resolution raised a completely new issue, basic to the National Health Service and possibly dangerous to negotiations on the charter. The Labour Government had removed charges to patients for certain services (which had been increased under the previous Conservative administration) and was committed to providing health services free to the whole population. It was clear that the Minister would refuse to consider patient payments as a basis for negotiation. Nevertheless the assembly not only passed it, against the advice of the GMSC chairman, but declared it to be a resignation issue; and this became BMA policy. The situation illustrated the confusion within the BMA system.

In the event, such fee-for-service was ignored by the negotiating team, whose discussions with the Ministry continued to focus on developing another detailed claim to present to the Review Body, for consideration at its three-year review in 1966. There was, however, a movement toward the fee-for-service concept in private practice in certain sections of the profession. In Birmingham, where there had been early talk of GP withdrawal, thirteen GPs had resigned from the National Health Service by mid-August 1965, of whom four set up in private practice.[32] The BMA established its

---

30. A constitutional difficulty was narrowly averted in these decisions. The GMSC had recommended that the resignations be destroyed, the BMA Council that they continue to be held. Enormous problems would have arisen if the Conference of Local Medical Committees had followed GMSC opinion and the Representative Body that of the BMA Council, since there was no machinery to determine what should be done in case of disagreement between the two bodies. In fact, however, the Conference followed the Council's view. See *Brit. Med. J. i* (1965), 1446, Suppl. *i* (1965), 258.

31. *Brit. Med. J.* Suppl. *ii* (1965), 67.

32. These doctors, spearheaded by Dr. Gilbert Smith, leader of the Birmingham Action Group, charge patients a weekly fee and fees for service; drugs are included

own committee on private insurance, which subsequently developed its own insurance company, "Independent Medical Services Ltd.," initially staffed from BMA headquarters, and primarily intended as an alternative scheme to the National Health Service should negotiations fail. The General Practitioners' Association encouraged support (including financial support) of the Birmingham group, and made available a firm of insurance brokers.[33] As yet there appeared to be no general movement to return to private practice.[34] But the existence of such machinery considerably strengthened the GPs' bargaining position.

Once again the Review Body was being asked to solve the GP's problems. Its position was not made easier in that its next report would also consider the incomes of hospital staffs, who had increasing problems of their own. The Central Consultants and Specialists Committee issued a memorandum in the summer of 1965 recommending increased salary scales for hospital junior staff and senior registrars, increments for postgraduate diplomas, and the abolition of residence charges where residence in the hospital was compulsory. Nor were GPs the only section of the profession who complained of being overworked. It was also time, it was claimed, for the long hours and alleged exploitation of junior hospital staff to come to an end. These points were developed by the Hospital Junior Staffs Group of the BMA and by an independent group from St. Bartholomew's Hospital, London, each issuing separate statements, the latter gaining considerable coverage in the public press.[35] At the same time alarm was expressed over the physical state of hospitals. The ambitious hospital plan of 1962 had been curtailed for lack of funds, and reports had begun to appear in the press of the poor condition of some hospitals after long years of financial neglect.[36] The GP's problems did not stand in isolation; in fact the National Health Service was at a crossroad. Decisions that should have been taken several years before on long-term development had become urgent, but the focus on GP incomes in this period probably contributed to their being ignored.

Once again there was a basic question of responsibility. General practitioners had sought to solve their problems through the income structure,

---

in the regular charges. The Ministry of Health brought in nine GPs with guaranteed incomes to replace them. Birmingham was in some respects atypical, and it did not appear that any large-scale movement toward private practice would result. Anne Lapping, *New Society,* 19 Aug. 1965, p. 18.

33. General Practitioners' Association, *Members' Newsletter,* July 27, 1965.

34. *The Times* reported in September 1965 that fewer than 2% of the 30,000 patients approached by the Birmingham Executive Council expressed a wish to withdraw from NHS lists. This was in the area on which the private practice movement was centered, and it was possible that those GPs who had left the NHS might lack patients. (Sept. 21, p. 6).

35. British Medical Association, Central Consultants and Specialists Committee, *An Appraisal of the Hospital Service* (June 1965); *Brit. Med. J.* Suppl. *ii* (1965), 70, 119; *Brit. Med. J., ii* (1965), 836; *The Times,* Oct. 11, 1965, p. 10.

36. For example, *The Times,* March 2, 1965, p. 4; March 10, pp. 14–15.

and in doing so had thrown an unfair burden on the Standing Review Body on Doctors' and Dentists' Remuneration, an inadequate vehicle for major health service planning decisions. Hospital staffs appeared to be following suit. As a result, the Review Body was being forced to become an arbitration tribunal. Although it was announced that the actual proceedings would remain secret, the Ministry of Health agreed to publish its own evidence in the 1966 decision, and the BMA was allowed its request (at least on this occasion) to present oral evidence through legal counsel. Since the members of the Review Body were not themselves experts in medical planning, the content of the evidence was of supreme importance. Meanwhile, negotiations continued between GP representatives and the Ministry of Health, engaged in developing a new pay structure which would form part of the Review Body evidence.

The second report of these joint discussions was published in October 1965. It bore evidence of a much more careful and comprehensive approach to GP problems than had distinguished earlier discussions.[37] Indeed, so radical were many of its proposals that it might be regarded (as it was by the *British Medical Journal*) as equal in importance to the original Spens report.[38] Negotiations had evidently moved away from the strictures imposed in the GP charter to attempts to link the needs of general practice with the payment structure. The system now proposed was almost as complex as the system it was to replace, but it had been reached for recognizable reasons. It followed the demand of general practitioners, expressed in the charter, that their practice be divided for payment purposes into work undertaken in regular hours and work relating to overtime or leave; that financial recognition be given to increased work loads; and that seniority payments be made. The proposal also recognized the government's desire (which had appeared in the previous Review Body report) for merit awards for GPs, and a common wish for financial incentives to improve GP organization and work.

The suggested system was based on two existing principles: the ubiquitous capitation fee and a new lump-sum allowance. Practitioners would receive a basic capitation fee for treatment of patients during working hours (8 a.m. to 7 p.m., with a half day on Saturday and an off-duty Sunday). They would also receive a basic practice allowance, of unspecified proportions, which would be uniform for GPs with lists of more than a thousand patients. For out-of-hours work a separate lump sum and supplementary capitation fees would be payable, together with item-of-service fees for calls in the small hours (midnight to 7 a.m.). GPs might, however, assign their out-of-hours work to another practitioner—only if one could be found to accept it. The capitation fee had a further element, also new, relating to different work loads in different types of practice: supplementary capitation fees would be paid for each person on the GP's list over the age of 65. The basic practice allowance would have further elements in respect to seniority, experience,

37. The text of the report is published in *Brit. Med. J. ii* (1965), 153–59.
38. Ibid., p. 889.

and special qualifications; to practice in groups; and to service in areas classified as "designated" or underdoctored by the Medical Practices Committee. These last might be regarded as an extension of the payment scheme to induce organizational change. Other separate fees, such as payments for postgraduate education and for certain services, would continue. The new system would also recognize a total of six weeks a year for vacation and study, and additional payments (as well as full pay) to provide a deputy during the GP's absence in case of sickness.

The chief merits of the proposals seemed to be the speed with which they were drawn up, and their inclusion of all the important current issues except choice of payment; the possible alternative of reimbursement by a fee-for-service system was reserved for experiment, and salaried contracts were to apply primarily to GPs working in health centers. In addition, progress was reported on a scheme of full direct payment of "reasonable" expenditure on rents and rates of surgery premises. Other matters still to be negotiated included terms of service, access to hospital diagnostic facilities, and superannuation; these, however, could be discussed apart from the new payment scheme.

In accord with the Minister's earlier insistence, the proposals contained no cost element. The Review Body was to be asked to price each item, and thus to weigh one factor in terms of another. The larger the basic allowance (first cousin to the attacked concept of a "fixed element" in GP pay proposed in the early day of NHS discussions), the smaller would be the capitation fee. There were as yet no clues as to how large each major component would be, or what guidelines the Review Body would follow in its pricing. How far, for example, the extra allowances for working in a group practice or in an underdoctored area would in fact act as inducements to GPs would depend largely on their size.

The profession seemed reasonably pleased. A BMA ballot of GPs in Britain in October 1965 revealed 17,602 in favor and only 2,660 against submitting the document to the Review Body—despite the fears of some members of the General Medical Services Committee that such a ballot might precipitate problems similar to those that beset the BMA in 1948.[39] A milestone had been reached. It was true that no assessment of the proposals could be made until the Review Body fixed prices to the major components, but there was at least a certain optimism in the outcome, based as it must be on the combined recommendations of the Ministry and the medical profession. Almost inevitably the claim would result in a general income rise for GPs, as well as the increased spread of incomes implicit in the new proposals.

Current Problems

Between 1963 and late 1965, the problems of the health service revolved around the claims and needs of general practitioners. The GPs' case had

39. *The Times,* Nov. 5, 1965, p. 5; *Brit. Med. J.* Suppl., *ii* (1965), 149–51.

rested on their being underpaid in relation to consultants and overworked in relation to what they were paid; the Review Body had disagreed. In terms of the differential it appeared that the GP had in fact gained under the National Health Service. The original Spens Committee reports on medical incomes of 1946 and 1948 had indicated that the average GP between 40 and 50 years old should receive a net income of £1,300 and that a specialist should receive at least £2,500 at about the age of 40. The £5.5 million award raised the average net income of the GP from official sources to about £3,000, while the top of the consultant basic scale was £4,445. According to these figures, the differential had narrowed from 92 per cent to 48 per cent by 1965. Nor did the GP appear to have been left behind in relation to other professional earnings. The prewar general practitioner earned a net income (after practice expenses) which corresponded, for example, with the salary of a principal in the administrative class of the civil service; in May 1964 the average GP had a greater net income than the top of the principal's scale.[40] The real question was whether GPs, because of enhanced skills, different functions, or scarcity were worth relatively more in 1966 than in 1939. This question had been largely ignored.

The question of overwork was also relative; it had been partly engendered by a declining ratio of GPs in relation to the population. A report published by the College of General Practitioners in July 1965 suggested that the problems of general practice were primarily administrative: "The general practitioner is providing an old-fashioned service often in out-of-date premises with inefficient organization." The actual time spent with patients, including traveling time, was estimated at thirty-nine hours a week.[41] This report, based on published sources of various kinds, was received cautiously by the BMA, which remarked their preliminary nature and stated that the last full-scale inquiry had been that carried out by the BMA in 1950.[42] Unfortunately, however, the BMA had made no further inquiries in the following fifteen years, and could thus neither approve nor disprove the data presented by the College.

The question of leadership was still paramount. With the publication of its report on the needs of general practice, the College of General Practitioners appeared temporarily as a candidate for spearheading action; but the College quickly announced that it had no wish to be involved in "medico-political" affairs.[43] The BMA was involved in a crisis in its organizational structure. The interrelationships among the autonomous committees (GMSC, CCSC) and their constituents, and the council and representatives of the BMA, needed urgent attention. The BMA had not established a full-time planning team. The Ministry of Health had appointed an outside planning

40. *Economist,* "Salaries, Are You Better Off?" (May 1964).

41. The College of General Practitioners, *Reports from General Practice II. Present State and Future Needs* (July 1965), pp. 25, 50.

42. British Medical Association, Circular Letter to doctors dated July 22, 1965.

43. *Brit. Med. J. ii* (1965), 358.

advisory group.[44] What was now required was the rapid development of full-time staff in the Ministry and the BMA who would deal specifically with the organization and development of different types of medical practice.

The incomes dispute was in the end a question of imaginative planning. The recurring crises were undermining the fabric of the National Health Service—and thus of medical care as a whole. Moreover, the pay claims, by encouraging other employment groups to break the national income guidelines, inevitably aggravated the national wage–price spiral. More appropriate planning mechanisms than the Standing Review Body were required. A major reappraisal of the long-term roles of the different branches of the profession was essential. The GP could no longer remain in isolation; practitioners as a whole could not remain lethargic; nor could the public afford to ignore the implications of the GP's position for the future efficiency of the whole health service.

Postscript

The Review Body's report was made public in May 1966, after this book went to press. It bore out the predictions made in this chapter, strengthening the Review Body's role as a major NHS planning authority. GPs were given substantial pay increases (an average net increase of over 30% in a two-year period), based on the Ministry–profession recommendations. Junior hospital doctors, whose organizations had become more effective, were also given substantial raises, greatest for house officers (35%). Consultants received only 10% (£3200–£4885), but the number and value of distinction awards was increased, to totals of 1,900 C awards (now £925), 950 B awards (£2,175), and 315 A awards (£3,700). A-plus awards (now £4,885) remained limited to 100. For GPs there would be a basic practice allowance of £1000 p.a. with a standard capitation fee of £1 (increased to £1 8s. for those over 65) up to 1,000 patients on the GP's list, plus another 2s. 6d. for those above 1,000. £200 was to be paid for "out-of-hours" duties, plus a £1 fee for any call between midnight and 7 A.M. Those in group practice would receive £200. There were also payments for vocational and postgraduate training, and for initial practice in a "designated" area. The Review Body capitulated in respect to seniority allowances: £200 p.a. after 5 years, increased to £400 after 15 years, and to £650 after 25 years. But it also added distinction awards: 2,500 GPs would receive an extra £750, and 100 would receive £2,500. Other additional fees would remain. The cost was estimated as up to £39 million. *Seventh Report of the Review Body on Doctors' and Dentists' Remuneration,* Cmnd. 2992. *The Times,* May 5, 1966.

44. *The Times,* July 6, 1965, p. 7.

VI

Specialization:
Problems at the Mid-1960s

22

Problems in
Medical Education and Training

By the beginning of the 1960s action was urgently required in two wide areas of medical education and training.[1] First, there was a need to review the purpose of each stage of medical education: the preclinical and clinical phases of the undergraduate curriculum, the graduate (preregistration) and postgraduate programs. From such review the content of each stage might be discussed in more concrete terms, changes made, and responsibility for standards assigned among the universities, the hospitals, and the professional Colleges. Second, there was a recognized and acute need for postgraduate education and training programs in the hospitals, particularly in those hospitals that were labeled "nonteaching," in which the great majority of specialist trainees were employed, and which, as the district hospitals of the future, might also be expected to provide the professional focus of medicine for public health and for general practitioners.

Educating the Doctor

While it was relatively simple to appreciate that undergraduate medical education ought to be regarded as a general base for specialization, it was difficult to work out a curriculum to replace the one that was the direct descendent of prespecialization apprenticeship days. Medical schools had developed around the voluntary general hospitals: around concepts of disease rather than health, and around acute physical disorders rather than mental or chronic illness or, indeed, any disorder that did not require hospital care. The teaching hospitals had become increasingly esoteric, as university research centers and as reference centers in certain specialties for a wide hospital area.

It had been taken for granted that undergraduates should be trained at teaching hospitals attached to universities, and that postgraduates, although not usually studying for a university degree, would also receive better training in the teaching hospital. The university had conflicting functions. Although the undergraduate stage was being recognized as a general training

1. See Chap. 12.

in basic principles, requiring a wide focus and including an increasing number of nonmedical and social sciences, some departments of the teaching hospital were better equipped to train senior registrars than undergraduates. Indeed, there were more senior registrars in the undergraduate teaching hospitals in 1964 than in all regional hospital units.[2]

One major question was where the foci of undergraduate and postgraduate education ought to be. Was there a valid difference between a hospital complex designed as a practical laboratory for the undergraduate—including, perhaps, a general practice center, a mental health unit, and a program in social medicine—and one more properly associated with specialist training? It could be argued (and has been, in different regional hospital areas) that regional specialist units ought to be developed in nonteaching hospitals rather than in the teaching centers, and that the primary responsibility for training in specialist skills should lie with the regional hospital board. Alternatively, there was a case for a reverse of tradition by teaching undergraduates in ordinary district hospitals. But there were compelling, and ultimately overriding, reasons for educating university students in an intellectual climate where research and advanced techniques in medical and associated fields (which range from molecular biology to the social sciences) were furthered and demonstrated. This pointed either to the expansion of medical schools as miniature universities, which could themselves offer the courses and facilities that might be included in a new medical curriculum— an impractical long-term aim—or their fuller incorporation into university life.

No clear trend had emerged by 1965. Again there was discussion rather than action. Medical schools continued to be regarded as adjuncts of the particular hospitals from which they sprang—particularly the London schools, which stand on the same site as the hospitals, isolated from the university, and bear the hospital rather than the university name. Yet as the undergraduate period began to shift from the old vocational training to general medical education, its focus moved away from hospitals to the medical schools and other university departments; and the internal structure of the individual hospital became less important. Changes were still called for in the teaching hospitals, for reasons of general function as well as for education, but these hospitals needed no longer to be a reflection—indeed could no longer reflect—the content of the medical curriculum. There was thus a strong case to tighten the link between medical schools and universities, while retaining the teaching hospitals as flexible teaching and research laboratories which might well be supplemented by practical teaching in other hospitals and in other spheres of practice.

Discussions of the undergraduate curriculum were highlighted in the report of an unofficial study group stimulated by Dr. Nicholas Malleson and

2. Of 1,375 senior registrars, 654 were in undergraduate groups and 518 in nonteaching hospitals. The remainder were attached to the postgraduate teaching groups in London. Source: Ministry of Health Statistics Division

others in 1963.[3] This developed the concept of a basic degree in "human biology" rather than in the traditional medical sciences of anatomy, physiology, and pharmacology. The course would include these basic disciplines, but it would also treat related skills such as genetics, statistics, principles of epidemiology, general practice, and social and preventive medicine, and all would be required for a B.Sc. degree. Under the scheme the student would go from this degree to a clinical course lasting twenty-seven months, culminating with the usual medical degrees of M.B. and B.S. He would then move to a preregistration post within the region in which the school was situated, where close supervision would be possible. Since one could already (for example at Oxford and Cambridge) take a university degree in physiology or another medical science at the end of the preclinical course, the human biology course offered little that could not be achieved within the existing educational structure. Its chief innovations were three. First it suggested the inclusion of certain subjects, such as statistics, which had not been generally thought of as part of medical training. Second, it emphasized that the preclinical and clinical parts of medical training might be geographically separated. Thus the human biology degree might be taken in a university which was without a medical school but was strong in other paramedical and social sciences: a point that was seized eagerly by the University of Keele which quickly announced plans to initiate a human biology degree.[4] Third, the Malleson Committee indicated that the human biology degree need not be limited to students who were planning a career in medicine. Thus the interrelationship of medicine and society might finally be brought within the university setting, and the medical student no longer isolated from his future colleagues in the other social and biological sciences. Would it be possible in the future for the doctor to receive his basic university education, as did the physician in the eighteenth century, in the same classroom as the future biologist, cleric, or philosopher?

The possibility of a new classicism was tempting, although some considered the suggested course both unrealistic and too long.[5] Nevertheless, the Malleson report provided a material symbol of change. Many universities were already wrestling with their curricula, even though some of the actual changes that emerged were relatively conservative. Thus Edinburgh University developed a three-year B.Sc. course in medical science, but it still contained five hundred hours of anatomy.[6] The need to include community medicine was generally recognized, and several schools introduced voluntary apprenticeships in general practice as part of the curriculum. The older schools were precluded from revolutionary change by their existing struc-

---

3. *School of Medicine and Human Biology,* Reports of the Working Parties (London, Nov. 1963).

4. *Guardian,* June 15, 1964, p. 3.

5. J. Anderson and F. J. Roberts, *A New Look at Medical Education* (London, 1965), pp. 47–48.

6. *Lancet i* (1964), 868–69.

ture, particularly in the powerful departments of anatomy, physiology, pharmacology, and pathology, which were wedded to the traditional concepts of medical training, and which the old curriculum particularly benefited.[7] In Nottingham, where a new school was planned, a committee under Sir George Pickering announced in June 1965 that the curriculum would be in three parts: three years' training in a biological science, two years of clinical work, and two preregistration years.[8]

A reduction in the length of the undergraduate curriculum and a corresponding increase from one to two years in the preregistration period had advantages from a staffing point of view. To extend the preregistration period to two years would give the hospitals twice as many housemen, even if they were rotated over three- instead of six-months periods, as Sir Charles Illingworth and others suggested.[9] University accreditation of preregistration posts had not in the past brought the universities into effective contact with nonteaching hospital conditions. If a two-year registration period were eventually agreed upon, with one year taken from the undergraduate period, a much greater degree of university participation and supervision would be called for in respect to actual work in hospitals.

Such structural changes were widely discussed. But there was still no definition of the kind of medical person required to practice, teach, or undertake research in the 1970s and 1980s—when today's medical students complete their postgraduate training. "We train them to be possible anatomists, physiologists, biochemists, hospital bed-side observers—but not doctors," two teachers commented on the proposed Nottingham curriculum.[10] Clarification of the purpose of the undergraduate phase of education had clearly to be related to the doctor's future role; and of even more importance, it was contingent on developments in postgraduate training. Yet, although efforts were also made by individuals to reappraise each stage of medical education in relation to the whole educational and training program, there was no one body with the power to reform education and training at the graduate stage.

Training the Specialist

Responsibility for postgraduate education is divided among the professional Colleges, the university medical faculties, and the Ministry of Health. The General Medical Council is concerned primarily with minimum standards of competence for public administrative purposes. It does not oversee the general standards and programs of postgraduate training, and there is no alternative licensing system for specialists; the standard of specialists is largely maintained by the competition for consultant posts. Recent developments in the postgraduate educational structure have indicated the desire of certain specialist groups for an examination to indicate specialist compe-

7. See Anderson and Roberts, pp. 45–46.
8. *The Times,* June 25, 1965, p. 8.
9. *Lancet i* (1964), 283.
10. J. Anderson, F. J. Roberts, *The Times,* June 29, 1965, p. 13.

tence, and it may be that slowly a postgraduate system will develop in parallel with the undergraduate system; that is, under a joint professional board.

A suggestion for the establishment of a voluntary board was made in a professional committee in 1962 (the Porritt report),[11] but so far no action has been taken. Instead, the profession's chief concern in the postgraduate field in the last few years has been skeleton training programs in the nonteaching hospitals: a problem that was finally discussed in practical terms at a special conference on postgraduate education held in Oxford in December 1961.[12] The participants came from all interested spheres—the Ministry of Health, the universities, the Colleges, and the regional and teaching hospital boards. Up to that time, the whole emphasis of hospital staffing had been moving away from the original Spens Committee idea (1948) of a continuous training ladder from house officer to consultant, to more immediate demands for providing service to patients under the impact of specialization. A generation of junior and middle-grade hospital doctors had grown up—and their numbers were increasing year by year—with little or no formal instruction provided within the hospital group. The consensus of the 1961 conference was to reverse this process. All posts, it was suggested, from the preregistration level up, should be recognized as training grades, and all should include an appropriate training program.

Since the teaching hospital had proved an insufficient source of postgraduates, a plan was suggested to shift the focus of postgraduate training onto nonteaching hospitals, in association with the regional university. Each hospital region would continue to have a university postgraduate dean, but his responsibility needed to be widened; he would deal with integration between the regional hospitals and the university, supervise teaching in the region, give career advice, place overseas graduates for training, and bring general practitioners into the training arrangements. As before, he would have a regional postgraduate committee, but it would have wider responsibility. The committee would include, it was thought, eventual responsibility for the rotation of junior staff between specialties and hospitals. The conference agreed that the basic postgraduate training unit of the future should be the all-purpose district (or so-called nonteaching) hospital or the equivalent hospital group. It was recommended that one consultant in each district hospital or group be designated as "clinical tutor" by the regional postgraduate committee. The clinical tutor would have overall responsibility for teaching arrangements, both for medical staff working in the hospital group and for local general practitioners. All consultants attached to the hospitals would be expected, as before, to recognize their own responsibility for train-

11. The report urged that a central independent professional body be established, representing all the professional Colleges, associations, and universities, "not only to co-ordinate training but also to provide accurate data on problems of manpower, and to devise and introduce new methods of training" (p. 147). This suggestion was previously made by Dr. J. R. Ellis, *Lancet i* (1956), 872.

12. *Lancet i* (1962), 367.

ing; but it was suggested that they have time "over and above service commitments" for this purpose. This recommendation was especially timely, as the Platt review committees were then considering the future needs of consultant services; many of these committees did recommend extra teaching time in their consideration of staffing needs. The aim of the conference was to produce an "educational atmosphere in the regional hospital unit." For the first time, it was suggested, a member of staff working solely in a non-teaching hospital would have a direct relationship with the regional university. This was to be an important principle in postgraduate development.

The 1961 conference marked a great step forward, for it set out a practical scheme for building up postgraduate programs. The Nuffield Provincial Hospitals Trust—an independent body—agreed to provide £250,000 to finance experimental regional and area schemes according to the outlined principles, and by 1964, it was financing twenty-two separate educational plans.[13]

The experimental schemes for postgraduate tutors and centers were greeted in certain areas with unprecedented local enthusiasm. The West Cumberland hospital group, in the Newcastle region, which appointed as clinical tutor one of the group's consultant surgeons, claimed in 1964 that 80 or 90 per cent of general practitioners in the area attended its monthly luncheon meetings.[14] The medical profession of the City of Stoke-on-Trent contributed £10,000 out of their own pockets for a professional center and raised £92,000 in contributions. "Their experience had been that in a large regional centre the will that training should be provided was so strong, and the need so keenly felt, that the consultant staff were prepared to provide suitable accommodation by voluntary contribution." [15] Some groups made do with existing accommodations; others put up buildings. Some created ambitious scientific programs; others concentrated initially on social and intellectual gatherings of local hospital doctors, general medical or dental practitioners, and public health officials.

A rather different but related pattern was developed at Exeter, where the university, which had no medical school, approved the establishment of a postgraduate medical institute in 1962.[16] This was planned as an institute of the university, in cooperation with the regional medical school at Bristol. Its function is to provide an initial course for overseas graduates and re-

13. The Nuffield Provincial Hospitals Trust, *Sixth Report 1961–1964* (London, 1964), p. 10.

14. Personal communication. See also references to the Portsmouth group, *Brit. Med. J. ii* (1963), 304 (E.M. Darmady); Postgraduate Centre at the Whittington Hospital, London *(Brit. Med. J. i* 1964, 1390); Kent Postgraduate Medical Centre at Canterbury (ibid., p. 1518); Postgraduate School of the Midlands, Birmingham *(Brit. Med. J. i* 1963, 254); Postgraduate Medical School of Warwickshire *(Lancet i,* 1964, 677); Kingston medical centre, St. Albans medical centre *(Brit. Med. J. ii,* 1962, 1759, R. S. Murley); etc.

15. *Brit. Med. J. ii* (1963), 304 (J. P. P. Stock).

16. *Lancet ii* (1962), 1038.

fresher courses for British graduates returning to practice (e.g. from overseas; or married women returning after a period of family responsibilities). The first staff consisted of a medical director (a consultant physician) with supporting services, and it was intended to add lecturers in various aspects of medicine. The need was long overdue for a center that would introduce foreign graduates to different aspects of British practice and give them supervised practical assignments. As the overseas relations officer of the Royal College of Physicians had remarked, "Some visitors went home as happy diplomates: others returned less contented, after exploitation in the less popular posts of the National Health Service." [17] A similar but smaller scheme was started in Birmingham in 1963.

These postgraduate schemes and centers offered enormous potential for training and research. One such possibility was forecast by the establishment of a research center at Stoke Mandeville (nonteaching) Hospital. A study at this hospital would include a survey of the medical and social needs of the elderly in the community, undertaken by GPs, a geriatrician, and the Medical Officer of Health.[18] Little has yet been done in interdisciplinary surveys or in cooperation between hospital and community personnel. How far this potential will be realized in the form of hospital clubs and centers remains to be seen. Many of the existing centers appear to be geared chiefly to the edification of general practitioners, who have—and this is a point of criticism—no formal attachment to the hospital unless they happen to spend a half day a week as a consultant's assistant in the outpatient department. The centers may prove to be more valuable in increasing informal relationships among doctors and in stimulating self-education than in actually conveying knowledge or mounting community research projects or organizational experiments. The real test will come when the scheme moves from the experimental areas, which were receptive and may not be typical, to all nonteaching hospital groups or group combinations—which, it is hoped, will eventually be done.

In the early stages of the experiment there was some question whether the Ministry of Health or the universities would be financially responsible for such schemes. At a conference at the Ministry of Health early in 1962, it was agreed that the development of a scheme for providing both formal medical teaching and continuous education in regional board hospitals was essential, but not until November 1963 did the Ministry accept financial responsibility for continuing the postgraduate scheme when the Nuffield Trust money ceased, the cost to be met by each regional board.[19] It was suggested that the organization include the university postgraduate dean at regional level and clinical tutors appointed from the hospital staff at group or hospital level. It was also agreed that there be a regional postgraduate

17. Ibid., p. 1049.
18. C. L. Greenbury, *Brit. Med. J. ii* (1964), 626.
19. *Annual Report of the Chief Medical Officer of the Ministry of Health,* 1962, p. 210. *Brit. Med. J.* Suppl. *i* (1964), 4.

committee composed of representatives of the university, the Royal Colleges, the College of General Practitioners and the regional hospital board. At last, regional coordination between the chief training bodies might be achieved.

Hospital boards had shown interest in the programs; some had included provision for a postgraduate medical education suite in their detailed building plans. The Ministry's decision was a landmark in principle. The regional hospital (as opposed to the undergraduate teaching hospital) was accepted as a center for postgraduate education of specialists and general practitioners. The Ministry of Health had accepted a further professional responsibility, thrust upon it (since the universities had been unable to establish effective programs) by the medical profession. In education as well as in manpower planning, such decisions were becoming more centralized; they were regarded as much the province of the administration (or more so) as of the professional bodies.

Whether the postgraduate schemes will in fact spread to each non-teaching hospital depends on local interest, and on sufficient funds being made available as an inducement to hospital staff that might not otherwise be motivated. The Ministry's first announcements indicated only limited financial support.[20] It remains to be seen how far and on what lines teaching centers will develop, and the nonteaching hospitals thereby earn the title of postgraduate teaching hospitals. The Ministry, the Colleges and the universities might also provide effective stimulation in other ways, such as including postgraduate participation as a condition of raised salaries for hospital staffs, organizing pooled facilities for teaching material (tapes, films, and so on) and for rosters of teachers, or accrediting hospitals which fulfill certain conditions for preregistration or other posts and for the various specialist examinations. Such possibilities emphasize the need for a strong national postgraduate board or council with certain mandatory powers.

While these experiments in establishing clinical tutors and institutes outside the teaching hospitals continued through joint voluntary, university, and National Health Service effort, the Royal College of Surgeons brought to fruition its own surgical postgraduate training scheme, also financed by the Nuffield Provincial Hospitals Trust but not an integral part of the NHS training programs. The plan came to light in the College's journal in January 1964, although it was the result of deliberations of the College's special advisory committee on surgical training set up nearly five years before.[21]

---

20. Ministry circular HM (64) no. 69 announced the adjustment of the revenue allocations of regional hospital boards to include allowances for honoraria to staff, for incidental expenses such as secretarial services, and for the work of postgraduate deans. Capital expenditure was, however, to be met from the boards' existing budgets. Under these proposals enthusiastic boards might build or upgrade facilities for teaching and provide money for good libraries, etc.; other boards might feel that there were more urgent calls on their limited budgets, and offer local groups only minimum support for developing teaching programs. See D. H. Patey et al. *Brit. Med. J. ii* (1965), 557–64.

21. *Annals of the Royal College of Surgeons of England, 34* (1964), 70.

The Royal College of Surgeons had appointed a consultant in each of the fifteen hospital regions in England and Wales, who, with the president and council members, sat as a College panel of advisers in surgical training. All major branches of surgery were represented, and the meetings were also attended by representatives from the Ministry of Health and from the Scottish and Irish Colleges of Surgery. These regional panel advisers formed a link between the College and the regional hospital board and the university's postgraduate medical dean. In addition to this, and on an experimental basis, surgical tutors were appointed in the regions, under the supervision of the regional panel adviser, to cover one hospital or a group of hospitals. By the beginning of 1964, twenty-six such tutors had been appointed in England and Wales. Duties of the surgical tutor were similar to those of the all-purpose clinical tutors. He was to arrange seminars, joint ward rounds, and other educational programs; to establish study facilities; to arrange time off for study; to encourage research; and to "organize the provision of educational facilities in his area." It was explained that the plan was exploratory, and various methods of approach were in fact envisaged.

The Surgeons' scheme was independent of the one being adopted by regional hospital boards. The group surgical tutor would be available to give advice to the board, but he would look via the panel adviser (a College appointee) to the Royal College of Surgeons instead of to the regional board or the university. The College foresaw no difficulty; their scheme would "in no way conflict" with the joint regional schemes but would complement them. Organizationally, it was a logical extension of the College's supervision of its fellowship program. The council of the College had decided to modify the examination requirements for the FRCS to include an additional year as registrar or equivalent in an approved hospital or post (i.e. the candidate would have to be qualified for at least four years before sitting for the final examination). The College's interest in postgraduate training was thus to be extended through a large part of junior-grade training—one year of preregistration, followed by at least three years in house officer and registrar posts. In the long run, the separation of the regional and the Surgeons' training schemes may be wasteful of facilities. New district hospitals may find themselves with a clinical tutor in sugery and a clinical tutor in medicine—possibly a retrogression in the progress toward union between the two old branches and the newer branches of medical science, and in the growing responsibility of the employing boards for organizing postgraduate training. But this would not occur for many years; meanwhile there is a need for the proliferation of such experiments.

While clinical and surgical tutors were being appointed, a closer relationship was being suggested for the specialist institutes—the postgraduate medical schools attached to certain eminent specialist hospitals or groups of hospitals in London. In the 1940s these schools were linked for teaching purposes under the British Postgraduate Medical Federation, a constituent of London University. The hospitals, like the undergraduate teaching hospitals, were brought into the National Health Service under boards of governors which were directly responsible to the Ministry of Health.

By the 1960s the thirteen specialist institutes with their associated NHS hospitals were sizable; each had a full range of services and associated specialties. Although the institutes were federated, their resources were not pooled. Each specialist hospital and institute had developed out of, or around, an arbitrary clinical specialty whose identity in most cases had been recognized in the very different medical climate of the nineteenth century. Each was located on a separate site, and each had its own budget and its own program. The institutes feared that a specialty might lose its identity if it were merged in an aggregation of hospitals or institutes, and hence fail to attract patients with obscure diseases, visitors in that specialty from abroad, and the best postgraduate students. But now the boundaries of the specialties could not always be confined within the old divisions. Major advances in the specialties in the previous quarter century had not, it was claimed in 1962, come mainly from the special hospitals. One instance of indirect development from extraneous sources was provided by the surgical approach to diseases of the central nervous system and the cardiovascular system. Intellectual isolation followed when the specialties were separated from general science and from general medicine and surgery. There appeared to be a growing need for links between them.

A committee of six eminent medical teachers set up in 1961 considered the various alternatives.[22] Each institute could move to an undergraduate teaching hospital with which it could be associated; but this would involve the danger of a loss of identity by the special hospital, and complicating factors included excessive size of the merged group, the conflicting duties of undergraduate and postgraduate education, and two boards of governors with opposing loyalties. Alternatively, some or all of the institutes could move to the Postgraduate Medical School at Hammersmith. This scheme again, however, entailed the difficulties of a possible loss of identity and excessive size. The only viable arrangement, according to the committee, was for the institutes to associate in groups of four to six around the periphery of a circle. A number of specialist hospitals situated near each other could share such services as a blood bank and a central sterile supply department; moreover, together they could provide social and recreational facilities which would ease the recruitment of nursing and other staff. On the perimeter would be the research departments and library peculiar to each specialty, with smaller seminar rooms and a lecture theater. Nearer the center would be such departments as pathology, microbiology, biochemistry, genetics, biometry, and medical physics. At the nucleus would be a central library, a large lecture theater, a department of medical illustration, and an animal house serving the group. By this method the ill effects of physical conglomeration might be avoided. Hospitals might retain their boards of governors and their own methods of recruiting medical staff, and each

22. University Grants Committee, *Postgraduate Medical Education and the Specialties* (HMSO, 1962).

specialist hospital would have its own wards and operating theaters. These recommendations were accepted by the Ministry of Health. It was agreed to put them into effect if and when rebuilding allowed.

Observable Trends and Future Problems

There are thus in 1966 three separate educational movements: one relating to undergraduate and preregistration education, the second to postgraduate training, and the third to reorganization of the national specialty institutes in London. All reflect the fragmentation of specialism in the past and the search for a new cohesion; and all raise questions of responsibility for action.

The need for coordination of medical practice and education at all levels is apparent. In some spheres this has been undertaken; but in neither the medical staffing structure nor the postgraduate examination system (the two major examples) is there as yet a similar scheme for organizational unity. One problem is the division of responsibility for various aspects of education and planning. Undergraduate programs fall to the university medical schools. The postgraduate period is the professional responsibility of the Colleges and specialty associations and the administrative responsibility of the Ministry of Health and the university postgraduate deans. In accepting major responsibility for training in hospitals, the Ministry of Health has opened the gate to a number of other related questions and possibilities for experiment. It would be possible, for example, to rotate all hospital and GP trainees through carefully defined posts in hospital specialties and general practice; or to exclude all middle-grade staff from teaching hospitals, so that all doctors spend part of their time in nonteaching units; or to concentrate the senior registrar program on major nonteaching centers, thus making them postgraduate teaching schools and freeing the university schools to develop undergraduate programs.

Conversely, it might be desirable under the new curricula for all undergraduates to spend at least part of their time in typical district hospitals. As teaching hospitals assume the responsibilities of a district hospital—that is, the provision of comprehensive hospital services for the immediate area—there should be a decreasing functional difference between them and nonteaching district hospitals of similar size. Eventually all NHS hospitals may be full teaching hospitals. Thus the educational system has direct relevance to questions of organization and structure. It would be possible through training links to improve relations between consultants and GPs, and between teaching and nonteaching hospitals, even though the formal structure remains unchanged.

Both the Royal College of Physicians and the Royal College of Surgeons have recently revised their criteria for postgraduate training, and the other specialist bodies will probably follow a similar pattern: about two years in a general subject or general aspects of a specialty after registration, followed by about five years of specialty training—an eight-year postgraduate training in all, including the preregistration year. The professional phase thus falls into two parts—a general training, for example in general medicine or general surgery, followed by a specialist attachment. Unfortunately, this pattern does not follow the divisions into grades of staff in the National Health Service, nor the requirements of the Colleges' own examinations. There are at present four grades of hospital staffing—including those with tenure—before appointment as a consultant: house officer (during and sometimes also after the preregistration or intern year), senior house officer, registrar, and senior registrar. The basic College examinations are usually taken while the doctor is a registrar, as a necessary stepping-stone along the way; the senior registrar grade of some four years provides the grooming for consultant responsibility.

With the acceptance of all grades of hospital staff as training grades, the existing rift between the registrar and the senior registrar grades becomes an anachronism. A more logical pattern for the future, and one under discussion, might be one registrar grade, covering (say) six years, and possibly with a proficiency bar to sort out those of consultant caliber. With the acceptance of the senior house officer and registrar grades as training posts, it would be possible to arrange for rotation of staff in these, as well as in the senior registrar grade, both between hospitals and between specialties. Specialist medical training would therefore at last be an organizational continuum. Nevertheless, this pattern alone would not solve the equally compelling need to integrate trainee general practitioners and trainee specialists into one staffing structure. A possible line of development here might be the extension of the registrar grades to include general practice as one of the training specialties, and the abolition in the GP administrative structure of either trainees or assistants.

Though social adjustment is being encouraged in undergraduate university courses, and professional interrelationships established through the hospital service in conjunction with the regional university, the professional bodies still have to bear the major responsibility for actual training requirements, and thus the basic standards of general and specialist practice. But as yet, little has been done to make the influence of professional bodies felt within the hospitals. The surgical tutor scheme of the Royal College of Surgeons is an extension of its role; and it is possible that in the future the Royal College of Physicians may reconsider accrediting hospitals for training for the MRCP. But the knotty problem of relating the postgraduate examination system to the hospital and general practice training ladder, or vice versa, remains unsolved. The answer to the question: "What is a specialist?" is still ambiguous, for consultant or specialist status bears no absolute relationship to the fulfillment of the criteria laid down by the professional bodies. Members of appointment committees supposedly receive copies of the relative criteria, but there is still no place for the fully trained "specialist" (according to the College definition) who has not been appointed to a consultant post. He must await his turn on the ladder, hoping for the best.

Definition of a fully trained general practitioner is equally vague. The new regional training schemes are attempting to educate the general practitioner in the latest hospital procedures and to bring him physically into the hospital. But it is not clear what specific aims the schemes should have—to pass examinations, to keep up to date with the latest discoveries, to undertake research, or to encourage morale? If every hospital is to become a teaching hospital, the relationship between regional hospitals and the university hospital might be strengthened if they were linked under one local administration. But such an alliance would not of itself clarify the position of either type of hospital in the local community, in relation to general practice or to the population as a whole.

The major problems of education are thus related to definition of medical practice at both undergraduate and postgraduate levels, the structure of the National Health Service, and the relative responsibilities of university, profession, and state. The universities and the hospitals, under the NHS, accepted extended (if lukewarm) responsibility for medical education in the regional hospital structure. The Colleges were in the unique position of being able to specify and, through their prestige, to control training in each specialty field, including general practice. But, like the universities, they had to contend with their own legacies from the past. While expert committees and individuals were pondering in the early 1960s the practical steps to be taken to review the whole structure of medicine—the result of rapid and recent scientific change—the Royal College of Physicians was being pressed by specialty groups for further fragmentation—the result of a movement that had gestated for fifty years or more.

23

Specialties in the 1960s: New Dimensions

There are recognizable stages in the emergence of a scientific field from the part-time or particular interest of one or more practitioners to a professional subgroup whose members practice exclusively in a well-defined field. Nineteenth and early twentieth century specialization—like the new and developing specialty fields today—was reflected in the special interest of individuals and in scientific societies rather than in the formation of specialist regulating bodies. More recently, there appears to have been a certain compulsion for relatively large groups of specialists to become self-regulating branches of medicine with their own postgraduate examinations and with a powerful interest in advancing the status of their specialty. Improvement in standards is a primary motivation, but this is inevitably linked with improving prestige. The Royal College of Physicians and the Royal College of Surgeons were very early examples. Two recent claimants for similar status are pathology and psychiatry, described in this chapter.

This development of specialties as professional groups imposes a degree of structural rigidity on the development of the specialites, and raises new questions of defining a specialty or specialist status. Is there a legitimate difference between a "branch" of medicine (organizationally signified by the establishment of a professional examining College or faculty); a specialty within that branch (such as ophthalmology within the body of surgery); or a subspecialty or special interest within a particular specialty? The question has implications which concern both the development of postgraduate training programs in specialties, and professional representation: the latter a result of the Colleges' role in relation to the National Health Service.

The Present State of Specialization: The Changing Structure of Hospital Practice

Medical specialties cannot readily be compartmentalized. Ear, nose, and throat specialists fall organizationally within the Royal College of Surgeons, although recent developments, particularly the introduction of antibiotics, have made the otolaryngologist a physician as much as he is a surgeon. Like other specialists he has close links with several related branches of practice;

336

through irradiation for malignant diseases of the larynx, for example, he is in close touch with the radiotherapist and physicist. Ophthalmology overlaps the sphere of the nasal surgeon, the dermatologist, the psychiatrist, and the allergist, as well as the diagnostic and ancillary specialties.

Endocrinology, pigeon-holed as a subspecialty of general medicine, in fact cuts across the biological sciences, medicine, surgery, and gynecology. Clinical endocrinologists may have a background training in physiology, internal medicine, or a specialty onto which endocrinology may be grafted. Similarly, anesthesiology, organizationally linked with surgery, is developing wide claims across a number of originally distinct areas. It was said as early as 1952 that "The anaesthetist of the future must be a physician, a pharmacologist, a physiologist, a biochemist, an electronic engineer and a toxicologist." [1]

Cardiology is a spectacular example of the trend to regroup various specialties around specific techniques or conditions. "The present stream of cardiology is so broad," wrote a specialist reviewing the position in 1958, "that no physician or surgeon can claim to have mastered all its reaches." [2] Heart surgery requires a team of experts from medical, surgical, and non-medical fields: surgery itself, anesthesiology, cardiology, cardiological techniques, the full range of laboratory specialties, physiology, radiology, physics, and engineering.

Pediatrics illustrates the impact of subspecialization on holistic fields. The pediatric physician has been joined by subspecialists from a number of different disciplines; there are now pediatric surgeons, child psychiatrists, and pediatric radiologists. As a result, the scope of general pediatrics has become so wide that its future development is in some doubt. New subjects were appearing by the 1960s on the curriculum of some medical schools which were not being taught even a decade before—child development and its delays and disorders, recurrent ailments with a powerful psychological component, chronic illnesses, neurological and intellectual handicaps, and behavior problems.

In one sense the new specialties facilitated teamwork, but they did so within areas that were regarded as specialties themselves. They cut across the traditional organizational structure of medicine, thus creating further fragmentation. Pediatrics, neurology, and cardiology had been subspecialties of general medicine. Would the pediatric surgeon of the future identify himself more closely with pediatrics or with surgery? Would he remain a general surgeon with an interest in children, or would he regard himself as a specialist in children? The old process of division reappeared, but now at the level of the specialties.

The subspecialties, like the specialties before them, were focused primarily on disease. The more esoteric they became the more clearly disease-oriented they tended to be; by 1963 there were rheumatologists, neuro-

1. Peter Orchard Williams, ed., *Careers in Medicine* (London, 1952), p. 27.
2. *Brit. Med. J. i* (1958), 955.

radiologists, neurological physiologists, and specialists in chemotherapy. Technologically, the disease focus required more rational hospital planning: regional centers for open heart surgery, for the treatment of major burns and other accidents, for neurological conditions, and so on. As medicine concentrated on advanced techniques and the use of interrelated skills, the specialist was moving farther away from the healthy person in society. The dilemma was one of continuing the advance in medical science while responding to the equally compelling human need for personal medical care. There was a basic conflict between the desirability (indeed, the necessity) for further specialization to advance knowledge, and the organizational problems that came in its wake; between the need for narrower and deeper training in the specialties, and relating the new specialties most effectively to all other expanding fields of medicine.

The issues were infinitely more complex than at previous controversial periods when the relationships of generalism and specialism were argued. In the late nineteenth century the underlying issue was competition for patients. In the 1930s, specialization was regarded as a necessary evil, but its full implications were not apparent. By the 1960s there was no illusion of a return to generalism. The abandonment of the undergraduate curriculum as training for general practice was merely a belated recognition of all doctors as specialists in one field or another.

There remained several schools of thought. One, already discussed, was the introduction of a new type of generalism into the undergraduate field, as part of an attempt to emphasize medicine as an art as well as a science—as a new humanism.[3] A second, represented in the continuation of the general MRCP and FRCS examinations, was resistance to pressures to begin specialist training until after a period of general postgraduate experience. Finally, there were those who believed that early specialization was beneficial and should be actively encouraged. There was evidence that candidates in some specialties did not receive sufficient background knowledge in their special fields. One specialist observed of the FRCS in otology (the most applicable examination in that specialty) that he had never met a candidate who had any real understanding of the modern hydrodynamic and electrostatic theories of the inner ear, nor one who could correctly define the various units of intensity and loudness: "as if an electrician did not know what a volt was." [4] The questions of competence in a special field and knowledge over a wide area were once more in conflict, this time at the postgraduate level.

In the end, the question was academic, for there was as yet no way of ascertaining from the point of view of patient care whether specialists trained in one way were better than specialists trained in another. The practical

3. On the renewal of emphasis on medicine as an art as well as a science, see Robert Platt, *Universities Quarterly, 17* (1963), 327; George Pickering, *Brit. Med. J. ii* (1963), 133.
4. *Brit. Med. J. ii* (1963), 867 (A. Tumarkin).

answers rested with the professional medical bodies and pertained to two important questions, one relating to the Colleges and the second to the expectations of specialist groups. First, how far would the two primary branches of medicine and surgery, represented in the two older Royal Colleges with their generalist traditions, feel able to adapt their own structures to the further demands for independence when they inevitably arose? And second, would the emerging groups seek to remain within the existing College structure? If they did, organizational flexibility as well as comprehensiveness within each branch of medicine might be maintained. On the other hand, obstetricians and general practitioners had shown the advantages to their members of separate Colleges.

Pathology and psychiatry—both of which had benefited from the process of subspecialization—provided the opportunity to test these questions in the 1960s.

Specialties as Professional Organizations: The Importance of the College System

Both pathology and psychiatry expanded rapidly under the National Health Service. In 1964 each branch contained 10 per cent of all NHS consultants. Each was exceeded in size only by general medicine and general surgery, with their related specialties, and by anesthesiology. Both psychiatrists and pathologists outnumbered obstetrician–gynecologists by five to three; yet the obstetricians had their own Royal College.[5] Thus in terms of size alone there was a clear incentive for each specialty to form its own examining body. In addition, both specialties, but particularly pathology, were developing into vast fields with their own problems of specialization. General pathology was becoming moribund even faster than was general medicine, and psychiatry was subdivided both by areas of practice (e.g. child psychiatry; the psychiatry of the subnormal) and types of treatment. Yet for both pathologists and psychiatrists the only diploma of prestige was that of the Royal College of Physicians, and this examination was retained until 1964 over all the specialties of general medicine. The aspiring cardiologist or dermatologist took the same MRCP examination as the child psychiatrist or hematologist.

For both pathologists and psychiatrists, the deficiencies of the general MRCP were quoted as primary motives for setting up their own specialist examining bodies. Indeed, it was claimed in the early 1950s that the lack of a suitable higher diploma in pathology, comparable to the MRCP or FRCS, definitely influenced high-quality graduates to reject pathology as a career.[6]

5. Of the 7,973 consultants in 1964, 799 were in psychiatry and 810 were in pathology. In contrast there were only 485 gynecologist–obstetricians. Ministry of Health *Annual Report for 1964*, p. 146.

6. *Lancet ii* (1960), 863. This feeling of inferiority, said one correspondent, was likely to be intensified "when a man has attended a few appointment committees and had to explain why he has no higher qualification." Ibid., *ii* (1962), 1320 (A. G. Signy).

The Conjoint Board of the Royal Colleges had instituted a diploma in pathology (D.Path.) in 1950, to be taken after three years' experience in clinical pathology; there was also a Diploma in Clinical Pathology from the University of London. But it was claimed by proponents of a new higher examination that the first was not popular and the second too easy for those who took the appropriate postgraduate course in London and too difficult for those who did not. As with certain other specialist diplomas, the university diploma had become the haven of students from abroad, who used it—although this was not the intention—as a mark of specialist skill when they returned to their own countries to practice.[7]

The Diploma in Psychological Medicine (DPM) was the usual postgraduate examination for psychiatrists. This diploma was awarded by nine separate institutions: six universities and the professional Conjoint Boards of England, Scotland, and Ireland. The standard of this diploma varied from one examining body to the next, ranging downward from the DPM of London University, which followed an intensive three-year course at the Institute of Psychiatry.[8] But even the London DPM did not have the cachet of the MRCP, which was thought to mark outstanding ability rather than acquired technique. Many eminent psychiatrists (and pathologists) were members of the Royal College of Physicians; some had been elected fellows. The ordinary psychiatrist or pathologist—the aspiring consultant or SHMO to a large nonteaching hospital group—remained, however, outside this elite, concentrating on the specialist diploma and moving as quickly as possible into the career field of his choice. To him the MRCP seemed irrelevant; nor was he inclined to delay learning in his own specialty while gaining the experience in general medicine that he would need to pass that examination.

The functional gap between the Royal College of Physicians and the Royal College of Surgeons had widened in the 1950s. The Surgeons appeared to be developing as a College of Surgical Sciences. The Physicians, with its one general postgraduate diploma, the MRCP, was in theory a College for all medical specialties. But general medicine as a consultant field was being increasingly limited to the practice of internal medicine, instead of being a practice including a range of medical skills. Sooner or later the College had to make a major decision to follow the Surgeons and become a multifaceted College of Medical Sciences. Otherwise it might find itself bereft of major groups that had developed within "general" medicine but did not regard themselves as subspecialties of "internal" medicine. Pathology and psychiatry were merely the largest of such groups; pediatrics was a third.

Size of specialty and the increasing divergence of the specialty from the subject matter offered by College examinations provided two cogent argu-

7. *Lancet* i (1956), 375 ('Peter Davey'). The international implications of British postgraduate medical diplomas deserve further study. See Additional Notes, p. 371–72.

8. The candidate for the DPM of the English Conjoint Board, in contrast, has to have had two years' experience in a recognized psychiatric hospital, but there are no stated requirements for courses of study or instruction.

ments for independent specialty colleges or faculties. A further inducement was the potential for raising professional status. Psychiatrists and pathologists had had an inauspicious history; both had developed outside the mainstream of prestige. With minor exceptions, neither had the ultimate accolade of beds in the old voluntary teaching hospitals. Mingled with the desire for an independent examining structure, which might be provided (following the example of the Royal College of Surgeons) by semiautonomous faculties within the Royal College of Physicians, there was therefore a strong interest in enhanced prestige.[9] The question of relative status had been one reason, perhaps the major reason, for the foundation of the College of Obstetricians and Gynaecologists, for the Faculty of Radiologists and, more recently, for the College of General Practitioners. The success of these bodies was self-evident. They had raised the competence and professional standing of their respective fields, and they had increased the prestige of their membership both within the medical profession and in relation to the Ministry of Health.

The central policy-making role of the Colleges in the National Health Service added a further and perhaps more material incentive to separate from them. The pathologist who wished to exert power within the Royal College of Physicians first had to gain his MRCP and then hope to be elected a fellow. In both cases he felt he was in unfavorable competition with specialists in the more fashionable fields of medicine. The psychiatrist was in a similar position. This was not necessarily true of the eminent pathologists and psychiatrists working in major teaching and nonteaching centers and in close contact with leading practitioners in other medical fields; but it was likely to be true of the younger consultants in these specialties, who were appointed under the National Health Service to general and mental hospitals away from the teaching hospital centers—and whose numbers and status rapidly increased under the impact of the NHS. If the pathologist or psychiatrist felt his interests were not sufficiently served within the Royal College of Physicians, it followed that he was not properly represented on the professional bodies in which the College had members: the Distinction Awards Committee, the Joint Consultants Committee, and the General Medical Council.

These various combined factors stimulated demands for separate Colleges. For both pathologists and psychiatrists the underlying arguments were similar. They concerned examinations, status, and professional representation. But in both groups there was considerable opposition to such changes. The older established consultants at the teaching hospitals and in London tended to favor continuing within the Royal College of Physicians; the younger nonteaching and provincial hospital men (products of the postwar period) tended to favor separation.

9. This was marked by a feeling of professional inferiority on the part of the separatists. "As the Pharisee thanked God he was not as other men," wrote one correspondent, "do not Physicians preen themselves ever so slightly on not being Paediatricians, Psychiatrists, or Pathologists?" *Lancet ii* (1959), 231 ('Peter Davey').

A College of Pathology: Diverging Views and Ultimate Solutions

Pathologists had two major professional organizations. The Association of Clinical Pathologists (ACP), with a membership of over 1,000 in 1961, was the more politically inclined. The Pathological Society of Great Britain and Ireland, from which the ACP had developed in the 1920s, was primarily an academic and educational body. It was larger and internationally better known than the ACP, but it was criticized by some for its "political nihilism." [10] The two societies were complementary and had an overlapping membership. The College movement was dependent on the goodwill of both organizations. It took nine years (from 1953 when the ACP held preliminary discussions) before the interests of both groups were finally reconciled.

The movement for a College gained momentum within the Association of Clinical Pathologists. The report of an ACP subcommittee of 1955 reflected the ambivalence over the various factors involved in setting up a new body. It was readily agreed that the MRCP was not a suitable diploma for pathologists, but there was a reluctance to embark on the major step a separate foundation would imply. Nevertheless the seed was germinating. After reviewing existing diplomas, particularly the possibility of modifying the diplomas offered by the London and Edinburgh Royal Colleges, another ACP committee in 1958 came out more clearly in favor of establishing a College of Pathology.

The Edinburgh MRCP, unlike its London counterpart, had included pathology as a special subject from its foundation in 1881. Candidates were, however, expected also to be proficient in general medicine, in which there were written, clinical, and oral examinations; and the College was reportedly not willing in the late 1950s to expand the section on pathology in its MRCP examination at the expense of clinical medicine and pharmacology.[11] In any event, the London MRCP was more highly esteemed; the "unnatural keenness of competition among physicians has given to the Edinburgh membership in medicine, merely because it is ever so slightly easier than the London one, an undeserved stigma as a soft option, and the reasonable and respectable Membership has suffered in consequence." [12] It was probable that pathologists, seeking to enhance their status as well as their skills, would prefer a solution within the London, rather than the Edinburgh, College. But the Royal College of Physicians of London, although apparently willing at this point to establish a Mastership in Pathology, would not include the opportunity for the successful candidate to qualify for subsequent election to College fellowship (FRCP)—a matter of utmost importance for improving specialty status.

The university M.D. and Ph.D. were also rejected by the ACP committee

10. *Lancet i* (1956), 375 ('Peter Davey').
11. *Lancet ii* (1960), 863.
12. *Lancet i* (1956), 375 ('Peter Davey').

as indications of consultant ability, even though nonmedical Ph.D.s, particularly biochemists, worked by the side of medical pathologists and in some instances replaced them. Except for academic appointments, said one correspondent, higher university degrees "probably still frightened more than they attracted the jungly fringes that still controlled most selection committees." [13] Most of all, university degrees would not give to pathologists as a group the sense of unity, strength, and status that might be conferred by an educational body which was under their own control. Short of a major change of policy by the Royal College of Physicians of London, only a separate foundation appeared to offer all hoped-for benefits.

Circulars among members both of the ACP and the Pathological Society in 1958 elicited a favorable response to founding a College, but there was still considerable doubt about the wisdom of such a step. It was argued that even if a separate examination were devised for pathologists, it would have to be similar to the MRCP; that is, an examination taken early in the career to pick out the best available candidate for further training, rather than a test of competence as a consultant. The stumbling block in this case was not the purpose but the existing bias of the MRCP toward the selection of clinicians rather than scientists. Nor could many see an overriding need for a separate college as a political organization, since the ACP had for several years spoken on behalf of hospital pathologists both directly to the Ministry of Health and through the mediation of the Joint Consultants Committee.[14] Connection with the Royal College, it was stressed by many, merely needed to be modified.

Such views were reinforced in mid-1959 when the Royal College of Physicians proposed granting certain concessions which accorded with conditions made by a working party of the ACP as an alternative to a separate college.[15] The working party had recommended that a faculty or division of pathology be set up within the Royal College of Physicians, under the administrative control of a self-elected council, and that admission be by an examination controlled by the faculty with generous provision for the foundation membership. These terms were similar to those granted by the Royal College of Surgeons to its constituent Faculties of Anaesthetists and Dental Surgeons. Members of a faculty of pathologists would be eligible for the full FRCP in the same way and by the same machinery as members of the College. This would not necessarily mean that more pathologists would become fellows, since no modifications were apparently suggested in the status and responsibility of fellows as a group. Nevertheless, the existence of this possibility and the opening of a reasonable alternative strengthened the hand of those who opposed a separate foundation. At a meeting of the ACP in September 1960, it was made clear that "many of the older or wiser heads"

13. Ibid.
14. See, for example, the presidential address of Dr. McMenemy to the Association of Clinical Pathologists in 1958: *Lancet ii* (1958), 843.
15. *Lancet ii* (1960), 863.

had decided for such a faculty. Many of the speeches from the floor, however, still "spoke hotly for the college." [16]

In the last months of 1960, intensive lobbying took place at society meetings, through the medical journals, and by private persuasion. Of those who voted in the ACP's postal ballot at the turn of the year (1960–61) 415 wanted a new institution; 350 favored a faculty within the Royal College of Physicians.[17] A similar referendum was put to the Pathological Society. The votes were indicative, if not conclusive, of a desire for a College and, after balloting, a joint committee of the ACP and the Pathological Society was set up to make practical recommendations on what to do next. The Joint Committee had no hesitation. In December 1961 it unanimously recommended the establishment of a separate College for pathologists, one of whose first tasks would be to establish a higher examination.[18] The recommendations were circulated to members of both societies, together with further questions to discover the degree of support. In May 1962 it was decided that there was "ample support" for the founding of a College. More than seven hundred senior pathologists said they intended to apply for founder-membership and had sent subscriptions of £50 per head. At a public meeting of three hundred of these subscribers the following month, the motion in favor of founding a College of Pathologists was passed unanimously.[19]

One immediate and controversial question was whether to include nonmedical laboratory workers in the new College. This applied specifically to biochemists, who were often designated as chemical pathologists. Was a medical biochemist to be included in the College, but a nonmedical biochemist to be left out? There were many implications in the decision, not least of which was how far pathology ought to be a distinct scientific branch, related to medicine but not necessarily subservient to it. The foundation of a separate College indicated a break between pathology and general postgraduate clinical medicine. The break might logically be extended to include those trained in related scientific disciplines. But these questions remained unanswered, since biochemists themselves expressed no desire to add a further examination to their own graduate degrees or diplomas in chemistry. "Let the pathologist stick to his microscope," wrote one correspondent, "and leave biochemistry to those qualified to practise the subject." [20]

The College of Pathologists was founded in 1962 after a long campaign that had been by no means harmonious. Many pathologists, it had been observed, including some of the older and more influential, "just frankly do not want to be organized." [21] Nevertheless the College grew quickly. A

16. Ibid., p. 921 ('Peter Davey').
17. *Lancet i* (1961), 382.
18. *Brit. Med. J. i* (1962), 1258.
19. Ibid., pp. 1550, 1820.
20. *Lancet ii* (1960), 985 (E. B. Hendry).
21. Ibid., *i* (1956), 375 ('Peter Davey').

postal ballot in 1963 for the election of officers and council was circulated to over 1,100 subscribers. All medically qualified pathologists of consultant or similar status were automatically eligible for membership without examination—a system that was to continue until April 1966. The first examination for membership was held in 1964. It was designed in two parts: a broadly based primary examination taken after at least two years' full-time work in pathology, and a final examination in one of the four main branches of pathology (hematology, morbid anatomy, bacteriology, biochemistry).

The College of Pathologists was the first to break away from the old Royal Colleges since the College of Obstetricians was founded in 1929. It could be argued that pathology had become clearly distinguished from both medicine and surgery. Indeed, with its widely diversified specialties, pathology had greater claims for separate treatment than the combined specialty of obstetrics and gynecology. Alternatively, the separation of the College could be viewed as a failure in adaptation by the Royal College of Physicians, professional home in their time of the father of vaccination, Edward Jenner, and a brilliant host of other laboratory workers. Inexorably the Physicians were being forced to modify their traditional generalist approach.

Psychiatrists and the Royal College of Physicians

The psychiatrists' general professional body was the Royal Medico-Psychological Association (RMPA). This had an open, noncompetitive membership like the other specialty associations; but, unlike others, it was interested in all matters connected with the specialty, including psychiatric nursing. In 1963 the RMPA had a membership of 2,200.[22] It had a royal charter, a distinguished lineage, and its own journal *(The British Journal of Psychiatry)*. Like the Pathological Society and the ACP, it possessed considerable standing in the eyes of the profession. Nevertheless, the voices of psychiatrists began to be raised in the 1950s in favor of founding their own College. The RMPA itself set up a special committee to consider the possibility in November 1960, and—again after long debates on the financial implications, the responsibility for postgraduate education, and the greatest benefits to prestige—the various alternatives were circulated to RMPA members in 1962.

In psychiatry, the gap between the teaching and provincial hospital was wider than in pathology; the dispute was much more clearly one between university teachers and the great body of practitioners. The consultant psychiatrist at a teaching hospital might well be dedicated to neuropsychiatric problems in which he was emotionally or intellectually nearer to his colleagues in neurology—who, of course, were members or fellows of the Royal College of Physicians—than to psychiatrists in the average mental hospital. One correspondent, reflecting some of the provincial consultant's

22. Royal Medico-Psychological Association, *Annual Report,* June 1962–May 1963; and see supplement to *Journal of Mental Science,* Jan. 1963.

isolation, wrote revealingly that to the Royal College of Physicians the concept of psychiatry was "still represented by the teaching hospital psychiatrist with the vague, rural figure of the asylum medical officer in the background." [23] It was claimed that psychiatrists were being forced into the position of considering a complete breakaway from the Royal College of Physicians because, like the pathologists, they were not receiving equal treatment with members of other specialties within the College. The complaints of psychiatrists were, however, refreshingly different from those of pathologists, who had claimed there was no room in the College for scientists; it was declared by some psychiatrists that obtaining the MRCP needed "extensive training in and dedication to clinical medicine, which was increasingly based on mechanistic disciplines like chemistry and physics and was in danger of becoming a technology." Another view was that application to the College for a faculty for psychiatrists would surrender control to a body whose very history and chief membership would tend to keep psychiatry as an "ancillary science to something they would call medicine;" and several claimed that it was "extremely rare" for a nonteaching hospital psychiatrist to be elected a fellow of the RCP.[24] These views were primarily questions of status or representation. Proponents of a solution within the Royal College of Physicians tended to stress the scientific view: that it was impossible to treat mind apart from body, and body apart from mind, and that psychiatry should not therefore be divorced from general medicine.

The RMPA held a debate in November 1963 on the possibility of founding a College of Psychiatry.[25] By this time the College of Pathologists was well underway. It provided a living example to psychiatrists of the practicability of separate status, and undoubtedly whetted the appetites of the separatists. Thus, although it was asserted that the Royal College of Physicians was about to change the regulations for the MRCP examination (the result, said one speaker, of "death bed repentance"), the meeting formally resolved to establish a separate College, subject to a favorable response to a postal ballot.

The Royal College of Physicians made its announcement in the middle of May 1964—only shortly before the RMPA ballot was due. After a long period of debate, the MRCP was to be radically changed. In future, part of the examination might be taken in special subjects instead of in general, or internal, medicine. This was the first major change in the examinations of the College since the MRCP had been introduced one hundred years before (1861). It was thus a landmark in the College's history, as well as an apparent attempt to restrain certain groups from separatist action.

The College announced a restructuring of the examination that could not fail to answer the chief criticisms leveled against it; preselection of candidates (by a multiple-choice test) prior to the clinical examination; the intro-

---

23. *Lancet ii* (1963), 1163 (J. Hutchinson).
24. *Lancet ii* (1962), 1320; *Brit. Med. J. ii* (1962), 1750.
25. *Lancet ii* (1963), 1332 (A. Pearce).

duction of a choice of questions in specialized fields; and failure in one part of the examination not to entail failing the whole. After candidates had been weeded out in Part I, the examination proceeded in two sections. Part II ranged over the whole of general medicine, with question choice. Part III was a specialist examination; candidates might choose to take it in internal medicine, psychiatry, or pediatrics. A fourth possibility, in doubt after the foundation of the College of Pathologists, was pathology. The London MRCP thus drew closer to its Edinburgh counterpart.[26] One peculiarity, however, and initially subject to confusion, was that candidates who did well enough in Part II might be exempt from Part III; an inborn ranking process might therefore result.

Details of the new regulations appeared in the journals, and the president of the RMPA promptly urged members of that association through the columns of the medical press, to "make use of the opportunity created for them to have access to this information before voting." [27] Some psychiatrists saw this move as an attempt to influence the vote. If so, it was too late. Of those who voted in the RMPA poll, over 72 per cent (49 per cent of the total membership) were in favor of their own College. The council of the RMPA agreed in June 1964 to recommend to the body of their membership that they petition the Privy Council to change the name of the Royal Medico-Psychological Association to the Royal College of Psychiatrists; and this resolution was ratified by a "large majority" at the annual general meeting the following month. "The change sought," said the *British Medical Journal,* "is not of name but of status, prestige, and what follows from these, of standards." [28]

Whereas pathologists had merely established a new organization, psychiatrists had the additional complication of their royal charter—which, it seemed, they were not prepared to forego. Just as the title of college had more status than that of faculty or association, the title of *Royal* College was far preferable to the term college alone. It was thus hoped to retain the Royal affix while changing the Association's name and function; and this involved Privy Council ratification and approval of new bye-laws. To the Privy Council, official body for charter matters, the request posed a dilemma. The granting of a Royal Charter had come to imply professional eminence. There were already three Royal Medical Colleges in England. Two other Colleges, the General Practitioners and Pathologists, had prior claims for a charter in terms of their founding dates. If the Privy Council acceded to the request of the RMPA, which had received its charter as a study association (not an examining body), and if more colleges were formed, it might find it had lessened the prestige of the Royal Charter, which was largely gained through exclusiveness. So far this question has not been resolved.

26. See Additional Notes, pp. 370–71.
27. *Brit. Med. J. i* (1964), 1311 (D. Curran).
28. Ibid., p. 1585; *ii,* 137–38.

Specialty Organizations at the Mid-1960s

By changing the regulations for the MRCP, the Royal College of Physicians tacitly admitted a need (whether primarily scientific or primarily political) for recognizing pathology, psychiatry, and the third broad-spectrum specialty of pediatrics to be distinct specialties within the branch of general medicine. But the changes came too late to prevent the formation of the College of Pathologists and agreement for a College of Psychiatrists. These two groups, representing 20 per cent of all consultants, had in effect removed their allegiance from the Royal College of Physicians. Since it may be assumed that pathologists will in future take the membership examination of their own College rather than the MRCP, and that a College of Psychiatrists will eventually set up its own examination, the Royal College of Physicians may develop as an examining body for internal medicine and pediatrics and their related specialties rather than as a college of medicine or of medical sciences.

Correspondence on the deficiencies of the FRCS in relation to otology, ophthalmology, and orthopedics has hinted at further specialist examinations in the surgical specialties. Gayer Morgan wrote in 1963: "It seems quite unacceptable that keen and capable aspiring ophthalmologists should be failed because they do not know the minute anatomy of the pudental nerve, the psoas major, the ext. pollicus longus, and the pubic bone." [29] John Charnley suggested a FRCS in orthopedics as a specialist examination along the lines of the American specialty boards; and he spoke of the "desperate attempt to get the Final Fellowship" by young specialists in orthopedic departments, who were learning parrot fashion instead of being able to immerse themselves in orthopedic surgery.[30] Some wanted separate faculties in the College for these specialties. Others were concerned lest any further changes in the FRCS create a new rash of qualifications in different subspecialties, for example thoracic or neurological surgery. The arguments were familiar. Which was immediately more important to the young graduate: the general view or the swift acquisition of technique? Or were these in fact exclusive aims? Was a general grasp of optics more important to the ophthalmologist than a general grasp of other medical specialties? Was it more beneficial to generalize from a specialty or to specialize after a postgraduate period of general experience—and, in the specialized world of the hospital, how was general experience ideally to be achieved?

Such questions tended to be raised in relation to individual specialties or Colleges, rather than to postgraduate medical education as a whole. Yet the need for decision was universal, and affected general practice as well as the consulting specialties. Answers needed to be related to the length of postgraduate training, the purpose of the preregistration year or years, the appropriate stage for taking a postgraduate diploma, and, by no means least, to the relative functions of GPs and specialists. The Royal College of Phy-

29. *Brit. Med. J. ii* (1963), 743.
30. *Brit. Med. J. i* (1964), 1249.

sicians, in a 1964 report on the training of consultants, recommended seven years or more of postgraduate training for the medical specialties, psychiatry and pathology, including the preregistration (intern) years; for most specialties suggested training included one year of general clinical medicine at the registrar level.[31] The desirability of postgraduate general experience for the future specialist was not clearly stated. Was it to widen the specialist's horizons; or perhaps to enable him more easily to make correct diagnoses? If the general practitioner developed into or was replaced by the equivalent of the consultant general physician, these questions might have different connotations.

There are now seven independent specialty bodies of College stature, shown in Figure 6. Among them they provide fourteen final examinations of membership or fellowship status. In addition, the Conjoint Board of the Royal Colleges of Physicians and Surgeons offers twelve specialist diplomas, such as the Diplomas in Anaesthetics or Child Health, which offer no College affiliation. These do not approach in prestige the diplomas of the membership examinations or, usually, their standards.

Each change moves farther away from the strong postgraduate generalist tradition embodied in the 1944 Goodenough report, and of which the general MRCP and the general FRCS are the last bastions. It is worth questioning where the trend may eventually lead. Both the Royal College of Surgeons and the Royal College of Physicians have now accepted that with the increasing number of hospital medical staff and the growing sophistication of individual specialties, many of which have developed strong ties with nonmedical fields, particular arrangements have become necessary for certain specialist groups. In effecting these, the emphasis has inevitably shifted from a broad educational beginning to the acquisition of particular skills. For many years the older Colleges and a number of specialty associations have issued training criteria to be observed by trainees and by consultant appointments committees, but these have had no mandatory power. Ideally, as the *Lancet* has suggested, the Colleges will extend their influence to the full specialist level, either through raising the level of their examinations or by making acceptance conditional on satisfactory subsequent experience.[32]

The difficulty, as the experience of the pathologists and psychiatrists has shown, is to reconcile the technical education now needed for specialists with whatever advantages there may be in a common postgraduate training. The specialty groups have emphasized the first factor, the Royal Colleges the second. At present the specialty groups appear to be in the ascendant as their fields become more clearly divorced from general medical and surgical practice; and as, in turn, general medicine and general surgery are themselves confined to a limited aspect of the whole general spectrum— general medicine to internal medicine, and general surgery to abdominal and urological surgery. General competence in a wide specialist field is facing a crisis

31. Royal College of Physicians of London, *Report on Training for Consultants* (London, 1964).

32. *Lancet ii* (1963), 561, 1103.

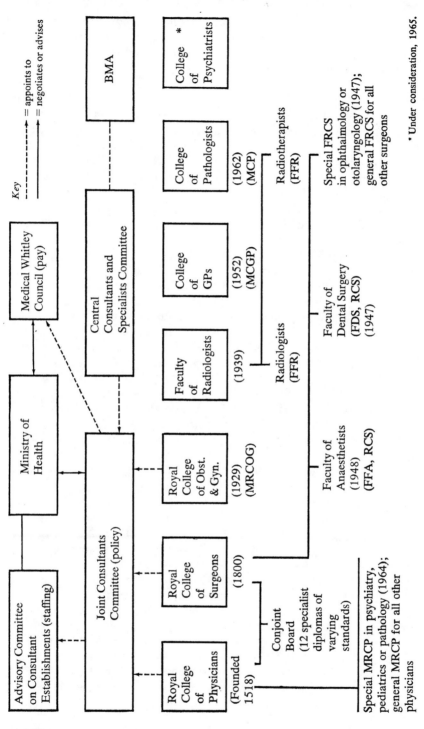

FIGURE 6. *Organization of Colleges and Faculties; England and Wales*

* Under consideration, 1965.

similar to that faced by general practitioner-specialists between the two world wars.

If the divisive movement in specialty examinations continues, the English system may well grow closer to that of the American specialty boards. The Royal College of Surgeons has accepted certain training (as well as examining) responsibilities through the FRCS; it has laid down certain basic requirements for surgical experience which must be fulfilled before the examination, and has developed a system of approving hospitals for such experience, according to recognized criteria.[33] In theory, the College thus wields considerable influence over the standard of surgical facilities; but in practice the approval scheme lacks teeth. Renewal is virtually automatic, the actual survey being made at intervals of ten years. There is no insistence on specific training programs, particular experience, or courses of study. Nor are there regulations for rotating programs, although the FRCS examination covers the whole of surgery. Under the system the individual candidate may spend his time in "general" surgery doing primarily abdominal and urological work, in "casualty" doing minor surgery with some orthopedics, and a varying period in a surgical subspecialty; and he may have little or no formal teaching.

The Royal College of Obstetricians and Gynaecologists approves posts for its membership examination, and the Faculty of Radiologists and the new College of Pathologists also demand specified experience as well as proficiency in their own examinations. The Royal College of Surgeons announced in January 1965 that in future, four years instead of three must elapse between basic qualification and sitting for the final examination for the FRCS, including one year as a full-time registrar.[34] Radiologists have gone farther; they demand at least four years of work in radiological practice and sciences as well as two years' general clinical experience, prior to the fellowship in their faculty (FFR). The College of General Practitioners, unlike the other Colleges, has accepted flexible membership criteria based primarily on experience, research, and evidence of postgraduate training.[35] The Royal College of Physicians, on the other hand, even with its revised arrangements, has kept as close as possible to its traditional pattern of assessment at a particular examination. Proponents claim the advantage of flexibility, pointing to the MRCP as an examination to be taken early in the consultant's career. The Royal College of Physicians has not instituted a system of specified training requirements for the MRCP; nor does it approve or accredit hospitals, although it did suggest in its report on consultant

33. Hospitals may be recognized individually or as a group, and must be of at least 100 beds. The number of surgical beds related to the particular post should be from 25 to 40, inclusive, and the consultant in charge take a "real interest" in providing training and experience. The assessor also confirms that the hospital has adequate departments of pathology and radiology, that the casualty department is supervised by a consultant, and that there are reasonable case records and a suitable library.

34. *Lancet i* (1965), 201.

35. Ibid., *ii* (1964), 1225.

training that training appointments should be in approved hospitals. Since no joint board yet exists for the examining bodies, there is no supervision of the primary function or purpose of each examination. The Colleges have the advantage of flexibility, but at the same time College membership means different things in relation to different specialties.

Whatever the ultimate solution, recent trends emphasize the necessity for combined action by the Colleges in the development of postgraduate education and training of all doctors, from the time of registration to the time of retirement. This is the most immediately important of all professional matters and central to all discussion on questions of staffing and of future manpower planning. Of all their functions, professional training is the one the Colleges are incomparably equipped to fulfill. As undergraduate programs develop as introductory courses, the postgraduate period assumes greater importance. As the sophistication of the specialties proliferates, and as the practice of medicine—such as certain aspects of chemotherapy—becomes potentially more dangerous, standards of competence become a question of acute concern.

The Colleges are in a position to exert necessary checks and balances. If they move before other specialty groups demand special treatment, further fragmentation of the professional bodies may be forestalled. Unified, the Colleges and faculties might form a postgraduate educational board responsible for all aspects of specialist and generalist skills, for sponsoring research, and for improving by effective accreditation and other means the standards of practice in hospitals and among general practitioners. In some respects the activities of the Colleges outside educational fields may have inhibited their educational influence. Medical representation on various NHS and professional committees could well have dissipated energy that might better have been applied in reviewing the purpose and structure of the doctor's training.

The announcement in June 1965 of a Royal Commission on Medical Education emphasized the interest of the public in professional standards.[36] Nineteenth-century medical reform, culminating in the Medical Act of 1858, had been encouraged by parliamentary committees of inquiry set up in 1834 and 1847. In a sense the wheel has come full circle, with the emphasis now on competence at the graduate stage. But the problems of reform are no longer of fusing separate streams of training into one combined program, as was achieved in 1858; they are much more complex. Scientific fragmentation—the increase of specialization—may be necessary to improve medical standards; in some respects it may need to be actively encouraged. The problems now concern the coordination of specialist skills so that the patient may reach the appropriate expert. Adequate educational programs are essential to this aim, developed in the context of a well-defined structure of medical practice. If the Colleges do not move of their own accord, the state may eventually be impelled to intervene.

36. *The Times,* June 30, 1965, p. 12.

24

Review and Prospect

From the patient's point of view the National Health Service Act was the culmination of a developing social philosophy. Gradually, the individualist philosophy of nineteenth-century laissez-faire had been replaced by governmental responsibility for those who were dependent or who were unprotected against certain economic risks; until finally, accelerated by the depression and two world wars, the concept of dependency changed into acceptance of a broad doctrine of social rights. The availability of free education for all, without a means test, was one such goal, achieved in 1944; comprehensive free medical care was another. The National Health Service could be regarded as one plank in the social platform of both the wartime Coalition and the Labour Government, crystallized out of the needs of the 1930s and brought to fruition after World War II. Over the same period, accelerated by the great advances in scientific techniques, the doctor became an essential public figure whose education, competence, availability and responsibility were matters of general concern.

The introduction of the National Health Service was not, however, merely the product of changing social demands: it was also an attempt to solve the major organizational problems implicit in the rapid expansion of medicine— and medical specialization—in the 1930s and early 1940s. The rising and potentially prohibitive cost of services to the patient was only one result of an increasingly complex medical technology and of increasingly effective diagnosis and treatment. Although free medical services in England removed the financial barrier between the doctor and the individual patient, the overall question of cost remained in the form of concern over the amount of money the nation as a whole was willing and able to spend, and in the development of services of maximum efficiency. Except for efforts to redistribute doctors geographically in relation to population needs, and partial regionalization of medical services, the English system provided no clearer answer to the basic economic and organizational issues than did that of any other country.

When the Act was passed in 1946, professional and organizational responses to specialization were incomplete. It was agreed that there should be a regionalized hospital and specialist service, but general practitioners and other personal health services were not included in this design. While it was apparent that the increase in specialized medicine would enhance the importance of the family doctor to give continuing care to the patient, existing GPs were brought into the health service on conditions that continued their historical role as junior partners to hospital consultants. In the twenty years that have elapsed, the pressures of specialization have intensified, and they will probably continue to do so. Indeed, the great era of medical specialism is probably just beginning. The beneficial changes specialization has already wrought, most spectacularly in the laboratory and surgical sciences, may be gauged by comparing the medicine of today with the pre-antibiotic days of only a generation ago. Within another generation spare-part surgery may be an everyday occurrence, discoveries concerning chemical and electrical reactions within the brain may have revolutionized modern neurology and psychiatry, and cancer may not only be cured but also prevented.

The speed of change means a continual, and perhaps increasing, time lag before the vast organization required to bring medical care to the patient adjusts to meet the new demands. A vital problem of medical care is to reduce this lag to a minimum by ensuring that the organization and availability of services, and the distribution and training of personnel, are sufficiently flexible to integrate new scientific developments as they arise. This need goes beyond the initial premises of the National Health Service Act. Despite the introduction of free health services provided through the government—albeit a historic landmark—the future development of medical services in England, as elsewhere, is as uncertain now as it was in the late 1930s.

Immediate problems within the National Health Service fall under three heads. The first concerns the relativities between general practitioners and consultants, in their function, facilities, organization, and income. The development of educational curricula and vocational training programs is a second important area; and third is the need to establish centralized planning techniques to initiate long-term policy. Obviously, the English solutions, whether they imply evolutionary or revolutionary change, must be found in relation to the professional history of English medicine. A distinction needs to be made, however, between unique traditions and the universal implications of specialized medicine. The problems of the National Health Service were generated not because of changes in the social structure, but because of changes in medical science. Certain questions, all of which raise problems of professional and public responsibility, are being asked in many countries: on the number, distribution, and quality of doctors; on the future of general practice; on the role of the hospital; and on the development of medical education and training. Although a different solution to these and other questions may be sought in countries with a different professional and social heritage, the approach is similar and the arguments familiar. The clearest answers will be found where professional traditions are used as a source of strength, not as a stranglehold; thus the careful review of history in this study. Nevertheless, it is probable that eventually, whatever the original differences, the demands of scientific medicine will bring the organizational structures of medical services closer together.

The Changing Balance of Medical Practice

One inescapable recent trend has been the shift from general into specialist practice. According to BMA figures, there were in 1929 in the whole of Britain (England, Wales, and Scotland) some 16,800 general practitioners engaged in practice under National Health Insurance and perhaps another 6,300 solely engaged in private general practice. About 2,400 consultants and specialists worked part time in voluntary and public hospitals and also conducted private practices; and there were another 2,200 whole-time hospital specialists and junior hospital staff.[1] The "general" focus of these services is overwhelming; GPs outnumbered consultants and hospital staff by at least four and perhaps five to one. By the 1960s the balance had shifted. Excluding house officers in their preregistration year, in 1964 there were 20,735 practitioners working in NHS hospitals, as against 21,903 in general practice. It seemed that in only a short time the majority of clinicians would be employed by hospitals. Indeed, if preregistration doctors were included, this situation had been reached in 1964.[2]

This was one aspect of the changing numerical balance between one career choice and another. A second was evident in the pattern of the hospital specialties. Increasing specialization in medicine not only channeled medical interest away from general and into specialized practice but also emphasized particular kinds of specialties; anesthesiology, radiology, pathology, and psychiatry emerged as substantial sectors of the profession. At the same time the old status patterns remained. General (internal) medicine was the first preference of almost a third of all first-year clinical (fourth-year) students in a study of five medical schools (1962).[3] Although by the final year of training the number choosing it had dropped to 17 per cent, this was still high compared with the opportunities for practice in that specialty, limited by the number of consultant posts. Obviously, general medicine had enhanced status in the eyes of aspirants to medical posts, as also had obstetrics and pediatrics. The same study noted that the groups with the most obvious laboratory orientation were by far the most unpopular, with a marked tendency toward rejection among clinical (fourth–sixth year) students. Yet such specialties had been among those with the fastest rate of growth under the National Health Service.

1. Figures kindly supplied by BMA Statistical Branch.
2. There were 1,521 preregistration house officers in 1964. Ministry of Health, *Annual Report for 1964*, pp. 71, 144.
3. The study also showed, however, an increasing acceptance of general practice; by the sixth or last year of undergraduate training 31% of students put general practice as a first career preference. F. M. Martin and F. A. Boddy, "Career Preferences of Medical Students," in *The Sociological Review Monograph No. 5* (Keele, 1962), pp. 21–32.

If all else were equal (if all branches of practice had been equally open), general practice might have dwindled as rapidly in England as it has in the United States, perhaps replaced by a larger number of specialists in internal medicine, obstetrics, and pediatrics. All else was not equal, however, because of the position of the GP in the English medical system.

The general practitioner held his own in a period of intense specialization largely because of the system of referral, evolved in the late nineteenth century out of intraprofessional demarcation disputes, and strengthened by the health legislation of 1911 and 1946. As a result, general practice is not only a special field but also a clearly defined administrative and professional function. On one side are all the hospital specialties, from general medicine and surgery to radiotherapy, with a monopoly of the hospitals; on the other, and professionally distinct, is the general practitioner, who as the doctor of first contact has a monopoly of patients.

Where the referral system did not exist in the same way, for example in the United States, there was no monopoly advantage in being a general practitioner, and there was every incentive to specialize; GPs and specialists were in direct competition for patients, and there was a natural desire on the part of the general public to bypass the GP and go straight to the specialist. In England, indeed in the whole of Britain, the GP's separate function contributed to the viability of general practice—despite the allure, the higher monetary rewards, and the expanding number of specialist openings. Disillusionment with the hospital staffing structure in the 1950s and the gloomy prospect of reaching the top may have drawn many young doctors to general practice as a more attractive alternative. Other aspiring GPs had no doubt which branch they preferred and did not seriously consider a specialist career.[4] But whatever the general motivation, until 1964 the absolute number of general practitioners increased under the National Health Service. Since 1964, their number has declined.

With this decline, the question of the GP's future has become more urgent; and the urgency has been intensified because, under a national service, effective choices can be made. The general practitioner could be allowed gradually to fade out by increasing the opportunities and inducements to specialize. Alternatively, he could be rejuvenated, upgraded, reorganized, and changed in function. The basic problems therefore deserve special attention. They resolve themselves into examining the present contribution of general practice, assessing its value and efficiency in relation to medicine as a whole, and in considering the possible alternatives.

Some effects of the retention of general practice on the distribution of full-time specialists can be observed by comparing England with the United States. The 1963 figures for both countries are shown in Table 29. The

4. One of the most interesting findings of the study by the General Practitioners' Association on GP remuneration (1964), conceived in the heat of the income dispute, was that job satisfaction was rated distinctly higher as a factor in general practice than for an average consultant in general medicine. *The GPA Report, Part 2.*, p. 48, and n. 11, Chap. 21 above.

TABLE 29. *Comparative Distribution of Medical Specialists and General Practitioners; England and Wales, and the United States, 1963*

	England and Wales		United States	
	Number	%	Number	%
All general practitioners and specialists	30,239	100.0	215,353	100.0
General practitioners and part-time specialists	21,020	69.5	75,987	35.3
Full-time specialists	9,219	30.5	139,366	64.7
Medical specialties	2,227	7.4	46,988	21.8
Internal medicine and related specialties	1,842	6.1	32,240	15.0
Pediatrics	233	0.8	11,840	5.5
Dermatology	152	0.5	2,908	1.4
Surgical specialties	2,481	8.2	44,845	20.8
General surgery and related specialties	1,171	3.9	23,778	11.0
Ophthalmology and otolaryngology	809	2.7	11,473	5.3
Orthopedics	461	1.5	5,636	2.6
Urology	40	0.1	3,958	1.8
Obstetrics and gynecology	517	1.7	13,269	6.2
Psychiatry and neurology	1,206	4.0	14,111	6.6
Other specialties	2,788	9.2	20,153	9.4
Pathology	909	3.0	5,501	2.6
Physical medicine	113	0.4	750	0.3
Radiology & radiotherapy	694	2.3	7,298	3.4
Anesthesiology	1,072	3.5	6,604	3.1

The figures for English GPs include principals only; there were also 947 assistants and 206 trainees in general practice in 1963. Full-time specialists include in the English data consultants and senior hospital medical officers employed under the NHS in all specialties classified by the Ministry of Health, except dentistry and orthodontics (517 specialists), social medicine (9), and unclassified (5). A relatively few SHMOs are also GPs, but it was not possible to separate them from the available figures.

United States figures, like the English data, exclude practitioners retired, not in medical practice, or status unknown (14,747), and those in training programs (38,519). They also exclude full-time specialists practicing in the fields of administrative medicine, aviation medicine, general preventive medicine, occupational medicine, and public health (17,858), whose counterparts do not appear in the English figures. With these exceptions, U.S. data include reported active MDs in private practice, federal service, or other nonfederal practice.

The term "full-time" implies a full-time specialist interest and does not refer to employment status.

Source: Ministry of Health, *Annual Report for 1963*, pp. 62, 136–37; U.S. Dept. of Health, Education and Welfare, *Health Manpower Source Book*, Section 18, *Manpower in the 1960's*, Table 16.

English figures include consultants and senior hospital medical officers, both of whom have tenure, and principals in general practice. The American figures represent specialists and nonspecialists in active practice, excluding those in training. Because of the difference in patterns of practice in the two countries, largely the result of different professional development, the two sets of data are not exactly comparable. Urology, for example, is in England frequently practiced by general surgeons rather than by specialists. Nevertheless, the figures at least indicate the difference in emphasis in the two countries, including some of the effects on other specialties of the presence or absence of the primary GP.

In England, taking those at the height of their careers, seven of ten doctors were in general practice in 1963. In the United States the balance was reversed; more than six of ten doctors were in full-time specialist practice, and many of the remaining four were specialists in a part-time capacity. As might be expected, hospital service specialties (pathology, physical medicine, radiology, and anesthesiology) accounted for comparable proportions of medical manpower in each country—somewhat over 9 per cent. Psychiatry showed comparatively little proportional difference. The major differences, and those in which it may reasonably be supposed that general practice in England had made its greatest impact, were in pediatrics, obstetrics, internal medicine, and general surgery. The proportion of doctors in these four specialties in England and Wales was 12 per cent; in the United States it was 38 per cent. If it is assumed that the real need for various specialist services is broadly similar in the two countries—a not unreasonable assumption, given the relatively high standard of living in both—it would appear that certain specialists in the United States are performing services that in England come within the purview of general practice; or conversely that the English GP acts as a part-time specialist in certain fields.

In 1962, for example, 34 per cent of all births in England and Wales occurred at home, under the supervision of a general practitioner. In addition, a substantial section of obstetric hospital beds (chiefly in small maternity centers) were under GPs. Almost 136,000 inpatients were discharged from GP obstetric beds in 1964, compared with almost 584,000 from consultant obstetric units.[5] Without these specialized services of general practitioners, there would have to be a marked increase in the number of consultant obstetricians. Similarly, in pediatrics, the English GP practices preventive medicine and treats minor and some major diseases of childhood in his own office. According to some sources, in any one year the GP might see as many as 74 per cent of the children in his practice.[6] It could therefore be argued that the GP is both part-time obstetrician and part-time pediatrician. He does not, however, compare with the American obstetrician,

5. Ministry of Health, *On the State of the Public Health 1963*, p. 89, *Annual Report for 1964*, p. 139.
6. A. A. Elder, quoted by Office of Health Economics, in *Personal Health Services* (London, 1963), p. 15.

pediatrician, or specialist in internal medicine (whose role is in some ways similar) in that the English GP lacks a similar background training.

The Future of General Practice

Such findings raise questions of whether specialists in obstetrics and pediatrics would provide a better service in the areas now covered by general practitioners, and of how far these specialties (as well as internal medicine and some aspects of general surgery) are central to the concept of family practice by a personal physician. If the number of GPs continues to decline in England relative to the population, decisions will have to be made on the most essential aspects of general practice as a specialty, and how far some of the GP's present duties can be organized more efficiently, undertaken by trained auxiliaries or removed to other medical specialists.

Professor T. McKeown has suggested that general practice be subdivided into four related fields: internal medicine, pediatrics, obstetrics, and geriatrics.[7] This would have two major advantages: it would retain the concept of personal medical care, while recognizing certain specialist functions within general practice; and it would have the advantage of enabling GPs to be directly linked to consultant "firms" or departments in hospitals. The GP might also be recognized as a specialist. Administrative fusion of the two branches of the profession would then become possible, and new combinations would be considered between general practitioners and consultants within broad specialty fields.

But there are also disadvantages in this approach. McKeown's suggestions might make the existing body of GPs better equipped scientifically and link them with hospital staffs, but it would not necessarily answer the need for a personal and family physician, now generally recognized as a complement to specialized medicine.[8] The referral system between a generalist who takes responsibility for the majority of illnesses and health problems, and a specialist who acts as a consultant and is responsible for hospital care, is still viable—even if not ideally applicable to the present training status of general practitioners. Indeed, as the focus of illness shifts from acute episodes to long-term and chronic sickness and to illnesses in which care involves the social or physical environment (carcinomas, cardiovascular disease, neuroses), a general practitioner of some kind becomes increasingly important. If the GP did not exist he (or someone like him) would have to be invented. Although the English referral system was not initially designed for such purposes, it provides one very relevant answer for the provision of personal medical care in a specialized environment.

The English general practitioner is, moreover, in a much stronger position than GPs in countries where there has been no similar history of a divided

7. *Lancet i* (1962), 923.

8. See, for example, World Health Organization, Technical Report Series No. 257, *Training of the Physician for Family Practice* (WHO, Geneva, 1963), pp. 10–14 and passim.

profession. His long history has been of advancing status in relation to that of the consultant, and there is every sign of this advance continuing at a stepped-up pace. He has numerical strength, professional cohesion in the College of General Practitioners, and acceptance as the patient's personal doctor. The Gillie report used the estimate that 90 per cent of all medical episodes were handled from start to finish by general practitioners, and it strongly recommended the retention of general practice with a generalist and community function.[9] All of this would argue for modifying the educational background and organizational structure of general practice, rather than altering or limiting the GP's activities.

Historically, the education and training for general practice was that undertaken by all doctors, some of whom went on to specialize. It has not yet progressed much beyond this level, nor will it until certain conditions are fulfilled. The first is a much more detailed definition of the kind of general practice desired than has yet appeared from the professional and public bodies. Second is a gauge of the importance of family practice in relation to other specialties and the standard of skill (and facilities) thus required. Third, and in some ways most important, there is the assignment of responsibility for making the definitions and setting the standards.

The organization of general practice, like the educational structure, has remained almost stationary while science has progressed. The Gillie report referred to general practice as a "cottage" industry.[10] Most general practitioners are in partnership with colleagues, but such partnerships are generally small: only 3 per cent of GP principals in 1964 were members of partnerships of six or more, and comprehensive group practice in the American sense, embracing both primary physicians and referral specialists, is unknown. The profession has endorsed the concept of GP partnerships to replace the initial NHS concept of health centers.[11] The Ministry claims that, without recourse to the erection of actual buildings, "the increase in partnerships and group practices has been ending the old isolation of the general practitioner which the health centers were designed to remedy." [12] But the large well-organized group practice as the norm of general practice lies in the future. General practitioners are still a largely unorganized or barely organized species, and, unless concerted action is taken, are likely to remain so within the next decade.

Such planning as there has been for general practice has been through the income structure: in the limited financial inducements to group practice from the early 1950s, which were offered through the group practice loans scheme and through the capitation system. The new payment scheme for GPs suggested in late 1965 (Chap. 21), follows in the same tradition. Recog-

9. Gillie report, p. 12.
10. Ibid., p. 56.
11. See Porritt report, p. 64; Gillie report, p. 32.
12. *Health and Welfare; The Development of Communiity Care*, Cmnd. 1973 (1963), p. 11.

nition of income manipulation as a potent instrument of planning only, however, re-emphasizes the basic problems of medical specialization. If career choice, training, and organization can be altered through the payment scheme (and to some degree this is clearly possible), those responsible for income structure and income determination must also accept responsibility for maintaining the balance of medical practice between generalists and specialists, among the specialties, and ultimately in the integration and focus of medical services in the hospital or in the GP's surgery.

Ultimate responsibility for planning has not yet been faced. The basic policy questions have been more usually approached in England through decisions of independent arbitrators, such as the Spens Committees, Mr. Justice Danckwerts, and (now) the Standing Review Body on Doctors' and Dentists' Remuneration, than through experimental designs with various forms of organization or manpower structures, or even through evaluation of existing differences. Until the Standing Review Body was appointed in 1962, the incomes of GPs and specialists were discussed on separate occasions. The long heritage of division in the medical profession, extending through the professional associations and the NHS structure, has made a comprehensive planning approach difficult to achieve. Yet the overriding need is to integrate the services of general practitioner and specialist so that the patient may benefit most from continuing association with a practitioner and the highest quality of specialist care.

The Role of the Hospital

Whereas general practice has been largely underdeveloped within the National Health Service, hospitals were brought together into a regional system. They too, however, have remained strongly influenced by pre-existing organizational patterns. By far the most deeply ingrained professional tradition, relict of the monopoly of large voluntary hospitals by consultants from the eighteenth century, is the separation of hospital from other kinds of medicine. The hospital has stayed at the fringe of medical care instead of becoming, as would have been possible under a national health service, the center from which other services sprang. The tendency has been to suggest a new environment for the GP or to give him a new label, rather than to look at medicine as one profession with interdependent component parts stretching over the whole field, in hospital and in community.

When the basic staffing patterns were established (chiefly in the eighteenth and nineteenth centuries), the hospital was only one aspect of medical practice. It provided a useful laboratory for teaching and research on the poor, but most of the techniques and skills of the profession could be used equally well, and often better, outside the hospital. Today, in contrast, many facilities offered by hospitals cannot be duplicated: the hospital has become an essential center for advanced techniques. The medical staffing structure, however, has remained much as before: a relatively few appointed consultants, seeing patients on referral, each with assigned junior medical staff and assigned hospital beds and outpatient clinics. As hospital medicine has become more highly specialized, consultants have also specialized, and the hospital has naturally provided the focus of the technical team. An equally viable alternative might have been the specialized group practice (e.g. a mixed group of specialists working within and out of common office facilities) such as exists in many places in the United States. But professional evolution in England did not lend itself to this type of extrahospital development.

The English system has certain practical advantages. Dependence on equipment, staffing, and facilities requires that a large proportion of the specialist's work be performed in the hospital. The introduction of salaried specialists based on hospitals has accelerated this process in England and has extended it to all hospital specialties; the specialist spends the great proportion of his working life in the hospital, and the trend is toward full-time hospital work. There are thus still relatively few doctors with access to hospital beds—relative, that is, to the American system, where the average specialist spends a much smaller proportion of his time in the hospital and where a much larger number of specialists uses hospital inpatient facilities. If the hospital is to be regarded as the center of medical technology, there is much to be said for concentrating in it a relatively small number of technological experts of the highest possible caliber for the maximum part of their time. There are also greater opportunities in the English pattern for informal communication and thus for operational teamwork among hospital specialists; and there are also scientific advantages, brought about by a more concentrated practice, which may affect the quality of hospital care.

The chief disadvantage of the English system as presently organized is the gulf between the hospital and other aspects of medicine. Nor are there immediate signs of change. The Platt report on hospital staffing (1961) stressed that the medical staffing structure in hospitals should continue to be based on consultants; that consultant responsibility was being excessively delegated and that more consultants were needed; and that the SHMO grade should be abolished in favor of a new permanent "medical assistant" grade to assist consultants.[13] Together, these not only suggested a need for substantial increases in hospital medical staff but also implied a continued schism between specialists and GPs. Although the medical assistant grade was intended to be sufficiently flexible to encourage GPs to re-enter hospital work, and from which hospital staff might enter general practice, the hospital staffing structure was to stay separate from that of general practice. To the GP the new grade might hold additional possibilities of part-time hospital work, but he would still be directly responsible in his hospital work to the consultant(s) to whom he was attached and he would continue to admit patients to hospital only on their behalf. From the first it appeared that the medical assistant grade would, if adequately filled, benefit the hospitals, which were desperately short of middle-grade staff, rather than solve the major dilemmas of medical practice.

13. See chap. 10.

The GP's relationship to the hospital has been increasingly ambiguous. The division of practice on which the administrative organization is based has not coincided with functional boundaries. Both consultants and the majority of general practitioners practice obstetrics; and the line between general practice and general medicine or general psychiatry—together with many other specialties—is difficult to draw. Pathologists and diagnostic radiologists, who in 1964 represented one of every six consultants, have a comparable relationship to each branch, as technical consultants, diagnosticians, and advisers, yet are ranged wholly on the side of hospital staffs.

In the absence of other facilities, the hospital is to the GP the center of diagnostic and specialist services. Whatever the attitude of individual general practitioners to their local hospitals, and whatever the prevailing traditions, the hospital has become the hub of scientific medicine. If the hospital with its great technical resources is to be integrated with other parts of medical care, one must ask whether it is possible to expand its dimensions to reduce, if not abolish, the present discontinuities between hospital and nonhospital practice. The rational approach would suggest reorganization of the professional and social structures of medicine around the hospital, with a coordinated personal medical service spreading throughout the surrounding community.

The idea of linking the arms of the National Health Service—hospital, GP, and local health services—at local or area level has been mooted since the service began. The medical profession's Porritt report (1962) recommended area health boards for this purpose, presumably somewhat similar in size, if not in form, to the joint authorities suggested in the 1944 White Paper.[14] But these would have the disadvantage of setting up a new layer of administration, without necessarily also improving communications and standards. A much more radical approach may be needed. Perhaps the most obvious would be the gradual conversion of the hospital into a complete medical center, which reaches out to embrace existing GP services, and through which specialists in the primary, referral, and "service" specialties work as equal partners and on similar terms. It is not suggested that the specialist in general or family practice should suddenly become a surgeon, or that he should have the same standing as the present specialist in internal medicine (although this would have much to commend it), or that he should have direct access to beds in general hospitals, or necessarily be employed at a consultant's salary. It is suggested only that the GP should be administratively integrated into the hospital service, organized under regional hospital boards to work in appropriate locations and with local hospital affiliations; and that the hospital service should be responsible for general practice of groups and individuals as well as for specialist services. Until some such system is introduced the potential of regionalization will remain unfulfilled, and the GP will not achieve final acceptance as a ranking specialist—nor attain the quality this implies.

14. Porritt report, p. 22 and passim; for the White Paper, see chap. 5.

The seeds of such change already exist. The district hospital concept envisages a community service area for hospital services, even for the teaching hospitals which have been in the past relatively isolated from local society.[15] The proposed new payment scheme for GPs, with more direct reimbursement of expenses, recognition of higher income for older doctors, and the possibility of distinction awards, will bring the general practitioner closer to the employment conditions of the specialist. There have been suggestions for appointing registrars and senior registrars in general practice, as well as in hospital practice, and this would be more easily achieved in relation to maintaining standards if all were under the hospital hierarchy.[16] These factors could precede an eventual change of emphasis, with the base hospital at the center of all community health services.

The advantages of attaching GPs to hospitals have been seen in the past as benefiting chiefly the general practitioner. If, as seems likely, the main disease hazards of the future will include larger proportions of a psychosocial origin or with important psychosocial elements, it will be the technical specialist in the hospital who will gain most from an increased contact with his GP colleagues. Administrative fusion would give much greater opportunities for flexibility between different types of practice than now exists, particularly in education and in choice of specialty; and the type of community practice that is most suitable to present-day needs could more easily be determined.[17] Experiments have been inhibited by the historical identification of consultant status with possession of beds in general hospitals. GPs have demanded beds rather than consultant status. They might ask whether if they gained the latter, they would need the former.

The general practitioner has never been accepted as professionally equal to the consultant. The next few years must see him attain a prestige status equivalent to that of a consultant by accepting additional training and

15. One of the first indications of actual change was the announcement in October 1965 that the board of governors of Guy's (teaching) Hospital, London, was to be responsible for providing the hospital and specialist services for its local area (Bermondsey and Southwark) *Lancet ii* (1965), 887.

16. College of General Practitioners, *Report on Special Vocational Training for General Practice* (May 1965), p. 18 and passim.

17. For example, group general practices, set up in association with the hospital, might agree to provide regular diagnostic services in the hospital's emergency department. Rotation of junior staff through general and hospital practice would be comparatively easy to arrange. Controlled experiments could be undertaken in "specialized group practice" (GP-specialists and specialists working together as one community team), and in various forms of diagnostic centers or health centers inside or outside the hospital. GPs could assist, as many now do, in specialized outpatient departments, and hold their own diagnostic and treatment clinics in their community offices. It should be easier to link community and hospital geriatric, pediatric, and obstetric services, and there might be advantages in attaching general practitioners with interests in these specialties to the appropriate hospital "firm," and specialists to group general practices. Finally, through fusion, it would be easier to consider objectively the future of the general practitioners.

organizational change; the cycle begun by the Apothecaries' Act will be finally complete. This prospect has major implications not only for the general practitioner but also for the consultant and the hospital. If, for example, the consultant branch is to continue as a full-time technological elite entirely based on referred hospital work, it must be supported by other physicians whose work is predominantly concerned with disease (and health) in the community at large. If the GP combines the present talents, if not all the skills, of the consultant in general medicine and pediatrics (to become the modern equivalent of the general physician who was GP to the upper classes at the beginning of this century), the status balance between the two branches might change, and the consultant in many specialties be regarded as the technical adviser to the GP rather than someone of generally superior ability. If the present GP were to vanish and there were not an adequate substitute to take his place, not only would more consultants need to be produced, but the whole referral system would break down. Decisions are largely, but not solely, in the hands of the medical profession.

Professional and Public Responsibility

The thread of responsibility for planning runs throughout the recent history of medical practice. The speed of scientific change demands no less than modification of established institutions, including the hospitals, medical schools, medical associations, and professional colleges. Experience so far has shown their relatively slow adjustment to changes in medicine that were already apparent before World War II, although there has been a trend toward more centralized machinery both in government and in the medical profession. The point has now been reached where questions have to be answered on the undergraduate medical curriculum; on the content, supervision, and place of training of postgraduates; on the number of doctors and other health personnel and their geographical and functional distribution; and on the interlocking of general medical care and the specialties. How should such decisions be reached, and who should make them?

One accompaniment of increased specialization, emphasized by the existence of the National Health Service, has been expanded government responsibility for medical care. This has increased in the years of the health service in such areas as responsibility for the number of doctors, for the hospital staffing structure, and for the organization of general practice. It can be expected to continue as the organizational problems become more complex. To imply, however, that government has been substituted for professional responsibility, is untrue; for there has also been a growing interdependence of the medical profession and the state, and increasing medical participation in the development and administration of national medical services. The impact of medical specialization is forcing the professional bodies of medicine to widen their horizons and to formulate their own policies on the general organizational development of medical care. There are compelling reasons to do so. The complex patterns of medical care under a system of specialization have raised questions of the most efficient method of providing medical services, and of the number and kinds of doctors—and their relevant training—appropriate to such developments. The efficiency of hospital medicine has emphasized the need to develop comparable programs for the prevention and alleviation of disease; and this includes consideration of the total social environment of modern living and the means through which the environment may be therapeutically manipulated. A new public health movement may be about to begin. The profession has become more dependent on social institutions and on other professions for the provision of good medical care: on hospitals and local health services, social workers, and technicians. Finally, the public itself has begun to express concern about the effective provision of medical care. All these factors—but perhaps especially the last—have brought the medical profession irrevocably into consideration of general social policy in relation to medicine, and into participation with public bodies in the development of medical services.

The National Health Service Act formalized the extended interest of the medical profession in matters which might formerly have been regarded as "social" rather than "medical." Doctors became concerned with the administration and development of the National Health Service at all levels and over all its aspects, so that the profession is largely responsible for its efficient operation. It may be argued that in England the pendulum has swung too far in the direction of professional involvement, and that the voice of neither the consumer nor the professional planner has been sufficiently heard. In any event, the English experience has indicated that by accepting increased participation in the provision of medical services—even in this case by accepting direct employment by the state—the medical profession does not necessarily endanger its autonomy, and its span of influence is almost inevitably widened.

In certain areas, neither the government nor the medical profession alone has been able to produce solutions. The single-handed general practitioner was appropriate to an age of individualism and relatively little medical knowledge; more complex medicine requires more elaborately and more effectively organized medical teamwork. The focus has shifted from the individual practitioner to the group or hospital, from the unit hospital to a hospital region, and then again upward to centralized planning in the crucial areas of education, manpower, and facilities. The trends appear to point to more central direction, whether from the profession or the government or both, and to sophisticated planning and the encouragement of experiments in all aspects of practice design.

One obvious deficiency in England has been the lack of basic information. The professional bodies have collected and published few studies of patterns of practice. The Ministry of Health is only beginning to enter the field of modern statistical method and still lacks a forward planning unit for comprehensive services. Both have been hampered by separate structures for hospital and nonhospital practices. Efforts were made by the profession to achieve a committee whose membership represented a cross section of medicine (the Porritt Committee), but this was unfortunately not retained once the committee's report was published. The Joint Consultants Committee might profitably be replaced by a central professional planning body which would act in conjunction with a Ministry planning unit. Whatever the machinery, however, government and professional action have become mutually dependent.

The need for combined public and professional action is seen most clearly in the development of medical education, key to the functions and balance of medical practice, and thus, ultimately, to the future of the hospital and of general practice, however they are organized. Recognition of minimum standards of medical competence and integrity has long been of public concern through the General Medical Council, a statutory professional committee. Admittance to the profession, medical education itself, and standards above the basic minimum have, however, been the responsibility of the medical profession and the universities. With the changing focus of medical education and training (particularly the deferment of specialist training to the postgraduate level), and the compelling need to identify the whole educational program with the organizational aims of medical care, the old distinctions have been blurred.

The Royal Colleges, which have historically provided the professional focus of consultant medicine, have not been able to reach or impose solutions to the problems of postgraduate and continuing education; nor have the universities, though they are strategically placed at the center of the regional hospital system. There is an obvious need for some kind of national educational board (perhaps a postgraduate equivalent to the General Medical Council). As presently organized, however, neither the professional structure nor the Ministry of Health has been able to set up such a body, nor to connect the educational pattern with the future demands for doctors in the various specialty areas. Questions have been deferred to the Royal Commission on Medical Education, set up in 1965. One cannot predict the recommendations of this commission, but they will inevitably demand further cohesion between the planning of health manpower and facilities (now primarily a Ministry of Health responsibility) and the development of undergraduate and specialty educational programs.

Manpower is no longer a question of overall numbers of students and practitioners but of geographical and functional deployment. The manpower problem of the early 1950s was an apparent excess of doctors; that of the early 1960s was an apparent general shortage. The middle 1960s look forward to a complete redefinition and rethinking of the basic concepts of general and specialist practice, and of the relation of both to hospitals and other medical facilities. Whether the present distribution of specialists (including general practice as one specialty) and the apparent trend toward fewer GPs and an increasing proportion of hospital doctors are satisfactory, in terms of providing optimum medical care, is an open question. It demands far-reaching studies of a kind and scope not so far attempted. But it also depends on more detailed and positive statements from the profession, government, and public on the kinds of doctor and facilities ideally required. Again, there is urgent need for the public and the profession to work in concert, using modern planning techniques.

The National Health Service Act recognized medicine as a social service, both as the culmination of a social philosophy and as the solution to some of the problems of specialized medicine in relation to availability and cost of services. Now the move from an individual to a collective philosophy is being seen in the organization of medical practice itself—and this is in considerable measure a result of the pressures of specialism. English experience has indicated three broad trends: in the changing role of the general practitioner, his need to work more closely with hospitals and specialists, and the requirement for postgraduate programs in a new type of generalism; in the central position of the hospital in providing specialist services and thus, increasingly, all kinds of medical services; and finally, in the development of professional organizations to control the standards of postgraduate education, which has now become the period of practical specialized professional training. In each of these areas, old structures are being modified. The pressures of medical specialization have become stronger than professional and social traditions.

Specialization has posed many complex questions, and undoubtedly more will arise. The National Health Service, product of a long evolutionary process, has provided some of the answers, including removal of the cost barrier from the patient and the regionalization of hospitals. The problems now facing medical education and organization cannot, however, await the slow readjustment of institutions to scientific change; they demand research, experiment, and comprehensive planning. Only a bold and imaginative partnership of the state, the public, and the medical profession—unafraid of rethinking the bases of medical practice and prepared to adjust with the times—will ensure the ready availability of good medical care to the whole population.

Additional Notes

The General Medical Council

The General Medical Council was established as a legal rather than an academic body; it supervises standards and issues training criteria but does not itself hold examinations. The examinations, the training, and the details of medical curricula remain with the universities, the conjoint boards of the professional colleges, and the Societies of Apothecaries, each of which is responsible for an examination which is recognized by the General Medical Council as of sufficient merit to allow the names of successful candidates to be inscribed in the Council's General Medical Register. Admittance to the register is equivalent to a license to practice. The university or other examinations are qualifying examinations for registration; the student is said to have "qualified," and the examinations are known as "qualifications." Until the Medical Act of 1950, the qualifying examination alone entitled the successful candidate to full registration. Now a compulsory year of hospital practice as a qualified doctor is also demanded—that is, after the university medical degree or legally equivalent professional diplomas but before a full entry in the General Medical Register. The educational picture is complicated in that the Royal Colleges of Physicians and Surgeons, although responsible for qualifying examinations (e.g. the LRCP and MRCS of the English Conjoint Board), do not have undergraduate training schools. The medical student attends a hospital medical school, which is now invariably also attached to a university, and is expected to take a university degree. He may, however, take a Conjoint Board diploma and become legally qualified to practice before he sits for the university final examination.

The Medical Register contains the names of all "duly qualified" practitioners. It is still legally possible to practice as a nonqualified or nonregistered doctor, but registration carries certain exclusive benefits, notably appointments in most hospitals and in other public services. Only registered doctors may give valid certificates of death and other statutory certificates, or prescribe dangerous drugs. The General Medical Council includes a disciplinary committee, which considers convictions of practitioners in the law courts and cases of "infamous conduct" that may require disciplinary action. The Council may order the offender's name erased from the Register, or suspension or probation. The full Council now consists of 47 members, of whom

8 are nominated by the Crown, 11 elected by postal votes of the profession in the three constituencies—England, Scotland, and Ireland (Northern Ireland and Eire, partition not having been professionally recognized)—and the remaining 28 from the universities, Royal Colleges, and Societies of Apothecaries (of London and Dublin) in the constituencies. (General Medical Council, *Functions, Procedure, and Disciplinary Jurisdiction,* London, 1965.)

Postgraduate Diplomas

Medical undergraduates in England qualify by one of two examination systems—university or Royal College—which exist in parallel. Postgraduate examinations, however, are chiefly the concern of the Royal Medical Colleges through the specialist diplomas of the Colleges' Conjoint examining board, their membership or fellowship examinations. The universities are responsible for a number of specialty diplomas, beside their academic Master's and Doctor's degrees. But because of the existence of the MRCP and FRCS as higher qualifications, the M.D. degree has not gained the pre-eminence that it has elsewhere. This degree and the M.S. tend to be taken by the specialist interested in research or particular experience, or who desires evidence of his ability in addition to the College examinations.

The MRCP. The membership examination of the Royal College of Physicians (London) is the major postgraduate examination for approximately one third of all those wishing to become consultants. In internal medicine, pediatrics, cardiology, neurology, and other specialties closely related to general medicine, the MRCP has been—and still is—an essential prerequisite of higher specialist posts. It has been subject to continued criticism of its structure, its function, and its efficiency. This stems from two apparently irreconcilable pressures: the historical purpose of the College in providing a corps of generally cultured and widely experienced physicians, and the demands of growing specialty groups for examinations to indicate specialist competence in a comparatively limited area of "general medicine."

Under regulations laid down in 1964, the MRCP includes three interconnected examinations. Part I consists of a preliminary written paper covering a wide field of medical knowledge and the basic sciences. Since Part I must be passed before the candidate may proceed to Part II, its purpose is largely to weed out those candidates who are clearly unprepared or unsuitable. Part II has a close resemblance to the original membership examination, although the written part is shorter and specialism has intruded. Each candidate takes one written paper divided into two sections: section I (1 hour) consists of questions in general medicine; section II (2.5 hours), questions covering the medical specialties including internal medicine, psychiatry, cardiology, pediatrics, neurology, dermatology, tropical medicine, pathology, geriatrics, social and preventive medicine, and epidemiology. From these the candidates may choose two questions. The written section is followed by an oral examination in which specialist examiners take part—although it was emphasized in 1964 that "specialised questions in both the paper and the oral will be so designed that candidates in general medicine could be expected to answer them satisfactorily." The intention was to "increase the range of the examination from a broad medical standpoint," and at the same time to admit specialist interests. Part II candidates are placed in one of three categories: if they pass outright they are awarded the MRCP and excused from further examinations; if they have done slightly less well, they are allowed to prove themselves in Part III; or they fail. Part III, taken at least three months after Part II, is a specialist examination with a choice of internal medicine, pediatrics, psychiatry, or pathology.

The FRCS. The present general fellowship examination of the Royal College of Surgeons is the direct descendant of the first fellowship examination held in December 1844. It includes two parts. The primary in anatomy and physiology was so named as early as the 1860s to distinguish it from the second part, which is an examination in surgery and surgical anatomy and includes examination of patients. Pathology was introduced into the primary as a subject in its own right in 1944.

Current regulations require the satisfactory completion of the 12-month period of service in preregistration hospital appointments before taking the primary. Thus the student who enters medical school at age 18, and obtains his basic qualification at 23, may sit the primary at age 24; if successful, he may enter for the final examination at age 26. There were 950 candidates for the final in general surgery in 1962. In addition, 67 candidates entered the final FRCS examination in ophthalmology, and 52 in otolaryngology: these candidates take the general primary examination, but a specialized final. Candidates in 1962 for the FFA (anesthesiology) and the FDS (dental surgery) numbered 290 and 96; each of these College faculties organizes its own primary and final examinations. Anesthesiologists may take the general primary instead of the primary in their field.

The primary has been held in certain countries abroad since 1927. The final may be taken only in London. About two thirds of the 200 successful candidates for the FRCS each year are from overseas. Those who leave Britain with their diploma move out of range of the continuing influence the Royal College of Surgeons expects to exert on its new fellows in British hospitals while they work in the senior registrar training grade and when they eventually come before consultant appointments committees. This problem is shared by all the Colleges, which expect candidates to sit for their examinations before they become senior registrars, and whose examinations are not therefore intended to signify consultant skills.

Specialist diplomas. The diplomas listed by consultants in the South-West Metropolitan hospital region in 1962 showed that 23% were members or fellows of the Royal College of Physicians of London or Edinburgh; 39% held the fellowship (including the Fellowship in the Faculty of Anaesthetists) in one of the Royal Colleges of Surgeons; 7% were members or fellows of the Royal College of Obstetricians and Gynaecologists; 2% were fellows of the Faculty of Radiologists. In all, 71% of the consultants belonged to at least one of these bodies. In the "medical" specialty group (excluding physical medicine, psychiatry, and pathology) 109 of the 133 consultants were members or fellows of a Royal College of Physicians, the exceptions being consultants in the older age groups or in the subspecialties which are most difficult to staff (venereology, dermatology, chest diseases). In all new appointments to this group the MRCP was essential for appointment. Similarly, the FRCS was held by 176 of the 194 members of the surgical group; all the most competitive surgical specialties (general surgery, neurosurgery, plastic and thoracic surgery) showed 100% FRCS membership. Only in a minority of specialties was the specialist diploma (given either by a conjoint board or a university) more popular than College association— notably psychiatry (Diploma in Psychological Medicine) and radiology (Diploma in Medical Radio-diagnosis).

When the Goodenough Committee reported in 1944, there were nearly 40 specialist diplomas available in Great Britain. The present disposition of diplomas by examining body is shown in Table 30. Some comparisons are given in Table 31. The English Conjoint Board is the largest single source of diplomas. It awards 12, ranging in alphabetical order from anaesthetics to tropical medicine, and has over 1,800 annual candidates.

The purpose these diplomas now serve is still debatable. As in College membership examinations, many candidates—reflecting the composition of junior and middle-grade hospital staffs—are of foreign nationality. For example, the majority of successful candidates in 1962 for the diploma in laryngology and otology (31 of 40) and the diploma in ophthalmology (54 of 93) of the English Conjoint Board were qualified outside the United Kingdom or Eire, and there were substantial proportions of foreign graduates in other specialties. As with other diplomas, however, these carry no connotation of specialist status in British terms; indeed, both the DLO and the DO, for example, require evidence of only one year of practice in the relevant specialty. (Material kindly supplied by Mr. Francis Stent, Secretary of the Examining Board in England.)

Many, if not most, of the foreign graduates eventually return to their own countries where the diplomas afford evidence of specialist training in Britain. It may be questioned whether the present diplomas are the best indications of such training, both to British and non-British graduates, and how far they imply specialist competence and at what level. In the absence of a national postgraduate board or unified administration of diplomas (as suggested by the Goodenough Committee), there has been no overall policy on the function and purpose of postgraduate examinations. This is clearly a field on which the Royal Commission on Medical Education will profitably focus.

Courses for Specialists in London

The 13 institutes attached to London special hospitals offer both apprenticeship programs and formal lectures. Apprenticeship training falls into

TABLE 30. *Postgraduate Diplomas, Great Britain* *

Specialty	Diploma	Examining Body			Total
		Conjoint Board †	Medical Corp. ‡	University	
Anaesthetics	DA	1			1
Obstetrics	D Obst. RCOG		1		1
Chest diseases	DTCD			1	1
Industrial health	DIH	1	2	1	4
	CIH			1	1
	DO Hyg			1	1
Biophysics				1	1
Medical jurisprudence	DMJ		1		1
Ophthalmology	DO	1			1
Otolaryngology	DLO	1			1
Paediatrics	DCH	1	1	1	3
Pathology	DCP			1	1
	D Path	1			1
Bacteriology	Dip Bact			2	2
Physical Medicine	D Phys Med	1			1
Psychiatry	DPM	2		4	6
	Dip Psych			1	1
Public Health	DPH	1		11	12
Medical administration	DMSA			1	1
Radio-diagnosis	DMRD	1		2	3
Radiotherapy	DMRT	1		2	3
Tropical medicine	DTM&H	1		2	3
	DCMT			1	1
	DTPH			1	1
Applied parasitology and entomology	DAP&E			1	1
Nutrition	DN			1	1
		13	5	36	54

* Excluding Northern Ireland and Eire.
† Includes the Scottish Triple Board and the English Conjoint Board.
‡ English and Scottish colleges and faculties, and Society of Apothecaries.

TABLE 31. *Qualifications for Selected Specialties, Great Britain*

Specialty	Qualification	Minimum specified time between qualifying and taking special diploma (months)	Required residence or period of study (months)
Medicine	MRCP, Lond.	18	0
	MRCP, Edin.	24	0
	FRFPS, Glas.	36	12
Surgery	FRCS, Eng.	36	24
	FRCS, Edin.	36	12
	FRFPS, Glas.	36	12
Obstet. & Gyn.	MRCOG	36	24
	FRCS, Edin.	36	12
Ophthalmology	FRCS, Eng.	36	12
	FRCS, Edin.	36	30
	FRFPS, Glas.	36	24
Ear-nose-throat	FRCS, Eng.	36	6
	FRCS, Edin.	36	12
	FRFPS, Glas.	36	24
Anaesthetics	FFA, RCS	36	18
Radio-diagnosis Radiotherapy	FFR	60	24 after recognized post-graduate diploma
Psychiatry	DPM, Conj.	36	24
	DPM, Lond.	54	42
Physical med.	D. Phys. Med.	36	24

Note: This table merely shows the time required to be spent in study of the specialty, not the total experience of medicine required. For example, the candidate for the FRCS in Ear-Nose-Throat must also have had 1.5 years' resident experience in medical and surgical posts.

three categories: appointment to the resident staff of the teaching hospital for a period usually of 1 to 3 years; appointment as a part-time clinical assistant; or a short period of attachment to the hospital. The Institute of Urology, for example, calls the last category "Practice of the Hospitals"; the student registers for a month at a time and is allowed to watch operations and to discuss cases and proposed lines of treatment. Special courses or lectures organized by the institutes range from outline courses to advanced study of a particular aspect of the specialty, and some may be used by candidates for higher qualifications: e.g. the Institute of Obstetrics and Gynaecology organizes an intensive 2-week course for the MRCOG, the Institute of Ophthalmology offers courses for the FRCS in ophthalmology and the Diploma in Ophthalmology, and the Institute of Laryngology and Otology gives courses for the FRCS in that subject as well as for diplomas and for higher surgical degrees. The Institute of Psychiatry offers an ambitious course of instruction covering up to 3 years, as preparation for the London University Diploma in Psychological Medicine.

Courses in the major specialties are also available in London through the Fellowship of Postgraduate Medicine, a nonprofit organization (set up to meet a recognized need after World War I), unconnected with either the University or any of the Colleges or associations. Some of the fellowship's courses are specifically designed to provide pre-examination experience, including courses for the MRCP and FRCS, and the Diploma in Child Health. The Royal College of Surgeons, through its Institute of Basic Medical Sciences (a joint faculty of the College and the British Postgraduate Medical Federation) organizes a comprehensive revision course, which, although carefully not so designated, is suitable for those embarking on the primary FRCS examination; and the College's full-time course in clinical surgery, held twice a year for 8 weeks, bears a similar relationship to the final FRCS. All these programs utilize NHS hospitals for practical teaching experience but are organized outside the NHS.

Bibliography

This bibliography includes the more important books referred to in the text. It is not intended to offer an exhaustive survey of material available on all aspects of the National Health Service, many of which are not covered in this book. An extended bibliography on the National Health Service may be found in Almont Lindsey, *Socialized Medicine in England and Wales.*

The bibliography is arranged in two sections. The first includes reports from the medical profession and material from government and other public agencies; the second all other books and documents. Journal articles are not included.

Reports and Official Documents

British Hospitals Association, *Report of the Voluntary Hospitals Commission* (London, BHA, 1937), "Sankey report"

British Medical Association, *The British Medical Association's Proposals for a General Medical Service for the Nation* (London, BMA, 1930)

————, *Interim Report by the Council of the Association on Health Centres* (London, BMA, July 1948)

————, *The Training of a Doctor,* Report of the Medical Curriculum Committee of the British Medical Association (London, BMA, 1948)

————, *General Practice and the Training of the General Practitioner,* The Report of a Committee of the Association (London, BMA, 1950)

Central Health Services Council, *Report of the Committee on the Internal Administration of Hospitals* (HMSO, 1954), "Bradbeer report"

————, *Committee of Enquiry into the Cost of the National Health Service, Report,* Cmd. 9663 (HMSO, 1956), "Guillebaud report"

————, *Accident and Emergency Services* (HMSO, 1962)

————, Standing Medical Advisory Committee, *The Field of Work of the Family Doctor,* Report of the Sub-Committee (HMSO, 1963), "Gillie report"

College of General Practitioners, *Reports from General Practice. I. Special Vocational Training for General Practice* (London, Council of the College of General Practitioners, May 1965); *II. Present State and Future Needs* (July 1965)

Committee on Higher Education, *Higher Education, Report of the Committee Appointed by the Prime Minister under the Chairmanship of Lord Robbins, 1961–1963,* Cmnd. 2154 (HMSO, 1963)

Consultative Council on Medical and Allied Services, *Interim Report on the Future Provision of Medical and Allied Services,* Cmd. 693 (London, 1920), "Dawson report"

Flexner, Abraham, *Medical Education in Europe—A Report to the Carnegie Foundation for the Advancement of Teaching* (New York, Carnegie Foundation, 1912)

General Medical Council, *Functions, Procedure, and Disciplinary Jurisdiction* (London, General Medical Council, 1965)

General Practitioners' Association, *The GPA Report, Part One* (London, GPA, May 1964); *The GPA Report, Part Two, Doctors' Remuneration* (London, GPA, Dec. 1964)

Gray, A. M. H., and A. Topping, *The Hospital Services of London and the Surrounding Area,* Hospital Survey (HMSO, 1945)

Medical Practitioners' Union (J. Sluglett), *Health Centre Report* (London, MPU, Oct. 1960)

Ministry of Health, *Annual Reports of the Ministry of Health* (HMSO). Part II of the report, *On the State of the Public Health,* the annual report of the Chief Medical Officer of the Ministry of Health, has appeared under this separate title since 1962.

———, *The Development of Specialist Services* (HMSO, 1950)

———, *Report of the Maternity Services Committee* (HMSO, 1959), "Cranbrook report"

———, *Report of the Joint Working Party on the Medical Staffing Structure in the Hospital Service* (HMSO, 1961), "Platt report"

Ministry of Health, Department of Health for Scotland, *A National Health Service,* Cmd. 6502 (HMSO, 1944), "The 1944 White Paper"

———, *Report of the Inter-departmental Committee on Medical Schools* (HMSO, 1944), "Goodenough report"

———, *Report of the Inter-departmental Committee on Remuneration of General Practitioners,* Cmd. 6810 (HMSO, 1946), "Spens Report on General Practitioners"

———, *Report of the Inter-departmental Committee on the Remuneration of Consultants and Specialists,* Cmd. 7420 (HMSO, 1948) "Spens Report on Consultants and Specialists"

———, *Report of the Committee to Consider the Future Numbers of Medical Practitioners and the Appropriate Intake of Medical Students* (HMSO, 1957), "Willink report"

National Health Service, *A Hospital Plan for England and Wales,* Cmnd. 1604 (HMSO, 1962)

———, *Health and Welfare—The Development of Community Care,* Cmnd. 1973 (HMSO, 1963), and *Revision to 1973–74* (HMSO, 1964)

Newman, George, *Some Notes on Medical Education in England,* Cd. 9124 (HMSO, 1918)

Nuffield Provincial Hospitals Trust, *The Hospital Surveys: The Domesday Book of the Hospital Services* (London, Oxford University Press for Nuffield Provincial Hospitals Trust, 1946)

PEP (Political and Economic Planning), *Report on the British Health Services* (London, PEP, 1937)

———— (Rehin, G. F., and F. M. Martin), *Psychiatric Services in 1975* (London, PEP, 1963)

A Review of the Medical Services in Great Britain, Report of a Committee sponsored by the Royal College of Physicians of London et al. (London, Social Assay, 1962), "Porritt report"

Review Body on Doctors' and Dentists' Remuneration, Third, Fourth, and Fifth Reports, Cmnd. 2585 (HMSO, 1965). The earlier reports were not published.

Royal Commission on Doctors' and Dentists' Remuneration 1957–1960, Report, Cmnd. 939 (HMSO, 1960); *Minutes of Evidence* (separately published, HMSO, 1958–60); *Written Evidence,* Vol. 1 (HMSO, 1957), Vol. 2 (HMSO, 1960)

Royal Commission on National Health Insurance, Report, Cmd. 2596 (HMSO, 1928)

Scottish Home and Health Department, *Medical Staffing Structure in Scottish Hospitals* (HMSO, 1964)

University Grants Committee, *Postgraduate Medical Education and the Specialties* (HMSO, 1962)

————, *University Development 1957–1962,* Cmnd. 2267 (HMSO, 1964)

Other Publications

Abel-Smith, Brian, *A History of the Nursing Profession* (London, Heinemann, 1960)

————, *The Hospitals 1800–1948* (London, Heinemann, 1964)

———— and Kathleen Gales, *British Doctors at Home and Abroad,* Occasional Papers on Social Administration No. 8, (Welwyn, Codicote Press for the Social Administration Research Trust, 1964)

Acton Society Trust, *Hospitals and the State: 1. Background and Blueprint* (London, Acton Society Trust, 1955); *2. The Impact of the Change* (1956); *3 and 4. Groups, Regions and Committees* (1957); *5. The Central Control of the Service* (1958); *6. Creative Leadership in a State Service* (1959)

Anderson, J., and F. J. Roberts, *A New Look at Medical Education* (London, Pitman Medical, 1965)

Birmingham University, *The History of the Birmingham Medical School* (Birmingham, Cornish Brothers, 1925)

British Medical Journal Symposium, *Fifty Years of Medicine* (London, BMA, 1950)

Brockbank, E. M., *The Foundation of Provincial Medical Education in England* (Manchester, Manchester University Press, 1936)

Brockbank, William, *The Honorary Medical Staff of the Manchester Royal Infirmary 1830–1948* (Manchester, Manchester University Press, 1965)

Cameron, Charles A., *History of the Royal College of Surgeons in Ireland* (Dublin, Fannin, 1886)

Cameron, H. C., *Mr. Guy's Hospital 1726–1948* (London, Longmans, Green, 1954)

——, *The British Paedriatric Association, 1928–52* (London, Metcalf & Cooper, 1955)

Carr-Saunders, A. M., and P. A. Wilson, *The Professions* (London, Oxford University Press, 1933)

Clark-Kennedy, A. E., *The London—A Study in the Voluntary Hospital System; Vol. I, The First Hundred Years 1740–1840* (London, Pitman Medical, 1962); *Vol. II, The Second Hundred Years 1840–1948* (London, Pitman Medical, 1963)

Clegg, H. A., and T. E. Chester, *Wage Policy and the Health Service* (Oxford, Basil Blackwell, 1957)

Comyns Carr, A. S., W. H. Stuart Garnett, and J. H. Taylor, *National Insurance* (London, Macmillan, 1912)

Cope, Zachary, *The History of St. Mary's Hospital Medical School* (London, Heinemann, 1954)

——, *The Royal College of Surgeons of England: A History* (London, Anthony Blond, 1959)

Creswell, Clarendon Hyde, *The Royal College of Surgeons of Edinburgh* (London, Oliver & Boyd, 1926)

Davidson, Maurice, *The Royal Society of Medicine* (London, Royal Society of Medicine, 1955)

Davies, D. L., and M. Shepherd (eds.), *Psychiatric Education* (London, Institute of Psychiatry, 1964)

Eckstein, Harry, *The English Health Service* (Cambridge, Harvard University Press, 1958)

——, *Pressure Group Politics, The Case of the British Medical Association* (London, Allen & Unwin, 1960)

Frazer, W. M., *A History of English Public Health 1834–1939* (London, Bailliere, Tindall & Cox, 1950)

Ginsberg, Morris (ed.), *Law and Opinion in England in the Twentieth Century* (London, Stevens, 1959)

Hardy, Horatio Nelson, *The State of the Medical Profession in Great Britain and Ireland in 1900* (Dublin, Fannin, 1901)

Hunter, W., *Historical Account of Charing Cross Hospital and Medical School* (London, Murray, 1914)

Jacob, Frank H., *A History of the General Hospital near Nottingham* (London, Marshall, 1951)

Jewkes, John and Sylvia, *The Genesis of the British National Health Service* (Oxford, Basil Blackwell, 1961)

Kershaw, Richard, *Special Hospitals* (London, Pulman, 1909)

Levy, Hermann, *National Health Insurance* (London, Cambridge University Press, 1944)

Lindsey, Almont, *Socialized Medicine in England and Wales* (Chapel Hill, University of North Carolina Press, 1962)

Little, E. M., *History of the British Medical Association, 1832–1932,* (London, BMA, 1932)

McCleary, G. F., *National Health Insurance* (London, Lewis, 1932)

McInnes, E. M., *St. Thomas' Hospital* (London, Allen & Unwin, 1963)

McLachlan, Gordon (ed.), *Problems and Progress in Medical Care* (London, Oxford University Press for Nuffield Provincial Hospitals Trust, 1964)

Newman, Charles, *The Evolution of Medical Education in the Nineteenth Century* (London, Oxford University Press, 1957)

Office of Health Economics, *The Personal Health Services* (London, Office of Health Economics, 1963)

Panton, Philip, *Leaves from a Doctor's Life* (London, Heinemann, 1951)

Platt, Robert, *Doctor and Patient—Ethics, Morale, Government* (London, Nuffield Provincial Hospitals Trust, 1963)

Poynter, F. N. L. (ed.), *The Evolution of Medical Practice in Britain* (London, Pitman Medical, 1961)

Puschmann, Theodor, *A History of Medical Education* (London, Lewis, 1891)

Revans, R. W., *Standards for Morale, Cause and Effect in Hospitals* (London, Oxford University Press for Nuffield Provincial Hospitals Trust, 1964)

Rosen, George, *The Specialization of Medicine with Particular Reference to Ophthalmology* (New York, Froben Press, 1944)

Royal College of Physicians of Edinburgh, *Historical Sketch and Laws* (Edinburgh, Royal College of Physicians, 1925)

Shaw, William Fletcher, *Twenty-five Years—The Story of the Royal College of Obstetricians and Gynaecologists 1929–1954* (London, Churchill, 1954)

Sprigge, S., *The Life and Times of Thomas Wakley* (London, Longmans, Green, 1897)

Titmuss, R. M., *Problems of Social Policy* (HMSO and Longmans, 1950)

———, *Essays on the Welfare State* (London, Allen & Unwin, 1958)

Webb, Sidney and Beatrice, *The State and The Doctor* (London, Longmans, Green, 1910)

Widdess, J. D. H., *A History of the Royal College of Physicians of Ireland 1654–1963* (Edinburgh, Livingstone, 1963)

Williams, Peter Orchard (ed.), *Careers in Medicine* (London, Hodder & Stoughton, 1952)

Index